Surgical Management of Movement Disorders

Surgical Management of Movement Disorders

edited by

Gordon H. Baltuch
University of Pennsylvania
Philadelphia, Pennsylvania, U.S.A.

Matthew B. Stern
University of Pennsylvania
Philadelphia, Pennsylvania, U.S.A.

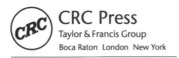 CRC Press
Taylor & Francis Group
Boca Raton London New York

CRC Press is an imprint of the
Taylor & Francis Group, an **informa** business

To our families, for their support

Preface

Movement disorders represent major causes of neurological disability and eventual mortality affecting millions of people across the globe. From Parkinson's disease to spasticity, these neurological disorders devastate young and old worldwide. While progress continues to be made toward effective treatment, many limitations remain.

The combination of the limitation of medical therapy and surgical technological advances have, however, led to an exponential growth in functional neurosurgery in the last 5 years. Surgery represents an alternative where there existed only finite treatment options before. This field is developing rapidly with emerging novel therapies as well as evolving indications for existing procedures.

We intended this book to be a thorough review of the surgical treatments currently available for various movement disorders, with an emphasis on surgical indications and results of surgery. It should be of utmost interest to practitioners and trainees in the clinical neurosciences (neurology/neurosurgery) who want a better understanding of candidates for movement disorder surgery, the current surgical procedures, the effected results of surgery, and the complication rate of these procedures. Our goal was to summarize the current status of the field as well as make projections for the next few years.

Gordon H. Baltuch
Matthew B. Stern

Contents

Contributors

Gordon H. Baltuch   Department of Neurosurgery, Penn Neurological Institute, University of Pennsylvania School of Medicine, Philadelphia, Pennsylvania, U.S.A.

Kelvin L. Chou   Department of Clinical Neurosciences, Brown University Medical School, Providence, Rhode Island, U.S.A.

Nicolas de Tribolet   Department of Neurosurgery, University of Geneva, Geneva, Switzerland

Habib E. Ellamushi   The Royal Hospital of St. Bartholomew and The Royal London Hospital, London, U.K.

Jean-Pierre Farmer   Division of Pediatric Neurosurgery, McGill University Health Centre, Montreal, Quebec, Canada

Santiago Figuereo   Department of Neurosurgery, Philadelphia Veterans Administration Hospital, University of Pennsylvania, Philadelphia, Pennsylvania, U.S.A.

Joseph Ghika   Neurology Service, Centre Hospitalier Universitaire Vaudois, Lausanne, Switzerland

Jeff D. Golan   Division of Neurosurgery, McGill University, Montreal, Quebec, Canada

Line Jacques   Division of Neurosurgery, McGill University, Montreal, Quebec, Canada

Galit Kleiner-Fisman   Parkinson's Disease Research Education and Clinical Center (PADRECC), Philadelphia Veterans Administration Hospital, University of Pennsylvania, Philadelphia, Pennsylvania, U.S.A.

Andres M. Lozano   Division of Neurosurgery, Toronto Western Hospital, University of Toronto and University Health Network, Toronto, Ontario, Canada

Michel R. Magistris   Department of Neurology, University of Geneva, Geneva, Switzerland

William J. Marks, Jr.   Department of Neurology, University of California, San Francisco and San Francisco Veterans Affairs Medical Center, San Francisco, California, U.S.A.

Sandeep Mittal   Division of Pediatric Neurosurgery, McGill University Health Centre, Montreal, Quebec, Canada

Jill L. Ostrem   Department of Neurology, University of California, San Francisco and San Francisco Veterans Affairs Medical Center, San Francisco, California, U.S.A.

Ali R. Rezai   Department of Neurosurgery, Cleveland Clinic Lerner College of Medicine, Cleveland, Ohio, U.S.A.

Joshua M. Rosenow   Department of Neurosurgery, Feinberg School of Medicine of Northwestern University, Chicago, Illinois, U.S.A.

Uzma Samadani   Department of Neurosurgery, University of Pennsylvania, Philadelphia, Pennsylvania, U.S.A.

Frédéric Schils   Department of Neurosurgery, University of Geneva, Geneva, Switzerland

Jason M. Schwalb   Division of Neurosurgery, Toronto Western Hospital, University of Toronto and University Health Network, Toronto, Ontario, Canada

Tanya Simuni   Department of Neurology, Feinberg School of Medicine, Northwestern University, Chicago, Illinois, U.S.A.

Philip A. Starr   Department of Neurosurgery, University of California, San Francisco and San Francisco Veterans Affairs Medical Center, San Francisco, California, U.S.A.

Matthew B. Stern   Parkinson's Disease and Movement Disorders Center, Pennsylvania Hospital, University of Pennsylvania School of Medicine, Philadelphia, Pennsylvania, U.S.A.

Atsushi Umemura   Department of Neurosurgery, Nagoya City University Medical School, Mizuho-ku, Nagoya, Japan

Jean-Guy Villemure   Neurosurgery Service, Centre Hospitalier Universitaire Vaudois, Lausanne, Switzerland

François Vingerhoets   Neurology Service, Centre Hospitalier Universitaire Vaudois, Lausanne, Switzerland

Eun-Kyung Won   Department of Neurosurgery, University of Minnesota, Minneapolis, Minnesota, U.S.A.

1

Overview

Kelvin L. Chou

Department of Clinical Neurosciences, Brown University Medical School, Providence, Rhode Island, U.S.A.

Gordon H. Baltuch

Department of Neurosurgery, Penn Neurological Institute, University of Pennsylvania School of Medicine, Philadelphia, Pennsylvania, U.S.A.

Matthew B. Stern

Parkinson's Disease and Movement Disorders Center, Pennsylvania Hospital, University of Pennsylvania School of Medicine, Philadelphia, Pennsylvania, U.S.A.

1. INTRODUCTION

From Parkinson's disease (PD) to dystonia, movement disorders are major neurologic causes of disability, causing not only physical handicap, but often social embarrassment as well. Although a plethora of pharmacologic options exists to treat these disorders, many limitations unfortunately remain. Functional neurosurgery now has the ability to reduce the severity of symptoms and improve the quality of life for patients with these devastating neurological disorders.

Surgery for the field of movement disorders has evolved significantly since Spiegel et al. first described stereotaxis in 1947 (1). Much of this progress has been made within the last decade with the development of techniques for precise targeting of brain structures and the discovery of new targets and indications for existing procedures such as deep brain stimulation (DBS). This chapter provides a general overview of the field of movement disorders surgery, including a brief summary of basal ganglia structure and function, as well as discussions of the major surgical treatments available for PD, essential tremor (ET), other tremor disorders, dystonia, and spasticity.

2. PATHOPHYSIOLOGY OF MOVEMENT DISORDERS

All movement disorders are believed to result from abnormalities of the basal ganglia. Our understanding of the organization and function of the basal ganglia has grown significantly in the modern era, largely as a result of recent experience with stereotactic neurosurgery in humans and animal models. Although current theories do not adequately account for the clinical findings seen with all disorders of involuntary movement, it is still essential for those interested in functional neurosurgical procedures to be familiar with the basic anatomy and functional organization of the basal ganglia.

2.1. Structure and Function of the Basal Ganglia

A detailed discussion of basal ganglia anatomy and function is beyond the scope of this chapter, but a brief summary follows. The basal ganglia are organized into several parallel circuits (associative, limbic, motor, and oculomotor) that connect cortical regions with thalamic and basal ganglia nuclei (2). Disturbances of the motor circuit are believed to manifest as movement disorders. In the classical model of basal ganglia function, a balance between two opposing pathways in the motor circuit, the direct and indirect pathways, regulates normal voluntary movement (3). Both pathways begin with neurons in cortical motor areas projecting to the putamen, which in turn sends signals that ultimately terminate in the internal segment of the globus pallidus (GPi). Putamenal output in the indirect pathway, however, travels through the external segment of the globus pallidus (GPe) and subthalamic nucleus (STN) before it reaches the GPi, whereas the direct pathway projects directly from the putamen to the GPi. The majority of GPi output is directed toward the thalamus, which sends projections to the supplementary motor area, the premotor cortical area, and the primary motor cortex. Activation of the direct pathway decreases the normal inhibitory outflow from the GPi to the thalamus, leading to increased cortical motor activation and the facilitation of voluntary movement. In contrast, stimulation of the indirect pathway causes inhibition of the GPe, disinhibition of STN excitatory fibers, and an increase in the inhibitory outflow from the GPi onto the thalamus, resulting in decreased output to the motor cortex and suppression of voluntary movement.

The exact mechanism by which the basal ganglia interpret the information flowing through these two opposing motor circuit pathways to control normal movement is unclear. Two theories have been proposed: *scaling* and *focusing* (2–4). In the *scaling* hypothesis, movement is controlled by temporally changing activity in the basal ganglia. For example, putamenal output would first facilitate a particular movement by disinhibiting the thalamus through the direct pathway, and subsequently stop the ongoing movement by causing the same GPi neurons to increase inhibition of the thalamus through the indirect pathway. In the *focusing* hypothesis, movement is allowed to proceed by stimulation of the direct pathway, whereas extra, unnecessary movements are suppressed by activity in the indirect pathway. Unfortunately, both models are likely oversimplifications of the true underlying mechanism, since they do not account for all experimental findings.

2.2. Pathophysiologic Models of Hypo- and Hyperkinetic Movement Disorders

Based on the model of basal ganglia function described above, an imbalance between the direct and indirect pathways accounts for the clinical manifestations of hypo- and hyperkinetic disorders. The release of dopamine from nerve terminals in the striatum appears to stimulate the direct pathway and inhibit the indirect pathway, thus effectively facilitating movement (5). Consequently, degeneration of the dopaminergic nigrostriatal pathway, as seen in parkinsonism, would result in decreased dopamine receptor activation and disinhibition of the indirect pathway, leading to increased activity in the STN and GPi. The increased inhibitory outflow from GPi on the thalamus would decrease cortical motor activation, with the end result being slowed movements, or bradykinesia. Conversely, hyperkinetic disorders such as Huntington's disease (HD) are thought to result from excess dopamine, causing overactivity of the direct pathway, less inhibitory activity from GPi on the thalamus, increased activity of the thalamocortical projections, and excessive involuntary movement.

2.2.1. Hypokinetic Movement Disorders

There is considerable evidence supporting the classical model for the parkinsonian state. For example, in 1-methyl-4-phenyl-1,2,3,6-tetrahydropyridine (MPTP)-treated monkeys, neuronal firing frequency is increased in the STN and GPi and reduced in the GPe, consistent with the predictions of the above model (6,7). Further support comes from advanced PD patients treated with STN and GPi DBS, where stimulation clearly improves parkinsonian symptoms (8–11) and increases activity in cortical motor areas as detected by positron emission tomography (PET) imaging (12).

There are many inconsistencies with this model, however. For instance, a lesion in the thalamus should worsen PD motor symptoms due to decreased activity of the thalamocortical projections, yet, thalamic lesioning and thalamic DBS have both been proven to suppress parkinsonian tremor (13,14). In addition, pallidotomy should result in excessive movement (i.e., dyskinesias) because of decreased inhibition on the thalamus, but in fact, the opposite is true (15).

This has led to a rethinking of the classical model, with some investigators proposing that it is the overall pattern of basal ganglia activity that is altered in PD, rather than the rate of activity of individual structures (16). Studies have suggested that in the normal brain, information flows through independent and parallel circuits within the basal ganglia, while in the parkinsonian brain, these circuits break down, and interconnections between these circuits become active and synchronized (17). This synchronization is believed to contribute to the parkinsonian state. Lesions of the STN and GPi may change this pattern back to a more "normal" pattern of neuronal transmission through the basal ganglia. Indirect evidence for this comes from human PET imaging studies that have shown a restoration of normal cortical activity after lesions of the STN or GPi (12,18).

2.2.2. Hyperkinetic Movement Disorders

As explained above, the classical model predicts that hyperkinetic movement disorders result from a reduction in GPi activity and an increase in thalamic and cortical activity. In fact, it has been shown that MPTP-treated monkeys given levodopa or apomorphine have a gradual reduction in GPi firing rate as the monkeys transition from an "off" state, to an "on" state without dyskinesias, to an "on" state with dyskinesias, supporting this model (19). GPi discharge rates are also reduced in other hyperkinetic disorders, such as dystonia and hemiballismus (16). However, decreased GPi activity cannot account for hyperkinetic movements by itself; otherwise, lesions of the globus pallidus would be expected to result in extra movements. As with the parkinsonian model, many experts now think that it is the pattern of GPi activity, rather than the rate of GPi activity, that is important in determining movement (16,20). It may be that the absence of activity is preferable to abnormal activity, which is why surgical lesioning improves clinical symptoms.

The pathophysiology of tremor, whether in PD, ET, or cerebellar tremor, is even less clear, and remains hotly debated. There may be some peripheral afferent component to the development of tremor, but it is more likely that a central mechanism is responsible. Evidence for this includes recordings of neuronal rhythmic activity in the thalamus that are synchronized with tremor activity in the limb in patients with ET and cerebellar tremor (21), and recordings of rhythmic activity in the STN that correlate with contralateral tremor in PD patients (22,23). Other supporting evidence includes the fact that thalamic stimulation improves tremor, whether for PD or ET (13). Whatever the true mechanism, however, it is clear that much work remains to be completed before we can fully comprehend the complex mechanisms underlying abnormal movements.

3. SURGICAL TREATMENT OF MOVEMENT DISORDERS

3.1. Parkinson's Disease

PD is a slowly progressive neurodegenerative disorder characterized by a clinical triad of motor features—tremor, bradykinesia, and rigidity. Ideal candidates for surgery should have a clear response to levodopa therapy, but continue to have severe motor fluctuations, dyskinesias, or intractable tremor despite optimal medical therapy. Older patients tend to fare worse after surgery, as do patients with cognitive impairment, so comprehensive neuropsychological testing should be performed prior to surgery (10,24). It is also being increasingly recognized that psychiatric symptoms such as depression worsen after DBS procedures (25), so more centers are incorporating a psychiatric screen into the DBS evaluation process. Patients with atypical parkinsonism, such as progressive supranuclear palsy and multiple system atrophy, are not candidates for surgery (26,27).

3.1.1. Ablative Procedures

Prior to the discovery of levodopa, thalamotomies were performed routinely for PD. However, they were only effective for tremor, and bilateral procedures resulted in a high incidence of dysarthria and cognitive side effects (28,29). Given the excellent results from pallidotomy in PD and the development of DBS, which holds the advantage of reversibility and fewer side effects with bilateral procedures, thalamotomies are no longer recommended for treatment of PD.

Laitinen et al. (30) revived the posteroventral pallidotomy for the treatment of PD in 1992. Of 38 patients followed for a mean of 28 months, 92% had "complete relief or almost complete relief" of bradykinesia and rigidity, and that 81% had "complete relief or almost complete relief" of tremor. While many authors have reported similar results from this procedure with short-term follow-up (15,31–34), other investigators, in contrast to Laitinen et al. (30), have reported a decline in surgical benefit from pallidotomy with long-term follow-up (35–37). Although these studies have consistently shown that pallidotomy's effects on tremor and dyskinesias are maintained at 3–5 years, other measures, such as the total off-period motor score, the ipsilateral motor score, the contralateral bradykinesia subscore, and the activities of daily living subscore, deteriorate with time. However, it should be noted that all of these studies have followed unilateral pallidotomy patients only, largely because of reports of unacceptable speech and neuro behavioral side effects from bilateral pallidotomy (38–41). As the natural history of PD suggests that the disease will eventually spread bilaterally, it is not surprising that the benefit of unilateral pallidotomy diminishes with time.

With regards to subthalamotomy, although animal studies had repeatedly shown that parkinsonian signs improved with ablative lesions of the STN, very few surgeons attempted to lesion the STN in humans for fear of causing hemiballismus (42). However, most clinical reports have shown that hemiballismus in subthalamotomy patients does not occur as often as previously thought (43–46). Unilateral subthalamotomy in patients with advanced PD has been demonstrated to decrease the Unified Parkinson's Disease Rating Scale (UPDRS) off-medication motor scores by about 30–50% (44–46). Persistent, lesion-induced dyskinesias have been problematic for only a few patients overall, with two requiring additional surgical procedures to control the choreic movements and another dying from aspiration pneumonia. The results of bilateral subthalamotomy have been reported for only two PD patients in the literature (43). Both patients showed an impressive reduction in UPDRS motor scores, with one patient going from 50 to 16, and the second improving from 64 to 16, without adverse effects.

3.1.2. Deep Brain Stimulation

Stimulation of the thalamic ventralis intermedius (VIM) nucleus for parkinsonian or other tremor of the limbs was the first Food and Drug Administration (FDA) approved indication for DBS, heralding a new era in functional neurosurgery. Thalamic DBS, in multiple long-term studies, has been shown to be safe and effective for parkinsonian tremor (47–49). Unfortunately, as with thalamotomy, other parkinsonian symptoms are unimproved and prevent this procedure from being useful in the long-term treatment of PD.

With reports of pallidotomy being effective for all the motor features of PD, and the gaining acceptance of thalamic stimulation for tremor, many surgical centers tried to see if stimulation of the GPi could help the parkinsonian symptoms not addressed by VIM stimulation, and the results have been positive. In one of the largest prospective double blind studies published, 38 PD patients underwent implantation of DBS electrodes bilaterally in the GPi (11). Stimulation produced a 37% median improvement in the off medication UPDRS score at 6 months. Furthermore, the amount of "on" time during the day without dyskinesias increased from 28% to 64%, while amount of "off" time decreased from 37% to 24%. The dyskinesia score improved by about 66%. Unfortunately, the mean daily levodopa dose was not significantly changed.

An increasing number of long-term studies evaluating GPi stimulation in patients with PD have been published in recent years, but it appears that the benefits seen early on may not endure. Visser-Vandewalle et al. (50) followed 26 patients with unilateral GPi electrodes for a mean of 32.7 months, and found that while GPi stimulation was beneficial at 3 months for symptoms both contralaterally and ipsilaterally, it was unsatisfactory at long-term follow-up, leading the authors to conclude that unilateral pallidal stimulation was not an effective treatment for advanced PD. Ghika et al. (51) followed six PD patients treated with bilateral pallidal stimulation for 2 years, and while there were still significant improvements in the UPDRS motor score and in the amount of "on" time at 2 years compared to baseline, a slight worsening after 1 year was observed. In the six patients with bilateral GPi electrodes for PD followed for a mean of 3 years by Durif et al. (52), the amount of time spent in the "off" state returned to the preoperative value after 2 years, even though improvements in UPDRS motor scores and severity of dyskinesias were sustained. Finally, Volkmann et al. (53) followed 11 patients treated with chronic bilateral pallidal stimulation for up to 5 years. Although there was a sustained reduction in dyskinesias at 5 years, UPDRS motor scores declined over time, despite continued levodopa responsiveness and changes in electrical stimulation parameters. Overall, the levodopa dose remained unchanged after surgery, but had to be increased in some patients. In all of these studies, complications were generally transient, and could be relieved by adjusting the stimulator. The hypophonia, dysarthria, and neuro-behavioral disturbances commonly reported with bilateral pallidotomy (38,40,41) were not seen with bilateral GPi stimulation.

In contrast, the benefits of DBS for PD appear to be longer lasting with STN stimulation, a technique that was pioneered by Benabid and his colleagues in the mid-1990s (54,55). Initial studies of subthalamic stimulation in patients with advanced PD demonstrated a reduction in the UPDRS motor score by 40–60%, as well as a decrease in dyskinesias and the daily levodopa dose by about 50% (8,10,11). STN DBS also decreased the amount of time in the off medication state, and other studies showed improvement in gait and balance (56), and even off-period dystonia (55). In the longest long-term follow-up study of STN stimulation in PD to date, Krack et al. reported that the UPDRS motor scores at 5 years while off medication were 54% better than preoperative scores (57). Furthermore, average daily levodopa dose and severity of dyskinesias continued to be significantly decreased compared to baseline. Unfortunately, speech, postural stability, and freezing continued to progress, which the authors concluded was consistent with the natural history of PD. Two other groups found similar results at 2 years (58,59), although the Toronto group (59) noticed that UPDRS axial subscores, as well as the UPDRS motor score, had diminished at the most recent follow-up. For all of these studies, most adverse events appeared to be transient; however, persistent events included cognitive decline, and mood changes such as depression and anxiety. One patient in the study by Krack et al. (57) committed suicide.

3.1.3. Comparison of Targets and Procedures

As mentioned above, the thalamus has fallen by the wayside as a target for PD because of its limited effects on bradykinesia and rigidity. The GPi and STN are clearly the two structures most commonly targeted today for PD, and most centers are using DBS rather than ablative procedures even though no double-blind, randomized, head-to-head comparison has been conducted between ablative therapy and DBS.

It is unclear whether GPi DBS or STN DBS is superior. Burchiel et al. (8) conducted a small randomized prospective trial comparing pallidal to subthalamic stimulation in 10 patients with advanced PD, and found no significant difference in off medication UPDRS motor scores between the two groups, although medications were able to be decreased in the STN group but not the GPi group. This trial was too small, however, to draw any solid conclusions. The Deep Brain Stimulation for Parkinson's Disease Study Group performed a large multicenter trial that enrolled 96 patients with STN DBS and 38 patients with GPi-DBS (11). Because patients were not randomized in this trial, it is difficult to compare the two groups, but the STN group appeared to have more favorable outcomes. Another prospective nonrandomized study carried out by Krause et al. (60) also suggested that the STN was the better target for all parkinsonian symptoms, but GPi stimulation was superior for reduction of dyskinesias.

One of the most consistent differences between the two sites is that STN stimulation allows patients to reduce dopaminergic medications, whereas daily levodopa equivalent doses in those undergoing pallidal stimulation remain largely unchanged. Many studies have also noted that STN stimulation requires less electrical energy than GPi-DBS (11,61), which allows for a longer battery life. GPi stimulation, however, does not seem to be associated as consistently with cognitive and psychiatric side effects as STN stimulation (51,53,57,59). Clearly, a large randomized comparison between the two targets needs to be completed before recommending one procedure over the other. The VA and NIH are currently supporting a multicenter trial of DBS in PD to address the comparative efficacy of GPi and STN stimulation.

3.1.4. Novel Surgical Strategies

Although DBS and surgical ablation are effective for the symptoms of PD, they may not interfere with the underlying neurodegenerative process and thus do not slow down or reverse the course of the illness. Consequently, much research is being conducted to evaluate alternative therapies and strategies that may alter the long-term outcome in these patients. One of these novel approaches is cell transplantation. Thus far, two human clinical trials of fetal nigral transplantation have been conducted, and although both studies showed uptake of the embryonic dopamine neurons in the basal ganglia on imaging and post-mortem examinations, both trials failed to meet statistical significance in their outcome measures (62,63). An unanticipated finding was the development of disabling off-medication dyskinesias in some transplanted patients. These findings, along with ethical concerns and the scarcity of human fetal tissue, currently limit the usefulness of fetal nigral transplantation as a viable clinical option for patients with PD. Other sources of cells for transplantation into patients include xenografts (from fetal pigs) (64) and embryonic stem cells, though these techniques still need to be refined and tried in small groups of patients before a large clinical trial can even be attempted (65).

Another top prospect for therapeutic trials in PD is glial derived neurotrophic factor (GDNF). GDNF has been extensively studied in animal models of PD and promotes dopamine neuron survival and growth (66). So far, a few clinical trials with GDNF have been undertaken in patients with PD. In the first trial, conducted by Nutt et al. (67), GDNF or placebo was administered through an intracerebroventricular catheter in 50 patients with advanced PD. The patients had multiple side effects, including nausea, vomiting, and anorexia, but did not have any improvement in UPDRS scores, likely because the GDNF did not reach the appropriate brain regions. Gill et al. (68) infused GDNF directly into the putamen of five PD patients, and reported a 39% improvement in the UPDRS off-medication motor score and a reduction in dyskinesias by about 64%. In addition, fluorodopa scans showed a 28% increase in putamenal uptake. However, a recent double-blind trial of intraputaminal GDNF was stopped because a six month analysis indicated no clinical benefit, causing the manufacturer, Amgen, to withdraw GDNF from all clinical trials.

3.2. Essential Tremor

Tremor is a rhythmic oscillation of a body part that is produced by alternating contractions of reciprocally innervated muscles (69). Of all the tremor syndromes, ET is the most common (70), yet fewer ET patients are referred for surgery than PD patients. One probable reason is that most ET patients suffer from a mild tremor which is either not severe enough to seek medical treatment, or can be controlled with medication (71). However, when tremor in ET is severe, it can be severely disabling, as well as cause significant social embarrassment. ET generally presents as a bilateral, symmetric postural and/or kinetic tremor of the hands, but it can commonly affect the head and voice as well (72). Primidone and propranolol are considered first-line therapy and should be tried alone or in combination before considering surgery (71).

The thalamus has been considered the optimal target for tremor ever since Hassler and colleagues reported better tremor control with thalamic lesions over 40 years ago (73,74). However, because of the success of STN stimulation in controlling parkinsonian tremor (8,11,22,23), some groups have begun to experiment with STN DBS for ET, with promising results in a small number of patients to date (75–78).

3.2.1. Ablative Procedures: Thalamotomy

Many investigators have reported successful suppression of tremor in ET with thalamotomy (79–86). In the majority of these studies, greater than 90% of patients had improvement of tremor in the limb contralateral to the lesion. Moreover, long-term studies indicate sustained benefit (80,81,83). In the largest long-term series published (81), of 65 patients with ET who were followed for a mean of 8.6 years, 80% continued to have contralateral tremor improvement. While adverse effects of thalamotomy are usually transient, persistent postoperative complications common to most of these studies include paresthesias, motor weakness, dysarthria, disequilibrium, and gait disturbance, occurring in approximately 10–20% of patients (80,81,83). It is important to note that almost all of the ET patients underwent unilateral thalamotomy, likely because of the data from the PD literature, which demonstrated a high occurrence of speech and cognitive disturbance from bilateral procedures (28,29).

3.2.2. Deep Brain Stimulation

Some ET patients cannot be adequately treated with unilateral thalamotomy, either because of midline tremor, such as head tremor, or severe bilateral hand tremors. However, due to the adverse effects associated with bilateral thalamotomies mentioned above, DBS of the VIM nucleus of the thalamus has become an increasingly popular surgical option. Benabid and colleagues were the first to report the successful treatment of limb tremor in ET using chronic VIM stimulation in a series of patients (87). Since then, a number of investigators have echoed Benabid et al.'s findings of the safety and efficacy of thalamic DBS in patients with ET, and many have published long-term results. Koller et al. (88) followed 25 patients with ET for a mean of 40 months after unilateral VIM DBS implantation, and found sustained tremor improvement (∼50% based on tremor rating scales) with little change in electrical stimulus parameters over time. Similar results were reported by a Swedish group (89) and a multicenter European group (90) for at least 6 years of follow-up. In all of these studies, adverse effects were minimal, and typically could be corrected by adjusting the stimulator, but required battery replacement every 3–6 years. Thalamic stimulation has also been shown to improve health-related quality of life for ET patients (91).

Fewer studies have focused on midline tremors, such as head or voice tremor, in patients with ET. Carpenter et al. (92) studied the effect of thalamic stimulation on voice tremor in seven patients undergoing DBS for hand tremor, and noticed mild improvement for four patients. Koller et al. (93) evaluated unilateral thalamic DBS in 38 patients with head tremor due to ET. At one year post implantation, 75% reported improvement in head tremor. Ondo et al. (94) studied 14 ET patients with head tremor and reported a 55% improvement at 3 months with unilateral thalamic stimulation. Obwegeser and colleagues found that although unilateral thalamic DBS resulted in a mild improvement in head tremor, there was an additional effect from bilateral stimulation (95). Furthermore, improvements in voice tremor (83%), tongue tremor (100%), and face tremor (100%) were noted with bilateral stimulation as well. Adverse effects from stimulation included dysarthria, disequilibrium, and paresthesias, similar to those reported in the long-term studies mentioned previously (88–90), but all resolved with stimulator adjustment. In the study conducted by Taha et al. (96), 9 of 10 patients with head tremor and 6 of 7 patients with voice tremor undergoing bilateral thalamic stimulation had greater than 50% improvement in tremor.

3.2.3. Thalamotomy vs. Thalamic DBS

A couple of studies have attempted to address whether thalamic ablative surgery or DBS implantation is better for the surgical treatment of ET. Tasker et al. (84) retrospectively compared 19 patients with DBS implants to 26 patients who underwent thalamotomy. Although most of the patients had PD tremor (only three patients in each group were diagnosed with ET), efficacy was similar in both groups. Thalamotomy had to be repeated in 15% of patients, while there were no revisions of DBS implants. Pahwa and colleagues (85) studied 34 ET patients retrospectively, 17 of whom were treated with thalamic stimulation, and 17 with thalamotomy. Again, there were no differences in efficacy, but the thalamotomy group had more surgical complications, including intracranial hemorrhages, cognitive abnormalities, hemiparesis, and aphasia. Finally, Schuurman et al. (86) conducted a prospective randomized study comparing thalamic DBS to thalamotomy, and concluded that both techniques were equally effective for tremor suppression, but that stimulation resulted in fewer adverse effects with improved function. As a result, DBS has virtually replaced thalamotomy for ET. However, there may still be a role for thalamotomy, especially if the patient is older or if there are barriers that prevent the patient from following up consistently postimplantation (97).

3.3. Other Tremor Disorders

Patients with tremors of other etiologies, such as cerebellar tremor due to multiple sclerosis (MS), posttraumatic tremor, or poststroke tremor tend not to respond to pharmacologic therapy (98), and may be candidates for stereotactic neurosurgery. Thalamic stimulation has been the most common surgical approach applied to these disorders, but success has been variable, and consists only of case reports or small case series. Among these other tremor disorders, cerebellar tremor secondary to MS has been the most studied (47,99–103), and results in general have shown that the postural component of the tremor in MS improves the most, whereas the action component responds variably and the cerebellar dysfunction remains unchanged. Unfortunately, it was impossible to predict which MS patients would respond to stimulation, based on clinical, radiological, or intraoperative grounds (100,103). Furthermore, those patients who responded to stimulation developed a "tolerance" to the treatment, and required frequent stimulator adjustments to maintain limb function (99,101–103). Stimulation was also less effective for tremor in long-term follow-up, likely due to the progression of MS (104).

3.4. Dystonia

Dystonia is an abnormal involuntary movement disorder characterized by sustained muscle contractions, which often result in twisting, writhing movements, or abnormal posturing (105). Dystonias can be classified by etiology (primary or secondary) or by body region (general, segmental or focal). Primary dystonias may be generalized, focal, or segmental. Generalized primary dystonia usually starts in childhood and has a genetic etiology (e.g., DYT-1) but may also be idiopathic. Focal primary dystonias, such as cervical dystonia (CD), hemifacial spasm, and blepharospasm, tend to occur in adulthood and are usually idiopathic. The causes of secondary dystonias are varied, and include birth trauma (cerebral palsy), multiple sclerosis, structural lesions (tumor or stroke), drugs (e.g., neuroleptics), metabolic disorders, and neurodegenerative processes such as PD.

Botulinum toxin is the preferred treatment for most focal and segmental dystonias. Too many different muscles are involved and too much botulinum toxin is needed to make this therapy practical for the treatment of generalized dystonia, for which anticholinergics and muscle relaxants are generally the first pharmacological agents prescribed. Stereotactic neurosurgery is reserved for those patients that have failed oral medications and/or botulinum toxin treatments. Although both ablative and deep brain stimulation techniques have been shown to be of benefit for most dystonias, the results vary widely between studies. This is likely due to the fact that there is significant clinical heterogeneity in the dystonia population, making it difficult to draw solid conclusions.

3.4.1. Chemodenervation

Botulinum toxin A (Botox®) was first shown to be effective for cervical dystonia by Tsui et al. in 1986 (106). Since then, Botox has been demonstrated to have long-term safety and efficacy for focal and segmental dystonias such as CD, blepharospasm, and hemifacial spasm (107–109). Botulinum toxin is a protein produced by the anaerobic bacterium, *Clostridium botulinum*, and exists as several immunological types, labeled A to G. Types A and B (Myobloc) are commercially available in the United States. The toxin is injected directly into the muscle and works by blocking the presynaptic release of acetylcholine at the neuromuscular junction. This results in decreased contraction of the muscle, thus relieving the involuntary movements and oftentimes the pain as well.

A clinical response from Botox usually occurs within 1 week after injection, and usually lasts 3–4 months. Common side effects include injection site pain, bruising, and focal weakness (107,110). Other side effects include a flu-like syndrome, and if injected into the neck muscles for CD, dysphagia (110). Some patients (5–10%) may experience diminishing effect from repeated treatments; this is often due to the development of antibodies to botulinum toxin (107,109,111,112).

3.4.2. Ablative Procedures

Early on, thalamotomy seemed to be the preferred procedure for dystonia, largely due to the results published by Cooper from the late 1950s to the 1970s (113). He performed thalamotomies on over 200 patients with primary generalized dystonia, and after an average follow-up of 7.9 years, approximately 70% had mild to marked improvement in their symptoms. Subsequent case series were also positive, although less favorable, with improvement seen in only 25–60% of all cases (114–117), and no significant overall difference in response between dystonias of primary or secondary etiologies. Though Cardoso et al. (117) noted better results for generalized dystonia (80% of patients improved) than other subgroups, and Andrew et al. (115) found that hemidystonia patients improved dramatically (100% showing fair to excellent improvement), the overall results of these studies suggest that there is no enhanced benefit from thalamotomy for any particular subgroup of dystonia patients. Furthermore, thalamotomy is associated with significant complications, notably dysarthria, especially if performed bilaterally (56–73% of patients) (115,116).

Pallidotomy was not widely performed for dystonia until studies of patients with PD undergoing pallidotomy reported a dramatic reduction in levodopa induced dyskinesias, both choreic and dystonic, and off-period dystonia (35,118,119). Seeing these encouraging results, many surgical centers then tried applying pallidotomy to patients with dystonia, and the GPi is now considered the target of choice for the treatment of dystonia (120). Overall, primary generalized dystonia patients seem to benefit more from pallidotomy (120–126), with mean reductions in the Burke–Marsden–Fahn dystonia rating scale (127) by 59–80% (122,124–126). Typically, the improvement is mild to moderate in the immediate postoperative period, but continues to show gradual improvement over the next few months (120–122). Most patients in the studies cited tolerated pallidotomy well, with minimal complications. In the study reported by Yoshor et al. (120), 6 of 18 patients undergoing thalamotomy had postoperative complications compared to 2 of 14 patients undergoing pallidotomy.

3.4.3. Deep Brain Stimulation

Though results from thalamic DBS were published as early as the late 1970s (128), most of the literature has focused instead on the globus pallidus as a stimulation target, likely because the data from ablative procedures suggested that GPi was a more effective site, but also because the few reports of thalamic DBS in dystonia have had generally poor results. The

Grenoble group, in reviewing their experience with thalamic stimulation for movement disorders, noted that their five patients with dystonia were "inconsistently, less significantly, or not improved" (129).

Vercueil et al. (130) implanted DBS leads into the thalamus of 12 patients, and although six of the patients rated their global functional outcome as satisfactory, dystonia rating scales and disability scales were not improved. Finally, Kupsch et al. (131) reported eight patients with heterogeneous causes of dystonia who underwent simultaneous bilateral GPi and VIM electrode implantation, with only two patients benefiting from stimulation of the VIM.

As with pallidotomy, the results from the pallidal DBS literature for dystonia are more encouraging. Indeed, in the few series where patients underwent both thalamic and GPi stimulation, the latter site seemed to result in greater improvement (130,131). Pallidal stimulation has been demonstrated to be effective for both primary (130,132–136) and secondary dystonia (130,134–136) although it appears to be most successful for generalized DYT-1 dystonia (132,136,137). The seven DYT-1 dystonia patients (six children, one adult) reported by Coubes et al. (132), had a mean improvement of 90.3% as measured by the Burke–Marsden–Fahn dystonia rating scale. This improvement appeared to be sustained after 2 years of follow-up (136). Primary DYT-1 negative dystonias, including idiopathic generalized dystonia as well as cervical dystonia, generally see between 20% and 80% improvement in their symptoms (133–136), while those with secondary dystonias, unfortunately, have even more variable results (134–136). This wide range in the amount clinical benefit is likely due to the heterogeneity of the dystonia population. Nevertheless, this provides intractable dystonia patients, whether primary or secondary, with another treatment option where before there was no palatable alternative. In contrast to DBS for PD, the effects from stimulation in dystonia tend to be more gradual, and the voltages and pulse widths used tend to be higher (131).

STN DBS is just starting to receive attention as a possible treatment for dystonia of either primary or secondary etiologies. The first clinical evidence to support studying the STN as a target for dystonia came from Limousin et al. (55), who found that off-period dystonia in PD patients disappeared with high-frequency stimulation of the STN. The same investigators then placed STN stimulators in four generalized dystonia patients in addition to 22 patients with PD who exhibited severe off-period dystonia (138). Although off-period dystonia was reduced by 70% in the PD patients, the generalized dystonia patients unfortunately had no benefit. This is in contrast to the case series reported by Sun et al. (139), in which four generalized dystonia patients all improved with STN stimulation, and the cervical dystonia patient reported by Chou et al. (75), whose pain and dystonic neck posture improved with stimulation of the STN. These results are encouraging, but further investigations are necessary before recommending the subthalamic nucleus as a target for the treatment of dystonia.

3.4.4. Comparison of Targets and Procedures

As mentioned earlier, most centers for movement disorders appear to be targeting the globus pallidus for dystonia, likely because the results from pallidotomy and pallidal DBS are more dramatic with fewer complications. Yet, there have been no prospective, head-to head trials comparing the globus pallidus to the thalamus, and thus, neither site has been proven to be superior to the other. Further, the STN needs to be further evaluated as a potential target for dystonia surgery. The retrospective study by Yoshor et al. (120) comparing thalamotomy versus pallidotomy suggests significantly better long-term improvement from pallidotomy, but comparisons between the two groups are limited because some had bilateral surgeries while others had unilateral. Further investigations comparing the two sites need to be performed in order to determine the optimal site. It also remains to be seen whether or not the subthalamic nucleus plays a role in the treatment of dystonia. Moreover, although the pendulum is swinging towards DBS over ablative surgery, no comparative study has been performed between DBS and ablation for dystonia. It is essential that such a study be conducted, assessing relative efficacy, complications, and cost-effectiveness so that optimal procedure can be recommended.

3.5. Spasticity

Spasticity is defined as an increase in muscle tone that is velocity dependent (140), and when severe, can manifest as painful muscle spasms and impair function. As with other movement disorders, surgery is indicated for severe spasticity only when noninvasive treatment with oral muscle relaxants, benzodiazepines, and physical therapy has failed. Historically, many different surgical approaches to spasticity have been attempted, including stereotactic brain surgery (141), cerebellar stimulation (142), and myelotomy (143). These procedures, however, ultimately proved unsuccessful and no longer play a role in the surgical treatment of spasticity. Instead, intrathecal baclofen and selective posterior rhizotomy have emerged as the most commonly recommended neurosurgical therapies. Intrathecal baclofen, because it is a reversible procedure that has been proven to be effective, is often considered before selective posterior rhizotomy, an irreversible neuroablative technique better suited for patients with focal spasticity.

Baclofen is a gamma-aminobutyric acid (GABA) agonist whose net effect is to inhibit spinal synaptic reflexes, and intrathecal infusion allows higher levels of the drug to be delivered in the central nervous system when compared to oral administration (144). The clinical effectiveness of intrathecal baclofen was first demonstrated by Penn and Kroin (144,145), and has since been substantiated by others (140,146–148). Potential candidates for intrathecal baclofen are first given a trial through a percutaneous catheter or access port. If candidates respond, an electronic pump is then implanted subcutaneously. Hardware complications often occur, including catheter occlusion, migration, disconnection, or infection (140,146). Baclofen itself is a central nervous system depressant, and can cause sedation and drowsiness, and in high doses can induce respiratory depression and coma (148).

Dorsal rhizotomy is one of the oldest surgical procedures for spasticity, but the technique has been refined over the years to what is now known as selective posterior rhizotomy (SPR). This procedure relieves spasticity by interrupting the peripheral stretch reflex, and can be performed in the cervical or lumbar areas. In the peripheral stretch reflex arc, impulses from muscle spindle fibers detecting a passive stretch are delivered through the posterior nerve roots and synapse on the alpha motor neuron, which then fires to contract the stretched muscle. In SPR, usually one quarter to one half of these posterior nerve roots are severed. SPR has been evaluated in three different prospective randomized trials for spasticity in cerebral palsy (149–151). A meta-analysis of these three trials concluded that SPR, along with physical therapy, reduces spasticity in children with cerebral palsy (152). Side effects of the procedure include sensory loss, weakness, and bowel or bladder dysfunction.

4. CONCLUSIONS

Functional neurosurgery for movement disorders has evolved considerably in recent years. Many patients with a variety of symptoms enjoy significantly improved quality of life with minimal side effects. There are now more treatment options for patients suffering with advanced PD, ET, cerebellar tremor, dystonia, and spasticity, and even more promising therapies are on the horizon. Nevertheless, surgical therapies for movement disorders as a whole still do not yet meet evidence-based standards. Further studies are essential in order to clarify the surgical targets and techniques that are optimally suited to treat patients with each of these devastating conditions.

REFERENCES

1. Spiegel EA, Wycis HT, Marks M, Lee AJ. Stereotaxic apparatus for operations on the human brain. Science 1947; 106:349–350.
2. Alexander GE, DeLong MR, Strick PL. Parallel organization of functionally segregated circuits linking basal ganglia and cortex. Annu Rev Neurosci 1986; 9:357–381.
3. Wichmann T, DeLong MR. Functional neuroanatomy of the basal ganglia in Parkinson's disease. Adv Neurol 2003; 91:9–18.

4. Albin RL, Young AB, Penney JB. The functional anatomy of basal ganglia disorders. Trends Neurosci 1989; 12(10):366–375.

5. Gerfen CR, Engber TM, Mahan LC, Susel Z, Chase TN, Monsma FJ, Jr., Sibley DR. D1 and D2 dopamine receptor-regulated gene expression of striatonigral and striatopallidal neurons. Science 1990; 250(4986):1429–1432.

6. Bergman H, Wichmann T, Karmon B, DeLong MR. The primate subthalamic nucleus. II. Neuronal activity in the MPTP model of parkinsonism. J Neurophysiol 1994; 72(2):507–520.

7. Filion M, Tremblay L. Abnormal spontaneous activity of globus pallidus neurons in monkeys with MPTP-induced parkinsonism. Brain Res 1991; 547(1): 142–151.

8. Burchiel KJ, Anderson VC, Favre J, Hammerstad JP. Comparison of pallidal and subthalamic nucleus deep brain stimulation for advanced Parkinson's disease: results of a randomized, blinded pilot study. Neurosurgery 1999; 45(6):1375–1382; discussion 1382–1384.

9. Kumar R, Lang AE, Rodriguez-Oroz MC, Lozano AM, Limousin P, Pollak P, Benabid AL, Guridi J, Ramos E, van der Linden C, Vandewalle A, Caemaert J, Lannoo E, van den Abbeele D, Vingerhoets G, Wolters M, Obeso JA. Deep brain stimulation of the globus pallidus pars interna in advanced Parkinson's disease. Neurology 2000; 55(12 suppl 6):S34–S39.

10. Limousin P, Krack P, Pollak P, Benazzouz A, Ardouin C, Hoffmann D, Benabid AL. Electrical stimulation of the subthalamic nucleus in advanced Parkinson's disease. N Engl J Med 1998; 339(16):1105–1111.

11. Deep Brain Stimulation for Parkinson's Disease Study Group. Deep-brain stimulation of the subthalamic nucleus or the pars interna of the globus pallidus in Parkinson's disease. N Engl J Med 2001; 345(13):956–963.

12. Limousin P, Greene J, Pollak P, Rothwell J, Benabid AL, Frackowiak R. Changes in cerebral activity pattern due to subthalamic nucleus or internal pallidum stimulation in Parkinson's disease. Ann Neurol 1997; 42(3):283–291.

13. Koller W, Pahwa R, Busenbark K, Hubble J, Wilkinson S, Lang A, Tuite P, Sime E, Lazano A, Hauser R, Malapira T, Smith D, Tarsy D, Miyawaki E, Norregaard T, Kormos T, Olanow CW. High-frequency unilateral thalamic stimulation in the treatment of essential and parkinsonian tremor. Ann Neurol 1997; 42(3):292–299.

14. Marsden CD, Obeso JA. The functions of the basal ganglia and the paradox of stereotaxic surgery in Parkinson's disease. Brain 1994; 117(Pt 4):877–897.

15. Lozano AM, Lang AE, Galvez-Jimenez N, Miyasaki J, Duff J, Hutchinson WD, Dostrovsky JO. Effect of GPi pallidotomy on motor function in Parkinson's disease. Lancet 1995; 346(8987):1383–1387.

16. Vitek JL, Giroux M. Physiology of hypokinetic and hyperkinetic movement disorders: model for dyskinesia. Ann Neurol 2000; 47(4 suppl 1):S131–S140.

17. Bergman H, Feingold A, Nini A, Raz A, Slovin H, Abeles M, Vaadia E. Physiological aspects of information processing in the basal ganglia of normal and parkinsonian primates. Trends Neurosci 1998; 21(1):32–38.

18. Davis KD, Taub E, Houle S, Lang AE, Dostrovsky JO, Tasker RR, Lozano AM. Globus pallidus stimulation activates the cortical motor system during alleviation of parkinsonian symptoms. Nat Med 1997; 3(6):671–674.

19. Papa SM, Desimone R, Fiorani M, Oldfield EH. Internal globus pallidus discharge is nearly suppressed during levodopa-induced dyskinesias. Ann Neurol 1999; 46(5):732–738.
20. Obeso JA, Rodriguez-Oroz MC, Rodriguez M, Lanciego JL, Artieda J, Gonzalo N, Olanow CW. Pathophysiology of the basal ganglia in Parkinson's disease. Trends Neurosci 2000; 23(10 suppl):S8–S19.
21. Kobayashi K, Katayama Y, Kasai M, Oshima H, Fukaya C, Yamamoto T. Localization of thalamic cells with tremor-frequency activity in Parkinson's disease and essential tremor. Acta Neurochir Suppl 2003; 87:137–139.
22. Rodriguez MC, Guridi OJ, Alvarez L, Mewes K, Macias R, Vitek J, DeLong MR, Obeso JA. The subthalamic nucleus and tremor in Parkinson's disease. Mov Disord 1998; 13(suppl 3):111–118.
23. Krack P, Benazzouz A, Pollak P, Limousin P, Piallat B, Hoffmann D, Xie J, Benabid AL. Treatment of tremor in Parkinson's disease by subthalamic nucleus stimulation. Mov Disord 1998; 13(6):907–914.
24. Lang AE, Widner H. Deep brain stimulation for Parkinson's disease: patient selection and evaluation. Mov Disord 2002; 17(suppl 3):S94–S101.
25. Berney A, Vingerhoets F, Perrin A, Guex P, Villemure JG, Burkhard PR, Benkelfat C, Ghika J. Effect on mood of subthalamic DBS for Parkinson's disease: a consecutive series of 24 patients. Neurology 2002; 59(9):1427–1429.
26. Chou KL, Forman MS, Trojanowski JQ, Hurtig HI, Baltuch GH. Subthalamic nucleus deep brain stimulation in a patient with levodopa-responsive multiple system atrophy. Case report. J Neurosurg 2004; 100(3):553–556.
27. Tarsy D, Apetauerova D, Ryan P, Norregaard T. Adverse effects of subthalamic nucleus DBS in a patient with multiple system atrophy. Neurology 2003; 61(2):247–249.
28. Selby G. Stereotactic surgery for the relief of Parkinson's disease. 2. An analysis of the results in a series of 303 patients (413 operations). J Neurol Sci 1967; 5(2):343–375.
29. Kelly PJ, Gillingham FJ. The long-term results of stereotaxic surgery and L-dopa therapy in patients with Parkinson's disease. A 10-year follow-up study. J Neurosurg 1980; 53(3):332–337.
30. Laitinen LV, Bergenheim AT, Hariz MI. Leksell's posteroventral pallidotomy in the treatment of Parkinson's disease. J Neurosurg 1992; 76(1):53–61.
31. Baron MS, Vitek JL, Bakay RA, Green J, Kaneoke Y, Hashimoto T, Turner RS, Woodard JL, Cole SA, McDonald WM, DeLong MR. Treatment of advanced Parkinson's disease by posterior GPi pallidotomy: 1-year results of a pilot study. Ann Neurol 1996; 40(3):355–366.
32. Kishore A, Turnbull IM, Snow BJ, de la Fuente-Fernandez R, Schulzer M, Mak E, Yardley S, Calne DB. Efficacy, stability and predictors of outcome of pallidotomy for Parkinson's disease. Six-month follow-up with additional 1-year observations. Brain 1997; 120(Pt 5):729–737.
33. Krauss JK, Desaloms JM, Lai EC, King DE, Jankovic J, Grossman RG. Microelectrode-guided posteroventral pallidotomy for treatment of Parkinson's disease: postoperative magnetic resonance imaging analysis. J Neurosurg 1997; 87(3):358–367.

34. Uitti RJ, Wharen RE Jr, Turk MF, Lucas JA, Finton MJ, Graff-Radford NR, Boylan KB, Goerss SJ, Kall BA, Adler CH, Caviness JN, Atkinson EJ. Unilateral pallidotomy for Parkinson's disease: comparison of outcome in younger versus elderly patients. Neurology 1997; 49(4):1072–1077.

35. Fine J, Duff J, Chen R, Chir B, Hutchison W, Lozano AM, Lang AE. Long-term follow-up of unilateral pallidotomy in advanced Parkinson's disease. N Engl J Med 2000; 342(23):1708–1714.

36. Baron MS, Vitek JL, Bakay RA, Green J, McDonald WM, Cole SA, DeLong MR. Treatment of advanced Parkinson's disease by unilateral posterior GPi pallidotomy: 4-year results of a pilot study. Mov Disord 2000; 15(2):230–237.

37. Pal PK, Samii A, Kishore A, Schulzer M, Mak E, Yardley S, Turnbull IM, Calne DB. Long term outcome of unilateral pallidotomy: follow up of 15 patients for 3 years. J Neurol Neurosurg Psychiatry 2000; 69(3):337–344.

38. Ghika J, Ghika-Schmid F, Fankhauser H, Assal G, Vingerhoets F, Albanese A, Bogousslavsky J, Favre J. Bilateral contemporaneous posteroventral pallidotomy for the treatment of Parkinson's disease: neuropsychological and neurological side effects. Report of four cases and review of the literature. J Neurosurg 1999; 91(2):313–321.

39. Lang AE, Duff J, Saint-Cyr JA, Trepanier L, Gross RE, Lombardi W, Montgomery E, Hutchinson W, Lozano AM. Posteroventral medial pallidotomy in Parkinson's disease. J Neurol 1999; 246(suppl 2):II28–II41.

40. Favre J, Burchiel KJ, Taha JM, Hammerstad J. Outcome of unilateral and bilateral pallidotomy for Parkinson's disease: patient assessment. Neurosurgery 2000; 46(2):344–353; discussion 353–355.

41. De Bie RM, Schuurman PR, Esselink RA, Bosch DA, Speelman JD. Bilateral pallidotomy in Parkinson's disease: a retrospective study. Mov Disord 2002; 17(3):533–538.

42. Bergman H, Wichmann T, DeLong MR. Reversal of experimental parkinsonism by lesions of the subthalamic nucleus. Science 1990; 249(4975): 1436–1438.

43. Gill SS, Heywood P. Bilateral dorsolateral subthalamotomy for advanced Parkinson's disease. Lancet 1997; 350(9086):1224.

44. Alvarez L, Macias R, Guridi J, Lopez G, Alvarez E, Maragoto C, Teijeiro J, Torres A, Pavon N, Rodriguez-Oroz MC, Ochoa L, Hetherington H, Juncos J, DeLong MR, Obeso JA. Dorsal subthalamotomy for Parkinson's disease. Mov Disord 2001; 16(1):72–78.

45. Patel NK, Heywood P, O'Sullivan K, McCarter R, Love S, Gill SS. Unilateral subthalamotomy in the treatment of Parkinson's disease. Brain 2003; 126(Pt 5): 1136–1145.

46. Su PC, Tseng HM, Liu HM, Yen RF, Liou HH. Treatment of advanced Parkinson's disease by subthalamotomy: one-year results. Mov Disord 2003; 18(5):531–538.

47. Benabid AL, Benazzouz A, Hoffmann D, Limousin P, Krack P, Pollak P. Long-term electrical inhibition of deep brain targets in movement disorders. Mov Disord 1998; 13(suppl 3):119–125.

48. Lyons KE, Koller WC, Wilkinson SB, Pahwa R. Long term safety and efficacy of unilateral deep brain stimulation of the thalamus for parkinsonian tremor. J Neurol Neurosurg Psychiatry 2001; 71(5):682–684.

49. Kumar R, Lozano AM, Sime E, Lang AE. Long-term follow-up of thalamic deep brain stimulation for essential and parkinsonian tremor. Neurology 2003; 61(11):1601–1604.

50. Visser-Vandewalle V, van der Linden C, Temel Y, Nieman F, Celik H, Beuls E. Long-term motor effect of unilateral pallidal stimulation in 26 patients with advanced Parkinson disease. J Neurosurg 2003; 99(4):701–707.

51. Ghika J, Villemure JG, Fankhauser H, Favre J, Assal G, Ghika-Schmid F. Efficiency and safety of bilateral contemporaneous pallidal stimulation (deep brain stimulation) in levodopa-responsive patients with Parkinson's disease with severe motor fluctuations: a 2-year follow-up review. J Neurosurg 1998; 89(5):713–718.

52. Durif F, Lemaire JJ, Debilly B, Dordain G. Long-term follow-up of globus pallidus chronic stimulation in advanced Parkinson's disease. Mov Disord 2002; 17(4):803–807.

53. Volkmann J, Allert N, Voges J, Sturm V, Schnitzler A, Freund HJ. Long-term results of bilateral pallidal stimulation in Parkinson's disease. Ann Neurol 2004; 55(6):871–875.

54. Benabid AL, Pollak P, Gross C, Hoffmann D, Benazzouz A, Gao DM, Laurent A, Gentil M, Perret J. Acute and long-term effects of subthalamic nucleus stimulation in Parkinson's disease. Stereotact Funct Neurosurg 1994; 62(1–4):76–84.

55. Limousin P, Pollak P, Benazzouz A, Hoffmann D, Le Bas JF, Broussolle E, Perret JE, Benabid AL. Effect of parkinsonian signs and symptoms of bilateral subthalamic nucleus stimulation. Lancet 1995; 345(8942):91–95.

56. Allert N, Volkmann J, Dotse S, Hefter H, Sturm V, Freund HJ. Effects of bilateral pallidal or subthalamic stimulation on gait in advanced Parkinson's disease. Mov Disord 2001; 16(6):1076–1085.

57. Krack P, Batir A, Van Blercom N, Chabardes S, Fraix V, Ardouin C, Koudsie A, Limousin PD, Benazzouz A, LeBas JF, Benabid AL, Pollak P. Five-year follow-up of bilateral stimulation of the subthalamic nucleus in advanced Parkinson's disease. N Engl J Med 2003; 349(20):1925–1934.

58. Herzog J, Volkmann J, Krack P, Kopper F, Potter M, Lorenz D, Steinbach M, Klebe S, Hamel W, Schrader B, Weinert D, Muller D, Mehdorn HM, Deuschl G. Two-year follow-up of subthalamic deep brain stimulation in Parkinson's disease. Mov Disord 2003; 18(11):1332–1337.

59. Kleiner-Fisman G, Fisman DN, Sime E, Saint-Cyr JA, Lozano AM, Lang AE. Long-term follow up of bilateral deep brain stimulation of the subthalamic nucleus in patients with advanced Parkinson disease. J Neurosurg 2003; 99(3):489–495.

60. Krause M, Fogel W, Heck A, Hacke W, Bonsanto M, Trenkwalder C, Tronnier V. Deep brain stimulation for the treatment of Parkinson's disease: subthalamic nucleus versus globus pallidus internus. J Neurol Neurosurg Psychiatry 2001; 70(4):464–470.

61. Volkmann J, Allert N, Voges J, Weiss PH, Freund HJ, Sturm V. Safety and efficacy of pallidal or subthalamic nucleus stimulation in advanced PD. Neurology 2001; 56(4):548–551.

62. Freed CR, Greene PE, Breeze RE, Tsai WY, DuMouchel W, Kao R, Dillon S, Winfield H, Culver S, Trojanowski JQ, Eidelberg D, Fahn S. Transplantation of embryonic dopamine neurons for severe Parkinson's disease. N Engl J Med 2001; 344(10):710–719.

63. Olanow CW, Goetz CG, Kordower JH, Stoessl AJ, Sossi V, Brin MF, Shannon KM, Nauert GM, Perl DP, Godbold J, Freeman TB. A double-blind controlled trial of bilateral fetal nigral transplantation in Parkinson's disease. Ann Neurol 2003; 54(3):403–414.

64. Schumacher JM, Ellias SA, Palmer EP, Kott HS, Dinsmore J, Dempsey PK, Fischman AJ, Thomas C, Feldman RG, Kassissieh S, Raineri R, Manhart C, Penney D, Fink JS, Isacson O. Transplantation of embryonic porcine mesencephalic tissue in patients with PD. Neurology 2000; 54(5):1042–1050.

65. Drucker-Colin R, Verdugo-Diaz L. Cell transplantation for Parkinson's disease: present status. Cell Mol Neurobiol 2004; 24(3):301–316.

66. Hurelbrink CB, Barker RA. The potential of GDNF as a treatment for Parkinson's disease. Exp Neurol 2004; 185(1):1–6.

67. Nutt JG, Burchiel KJ, Comella CL, Jankovic J, Lang AE, Laws ER, Jr., Lozano AM, Penn RD, Simpson RK, Jr., Stacy M, Wooten GF. Randomized, double-blind trial of glial cell line-derived neurotrophic factor (GDNF) in PD. Neurology 2003; 60(1):69–73.

68. Gill SS, Patel NK, Hotton GR, O'Sullivan K, McCarter R, Bunnage M, Brooks DJ, Svendsen CN, Heywood P. Direct brain infusion of glial cell line-derived neurotrophic factor in Parkinson disease. Nat Med 2003; 9(5): 589–595.

69. Wasielewski PG, Burns JM, Koller WC. Pharmacologic treatment of tremor. Mov Disord 1998; 13(suppl 3):90–100.

70. Zesiewicz TA, Hauser RA. Phenomenology and treatment of tremor disorders. Neurol Clin 2001; 19(3):651–680.

71. Deuschl G, Bain P. Deep brain stimulation for tremor: patient selection and evaluation. Mov Disord 2002; 17(suppl 3):S102–S111.

72. Elble RJ. Diagnostic criteria for essential tremor and differential diagnosis. Neurology 2000; 54(11 suppl 4):S2–S6.

73. Hassler R, Riechert T. [Indications localization of stereotactic brain operations]. Der Nervenarzt 1954; 25(11):441–447.

74. Hassler R, Riechert T, Mundinger F, Umbach W, Ganglberger JA. Physiological observations in stereotaxic operations in extrapyramidal motor disturbances. Brain 1960; 83:337–350.

75. Chou KL, Hurtig HI, Jaggi JL, Baltuch GH. Bilateral subthalamic nucleus deep brain stimulation in a patient with cervical dystonia and essential tremor. Mov Disord 2005; 20(3):377–380.

76. Plaha P, Patel NK, Gill SS. Stimulation of the subthalamic region for essential tremor. J Neurosurg 2004; 101(1):48–54.

77. Murata J, Kitagawa M, Uesugi H, Saito H, Iwasaki Y, Kikuchi S, Tashiro K, Sawamura Y. Electrical stimulation of the posterior subthalamic area for the treatment of intractable proximal tremor. J Neurosurg 2003; 99(4):708–715.

78. Kitagawa M, Murata J, Kikuchi S, Sawamura Y, Saito H, Sasaki H, Tashiro K. Deep brain stimulation of subthalamic area for severe proximal tremor. Neurology 2000; 55(1):114–116.

79. Ohye C, Hirai T, Miyazaki M, Shibazaki T, Nakajima H. VIM thalamotomy for the treatment of various kinds of tremor. Appl Neurophysiol 1982; 45(3):275–280.

80. Nagaseki Y, Shibazaki T, Hirai T, Kawashima Y, Hirato M, Wada H, Miyazaki M, Ohye C. Long-term follow-up results of selective VIM-thalamotomy. J Neurosurg 1986; 65(3):296–302.

81. Mohadjer M, Goerke H, Milios E, Etou A, Mundinger F. Long-term results of stereotaxy in the treatment of essential tremor. Stereotact Funct Neurosurg 1990; 54–55:125–129.

82. Goldman MS, Ahlskog JE, Kelly PJ. The symptomatic and functional outcome of stereotactic thalamotomy for medically intractable essential tremor. J Neurosurg 1992; 76(6):924–928.

83. Jankovic J, Cardoso F, Grossman RG, Hamilton WJ. Outcome after stereotactic thalamotomy for parkinsonian, essential, and other types of tremor. Neurosurgery 1995; 37(4):680–686; discussion 686–687.

84. Tasker RR. Deep brain stimulation is preferable to thalamotomy for tremor suppression. Surg Neurol 1998; 49(2):145–153; discussion 153–154.

85. Pahwa R, Lyons KE, Wilkinson SB, Troster AI, Overman J, Kieltyka J, Koller WC. Comparison of thalamotomy to deep brain stimulation of the thalamus in essential tremor. Mov Disord 2001; 16(1):140–143.

86. Schuurman PR, Bosch DA, Bossuyt PM, Bonsel GJ, van Someren EJ, de Bie RM, Merkus MP, Speelman JD. A comparison of continuous thalamic stimulation and thalamotomy for suppression of severe tremor. N Engl J Med 2000; 342(7):461–468.

87. Benabid AL, Pollak P, Gervason C, Hoffmann D, Gao DM, Hommel M, Perret JE, de Rougemont J. Long-term suppression of tremor by chronic stimulation of the ventral intermediate thalamic nucleus. Lancet 1991; 337(8738): 403–406.

88. Koller WC, Lyons KE, Wilkinson SB, Troster AI, Pahwa R. Long-term safety and efficacy of unilateral deep brain stimulation of the thalamus in essential tremor. Mov Disord 2001; 16(3):464–468.

89. Rehncrona S, Johnels B, Widner H, Tornqvist AL, Hariz M, Sydow O. Long-term efficacy of thalamic deep brain stimulation for tremor: double-blind assessments. Mov Disord 2003; 18(2):163–170.

90. Sydow O, Thobois S, Alesch F, Speelman JD. Multicentre European study of thalamic stimulation in essential tremor: a six year follow up. J Neurol Neurosurg Psychiatry 2003; 74(10):1387–1391.

91. Hariz GM, Lindberg M, Bergenheim AT. Impact of thalamic deep brain stimulation on disability and health-related quality of life in patients with essential tremor. J Neurol Neurosurg Psychiatry 2002; 72(1):47–52.

92. Carpenter MA, Pahwa R, Miyawaki KL, Wilkinson SB, Searl JP, Koller WC. Reduction in voice tremor under thalamic stimulation. Neurology 1998; 50(3):796–798.

93. Koller WC, Lyons KE, Wilkinson SB, Pahwa R. Efficacy of unilateral deep brain stimulation of the VIM nucleus of the thalamus for essential head tremor. Mov Disord 1999; 14(5):847–850.

94. Ondo W, Jankovic J, Schwartz K, Almaguer M, Simpson RK. Unilateral thalamic deep brain stimulation for refractory essential tremor and Parkinson's disease tremor. Neurology 1998; 51(4):1063–1069.

95. Obwegeser AA, Uitti RJ, Turk MF, Strongosky AJ, Wharen RE. Thalamic stimulation for the treatment of midline tremors in essential tremor patients. Neurology 2000; 54(12):2342–2344.

96. Taha JM, Janszen MA, Favre J. Thalamic deep brain stimulation for the treatment of head, voice, and bilateral limb tremor. J Neurosurg 1999; 91(1):68–72.

97. Speelman JD, Schuurman R, de Bie RM, Esselink RA, Bosch DA. Stereotactic neurosurgery for tremor. Mov Disord 2002; 17(suppl 3):S84–S88.

98. Alusi SH, Worthington J, Glickman S, Bain PG. A study of tremor in multiple sclerosis. Brain 2001; 124(Pt 4):720–730.

99. Geny C, Nguyen JP, Pollin B, Feve A, Ricolfi F, Cesaro P, Degos JD. Improvement of severe postural cerebellar tremor in multiple sclerosis by chronic thalamic stimulation. Mov Disord 1996; 11(5):489–494.

100. Whittle IR, Hooper J, Pentland B. Thalamic deep-brain stimulation for movement disorders due to multiple sclerosis. Lancet 1998; 351(9096):109–110.

101. Montgomery EB, Jr., Baker KB, Kinkel RP, Barnett G. Chronic thalamic stimulation for the tremor of multiple sclerosis. Neurology 1999; 53(3):625–628.

102. Alusi SH, Aziz TZ, Glickman S, Jahanshahi M, Stein JF, Bain PG. Stereotactic lesional surgery for the treatment of tremor in multiple sclerosis: a prospective case-controlled study. Brain 2001; 124(Pt 8):1576–1589.

103. Hooper J, Taylor R, Pentland B, Whittle IR. A prospective study of thalamic deep brain stimulation for the treatment of movement disorders in multiple sclerosis. Br J Neurosurg 2002; 16(2):102–109.

104. Schulder M, Sernas TJ, Karimi R. Thalamic stimulation in patients with multiple sclerosis: long-term follow-up. Stereotact Funct Neurosurg 2003; 80(1–4):48–55.

105. Fahn S, Bressman SB, Marsden CD. Classification of dystonia. Adv Neurol 1998; 78:1–10.

106. Tsui JK, Eisen A, Stoessl AJ, Calne S, Calne DB. Double-blind study of botulinum toxin in spasmodic torticollis. Lancet 1986; 2(8501):245–247.

107. Hsiung GY, Das SK, Ranawaya R, Lafontaine AL, Suchowersky O. Long-term efficacy of botulinum toxin A in treatment of various movement disorders over a 10-year period. Mov Disord 2002; 17(6):1288–1293.

108. Lew MF, Brashear A, Factor S. The safety and efficacy of botulinum toxin type B in the treatment of patients with cervical dystonia: summary of three controlled clinical trials. Neurology 2000; 55(12 suppl 5):S29–S35.

109. Kessler KR, Skutta M, Benecke R. Long-term treatment of cervical dystonia with botulinum toxin A: efficacy, safety, and antibody frequency. German Dystonia Study Group. J Neurol 1999; 246(4):265–274.

110. Dauer WT, Burke RE, Greene P, Fahn S. Current concepts on the clinical features, aetiology and management of idiopathic cervical dystonia. Brain 1998; 121(Pt 4):547–560.

111. Rollnik JD, Wohlfarth K, Dengler R, Bigalke H. Neutralizing botulinum toxin type a antibodies: clinical observations in patients with cervical dystonia. Neurol Clin Neurophysiol 2001; 2001(3):2–4.

112. Jankovic J, Schwartz K. Botulinum toxin injections for cervical dystonia. Neurology 1990; 40(2):277–280.

113. Cooper IS. 20-year followup study of the neurosurgical treatment of dystonia musculorum deformans. Adv Neurol 1976; 14:423–452.

114. Gros C, Frerebeau P, Perez-Dominguez E, Bazin M, Privat JM. Long term results of stereotaxic surgery for infantile dystonia and dyskinesia. Neurochirurgia 1976; 19(4):171–178.

115. Andrew J, Fowler CJ, Harrison MJ. Stereotaxic thalamotomy in 55 cases of dystonia. Brain 1983; 106(Pt 4):981–1000.

116. Tasker RR, Doorly T, Yamashiro K. Thalamotomy in generalized dystonia. Adv Neurol 1988; 50:615–631.

117. Cardoso F, Jankovic J, Grossman RG, Hamilton WJ. Outcome after stereotactic thalamotomy for dystonia and hemiballismus. Neurosurgery 1995; 36(3): 501–507; discussion 507–508.

118. Kondziolka D, Bonaroti E, Baser S, Brandt F, Kim YS, Lunsford LD. Outcomes after stereotactically guided pallidotomy for advanced Parkinson's disease. J Neurosurg 1999; 90(2):197–202.

119. de Bie RM, Schuurman PR, de Haan PS, Bosch DA, Speelman JD. Unilateral pallidotomy in advanced Parkinson's disease: a retrospective study of 26 patients. Mov Disord 1999; 14(6):951–957.

120. Yoshor D, Hamilton WJ, Ondo W, Jankovic J, Grossman RG. Comparison of thalamotomy and pallidotomy for the treatment of dystonia. Neurosurgery 2001; 48(4):818–824; discussion 824–826.

121. Eltahawy HA, Saint-Cyr J, Giladi N, Lang AE, Lozano AM. Primary dystonia is more responsive than secondary dystonia to pallidal interventions: outcome after pallidotomy or pallidal deep brain stimulation. Neurosurgery 2004; 54(3):613–619; discussion 619–621.

122. Ondo WG, Desaloms JM, Jankovic J, Grossman RG. Pallidotomy for generalized dystonia. Mov Disord 1998; 13(4):693–698.

123. Iacono RP, Kuniyoshi SM, Lonser RR, Maeda G, Inae AM, Ashwal S. Simultaneous bilateral pallidoansotomy for idiopathic dystonia musculorum deformans. Pediatr Neurol 1996; 14(2):145–148.

124. Lozano AM, Kumar R, Gross RE, Giladi N, Hutchison WD, Dostrovsky JO, Lang AE. Globus pallidus internus pallidotomy for generalized dystonia. Mov Disord 1997; 12(6):865–870.

125. Teive HA, Sa DS, Grande CV, Antoniuk A, Werneck LC. Bilateral pallidotomy for generalized dystonia. Arq Neuropsiquiatr 2001; 59(2-B):353–357.

126. Lin JJ, Lin SZ, Lin GY, Chang DC, Lee CC. Treatment of intractable generalized dystonia by bilateral posteroventral pallidotomy—one-year results. Zhonghua Yi Xue Za Zhi (Taipei) 2001; 64(4):231–238.

127. Burke RE, Fahn S, Marsden CD, Bressman SB, Moskowitz C, Friedman J. Validity and reliability of a rating scale for the primary torsion dystonias. Neurology 1985; 35(1):73–77.
128. Mundinger F. [New stereotactic treatment of spasmodic torticollis with a brain stimulation system (author's transl.)]. Med Klin 1977; 72(46):1982–1986.
129. Benabid AL, Pollak P, Gao D, Hoffmann D, Limousin P, Gay E, Payen I, Benazzouz A. Chronic electrical stimulation of the ventralis intermedius nucleus of the thalamus as a treatment of movement disorders. J Neurosurg 1996; 84(2):203–214.
130. Vercueil L, Pollak P, Fraix V, Caputo E, Moro E, Benazzouz A, Xie J, Koudsie A, Benabid AL. Deep brain stimulation in the treatment of severe dystonia. J Neurol 2001; 248(8):695–700.
131. Kupsch A, Kuehn A, Klaffke S, Meissner W, Harnack D, Winter C, Haelbig TD, Kivi A, Arnold G, Einhaupl KM, Schneider GH, Trottenberg T. Deep brain stimulation in dystonia. J Neurol 2003; 250(suppl 1):I47–I52.
132. Coubes P, Roubertie A, Vayssiere N, Hemm S, Echenne B. Treatment of DYT1-generalised dystonia by stimulation of the internal globus pallidus. Lancet 2000; 355(9222):2220–2221.
133. Bereznai B, Steude U, Seelos K, Botzel K. Chronic high-frequency globus pallidus internus stimulation in different types of dystonia: a clinical, video, and MRI report of six patients presenting with segmental, cervical, and generalized dystonia. Mov Disord 2002; 17(1):138–144.
134. Yianni J, Bain P, Giladi N, Auca M, Gregory R, Joint C, Nandi D, Stein J, Scott R, Aziz T. Globus pallidus internus deep brain stimulation for dystonic conditions: a prospective audit. Mov Disord 2003; 18(4):436–442.
135. Krauss JK, Pohle T, Weber S, Ozdoba C, Burgunder JM. Bilateral stimulation of globus pallidus internus for treatment of cervical dystonia. Lancet 1999; 354(9181):837–838.
136. Cif L, El Fertit H, Vayssiere N, Hemm S, Hardouin E, Gannau A, Tuffery S, Coubes P. Treatment of dystonic syndromes by chronic electrical stimulation of the internal globus pallidus. J Neurosurg Sci 2003; 47(1):52–55.
137. Tronnier VM, Fogel W. Pallidal stimulation for generalized dystonia. Report of three cases. J Neurosurg 2000; 92(3):453–456.
138. Detante O, Vercueil L, Krack P, Chabardes S, Benabid AL, Pollak P. Off-period dystonia in Parkinson's disease but not generalized dystonia is improved by high-frequency stimulation of the subthalamic nucleus. Adv Neurol 2004; 94: 309–314.
139. Sun B, Li D, Sun C, Liu D, Zhao Y, Shen J, Chen S. Target selection for primary dystonia deep brain stimulation: GPi or STN [abstr]. Proceedings from the American Society for Stereotactic and Functional Neurosurgery 2003 Quadrennial Meeting. New York City, NY, 2003, pp 91.
140. Ordia JI, Fischer E, Adamski E, Spatz EL. Chronic intrathecal delivery of baclofen by a programmable pump for the treatment of severe spasticity. J Neurosurg 1996; 85(3):452–457.
141. Speelman D, van Manen J. Cerebral palsy and stereotactic neurosurgery: long term results. J Neurol Neurosurg Psychiatry 1989; 52(1):23–30.

142. Gahm NH, Russman BS, Cerciello RL, Fiorentino MR, McGrath DM. Chronic cerebellar stimulation for cerebral palsy: a double-blind study. Neurology 1981; 31(1):87–90.
143. Laitinen L, Singounas E. Longitudinal myelotomy in the treatment of spasticity of the legs. J Neurosurg 1971; 35(5):536–540.
144. Penn RD, Kroin JS. Continuous intrathecal baclofen for severe spasticity. Lancet 1985; 2(8447):125–127.
145. Penn RD, Kroin JS. Intrathecal baclofen alleviates spinal cord spasticity. Lancet 1984; 1(8385):1078.
146. Van Schaeybroeck P, Nuttin B, Lagae L, Schrijvers E, Borghgraef C, Feys P. Intrathecal baclofen for intractable cerebral spasticity: a prospective placebo-controlled, double-blind study. Neurosurgery 2000; 46(3):603–609; discussion 609–612.
147. Penn RD. Intrathecal baclofen for spasticity of spinal origin: seven years of experience. J Neurosurg 1992; 77(2):236–240.
148. Lazorthes Y, Sallerin-Caute B, Verdie JC, Bastide R, Carillo JP. Chronic intrathecal baclofen administration for control of severe spasticity. J Neurosurg 1990; 72(3):393–402.
149. Wright FV, Sheil EM, Drake JM, Wedge JH, Naumann S. Evaluation of selective dorsal rhizotomy for the reduction of spasticity in cerebral palsy: a randomized controlled trial. Dev Med Child Neurol 1998; 40(4):239–247.
150. Steinbok P, Reiner AM, Beauchamp R, Armstrong RW, Cochrane DD, Kestle J. A randomized clinical trial to compare selective posterior rhizotomy plus physiotherapy with physiotherapy alone in children with spastic diplegic cerebral palsy. Dev Med Child Neurol 1997; 39(3):178–184.
151. McLaughlin JF, Bjornson KF, Astley SJ, Graubert C, Hays RM, Roberts TS, Price R, Temkin N. Selective dorsal rhizotomy: efficacy and safety in an investigator-masked randomized clinical trial. Dev Med Child Neurol 1998; 40(4):220–232.
152. McLaughlin J, Bjornson K, Temkin N, Steinbok P, Wright V, Reiner A, Roberts T, Drake J, O'Donnell M, Rosenbaum P, Barber J, Ferrel A. Selective dorsal rhizotomy: meta-analysis of three randomized controlled trials. Dev Med Child Neurol 2002; 44(1):17–25.

2

Patient Selection and Indications for Surgery

Jill L. Ostrem

Department of Neurology, University of California, San Francisco and San Francisco Veterans Affairs Medical Center, San Francisco, California, U.S.A.

Philip A. Starr

Department of Neurosurgery, University of California, San Francisco and San Francisco Veterans Affairs Medical Center, San Francisco, California, U.S.A.

William J. Marks, Jr.

Department of Neurology, University of California, San Francisco and San Francisco Veterans Affairs Medical Center, San Francisco, California, U.S.A.

1. INTRODUCTION

Parkinson's disease is a complex neurological disorder, painting a variety of clinical pictures. Age of onset, specific features and distribution of motor symptomatology, rate of disease progression, and presence of nonmotor signs and symptoms span a diverse spectrum among patients with the disorder. An array of modern therapeutic options enables clinicians to control many parkinsonian symptoms effectively for years. The challenge facing clinicians with regard to surgical treatment is determining which patients are likely to realize meaningful benefit from surgery and when along the course of each patient's disease to intervene. Since all surgical procedures are associated with the potential, though relatively small, for serious complication, anticipated benefit from surgical intervention must always be balanced against possible risks.

Though surgical procedures have been employed for decades to treat Parkinson's disease, practices in the modern era of surgical treatment are certainly not standardized, and they continue to evolve. Despite the absence of rigorously established guidelines informing the indications for surgery and selection of patients for such treatment, a general consensus is emerging that is useful in guiding clinical practice. Particularly with the availability of the nondestructive technique of deep brain stimulation, the role of surgery is now viewed as a means of maintaining motor function before significant disability ensues, rather than a last-resort intervention for end-stage parkinsonian patients with no other treatment options.

2. IMPORTANCE OF PATIENT SELECTION

Appropriate patient selection is a major determinant of successful postoperative outcome. The following sections of this chapter detail the factors that need to be considered when evaluating each patient's candidacy for deep brain stimulation or ablative surgery. Evaluation of patient suitability for surgery is probably best accomplished using a multidisciplinary approach in which neurological, medical, cognitive/psychiatric, and social issues are assessed by a team of clinicians. This team is typically comprised of neurologists, neurosurgeons, neuropsychologists, nurses, and others who work together to evaluate and educate patients and their families.

3. INDICATIONS FOR SURGERY

When patients with advanced Parkinson's disease develop moderate to severe motor fluctuation, medication-induced dyskinesia, medication refractory tremor, or significant intolerance to medications, surgery should be considered. A number of factors need to be assessed in a systematic manner to determine each patient's candidacy for surgical treatment.

3.1. Certainty of Diagnosis

Surgical treatment is most effective and appropriate for patients with idiopathic Parkinson's disease, and it is generally not helpful for patients with other parkinsonian syndromes. Thus, verification of the diagnosis of idiopathic Parkinson's disease is the first step in assessing a patient for possible surgery. Table 1 summarizes the clinical features of idiopathic Parkinson's disease.

Not uncommonly, patients initially diagnosed with Parkinson's disease are later found to have another type of parkinsonism, such as diffuse Lewy body disease, vascular parkinsonism, or a Parkinson's plus syndrome. A thorough neurological history and examination focused on the patient's initial and present symptoms and signs, rate of disease progression, response to dopaminergic therapy, and presence or absence of atypical symptoms or signs allows solidification or refutation of the diagnosis of idiopathic Parkinson's disease.

Table 1 Features Characteristic of Idiopathic Parkinson's Disease

- Presence of at least two of the three cardinal features of parkinsonism (rest tremor, rigidity, bradykinesia)
- Asymmetric onset of signs/symptoms
- Substantial response to levodopa or dopamine agonist
- Absence of features suggesting alternative diagnoses
  - Prominent postural instability in the first 3 years after symptom onset
  - Freezing phenomena in the first 3 years
  - Hallucinations unrelated to medication in the first 3 years of disease
  - Dementia preceding motor symptoms or in the first year
  - Supranuclear gaze palsy
  - Severe, symptomatic dysautonomia unrelated to medications
  - Documentation of a condition known to produce parkinsonism and plausibly connected to the patient's symptoms

Source: From Ref. 51.

3.2. Identification of Motor Symptoms and Their Disability

Once the diagnosis of Parkinson's disease is clinically certain, clinicians should ascertain which symptoms and signs are most troublesome or disabling for each patient to determine whether those particular problems are likely to be improved by surgery. Many surgical trials have now demonstrated the ability of surgical treatments, particularly deep brain stimulation of the subthalamic nucleus or globus pallidus, to improve the cardinal motor features of Parkinson's disease, including rigidity, tremor, bradykinesia, and disturbances of gait. In addition, a reduction in motor fluctuation is commonly seen following surgery. Patients experience high quality motor function ("on" time) consistently throughout their day, with fewer episodes of troubling motor symptomatology ("off" periods) and less hyperkinetic movement (dyskinesia) (1–13).

Features of Parkinson's disease that appear to be less responsive to surgical intervention include speech dysfunction and swallowing difficulty. In addition, patients who experience severe postural instability or freezing of gait deserve special mention. These symptoms can be two of the most disabling problems, and they often become more difficult to treat pharmacologically as Parkinson's disease progresses. Thus, patients with these symptoms may be referred for surgery when medications have failed. Severe disturbance of balance or gait unimproved by medication or that occurs when the patient is otherwise in a good state of medication-responsiveness (during the "on" period) appears to be resistant to improvement by surgery. Though not well studied, many nonmotor manifestations of Parkinson's disease (e.g., cognitive dysfunction, dysautonomia) also do not appear to benefit from surgical intervention. Recognizing the factors that contribute to each patient's disability, and the extent to which the patient's troubling symptoms are those that tend

Table 2 Questions for Patients to Assess Their Motor Symptomatology and Disability

---

1. What are the symptoms from your Parkinson's disease that bother you the most, beginning with the most troublesome problem, in order of severity?
2. During what percent of your waking day are you "off," that is, experiencing significant symptoms from your Parkinson's disease, despite taking your medication?
3. How would you describe the most severe "off" state on a typical day?
4. During what percent of your waking day do you experience troublesome dyskinesia, that is excessive and uncontrolled movements that bother you?
5. Do you have rigidity or muscle stiffness, and how much of a problem is it for you?
6. Do you have tremor or shaking, and how much of a problem is it for you?
7. Do you have slowness of movement or difficulty initiating movement, and how much of a problem is it for you?
8. Do you have trouble with walking, and how much of a problem is it for you?
9. Do you have problems with balance, and how much of a problem is it for you?
10. Do you fall? If so, why and how often?
11. What activities previously performed are now difficult or impossible due to your Parkinson's disease?

---

to respond to surgical intervention, will help identify those patients who will experience the greatest benefit from surgery. Table 2 lists helpful questions to be used in assessing the presence and extent of various motor symptoms preoperatively.

From the patient history and examination (particularly with the patient examined in their off-medication and on-medication states), as well as from the responses to the focused questions outlined in Table 2, one can develop an appreciation for the level of disability experienced by each patient. In order to justify the potential risk of surgical intervention, patients should be at a stage in their Parkinson's disease in which they are experiencing significant disability. Determining what constitutes significant disability is subjective and should be individualized for each patient. The goal is to intervene, if possible, just when the patient reaches a stage where the daily burden of parkinsonian motor symptomatology begins to cause significant interference with daily function, occupational activities, important leisure time pursuits, and/or basic activities of daily living.

A useful tool in gauging daily function is the motor fluctuation diary, a chart in which patients record their level of motor function periodically throughout their day. Typically patients are asked to rate their motor function every 30–60 min during wakefulness as to whether they are "off" (slow and/or experiencing other troublesome symptoms), "on" (functioning reasonably well), or "on with troublesome dyskinesia" (experiencing excessive, involuntary movements that impede function). Patients are also asked to indicate when medications were taken, allowing interpretation by the clinician of relationships between motor function and medication timing. Such "real time" ratings by patients and their family members provide extremely helpful information to clinicians in understanding the cumulative quantity and patterns of motor disability throughout each patient's day. Some surgical research protocols require that patients experience a minimum amount (e.g., 3 or more hours) of cumulative "off" and/or dyskinetic time each day to justify surgery. Other useful tools to document the extent of dyskinesia include the Unified Parkinson's Disease Rating Scale (UPDRS) Part IVa (dyskinesia) score, the Abnormal Involuntary Movement Scale (AIMS), or the Rush Dyskinesia Scale (14). To assess health-related quality of life, the Parkinson's Disease Questionnaire (PDQ-39) is most commonly used (15). To date, quality of life scores typically do not play a major role in the clinical assessment of surgical candidacy, though they are commonly incorporated into clinical studies.

3.3. Status of Pharmacological Treatment

Since currently available surgical treatments suppress symptoms but do not clearly alter disease progression, they are used to control symptoms when pharmacotherapy fails to provide adequate and consistent symptom relief. To deem medication treatment sufficiently ineffective before proceeding to surgery, one needs to ensure that the patients' medication regimen has been optimized for their particular symptoms. The patients' current and past medications and their dosing schemes should be carefully reviewed, as there are several strategies that can be used to improve control of symptoms, motor fluctuation, and dyskinesia. If not already undertaken, the strategies in Table 3 can be considered in an attempt to optimize pharmacological

Table 3 Strategies for Optimizing Pharmacological Treatment of Motor Symptoms in Advanced Parkinson's Disease

---

- Administer immediate-release levodopa at the appropriate dose and frequency tailored to the patient's wake/sleep, meal, and activity schedule (note that in advanced patients, controlled-release preparations of levodopa are often less consistent in their effect)
- Use a dopamine agonist at appropriate doses in conjunction with levodopa as tolerated; if one agonist is ineffective or poorly tolerated, consider a trial of another agonist
- Use a catechol-*O*-methyltransferase (COMT) inhibitor to maximize the duration of effect from levodopa
- Use an anticholinergic medication if the patient has severe tremor or dystonic dyskinesia
- Use amantadine to treat troublesome dyskinesia
- Use injectable apomorphine to rescue patients from severe "off" periods

---

treatment. Note that most of these strategies can be employed relatively quickly to determine whether symptoms can be brought under adequate control and surgery can be deferred. In some patients, medications are poorly tolerated and it may be best to proceed to surgery without exhausting trials of all medication options.

3.4. Extent of Dopaminergic Responsiveness

The degree to which a patient is responsive to dopaminergic medication, particularly levodopa, generally predicts how responsive motor symptoms will be to surgical treatment, especially treatment with deep brain stimulation (16). Levodopa responsiveness can sometimes be inferred from a careful history, but having objective confirmation of levodopa responsiveness and its extent can be helpful when evaluating a patient for surgery. The most widely used scale to assess motor signs and function in patients with Parkinson's disease is the motor subscale (part III) of the UPDRS (17). Many clinicians assess the UPDRS III score with the patients in their most symptomatic ("off") state and then again once the patient has responded to their antiparkinsonian medication and has achieved their best motor function ("on" state). This is practically achieved by assessing the patients in the morning, following cessation of antiparkinsonian medication for about 12 hr overnight, and then again after the patient has ingested their usual morning dose of medication (with or without extra levodopa) and derived a good response. Evaluation of the patients in the "off" state provides an instructive glimpse into their motor symptoms and associated disability at its most severe (not often appreciated in a routine office visit), and comparison of the "off" and "on" UPDRS III scores indicates the degree of responsiveness to dopaminergic medication. In order for patients to be considered for surgical treatment, some clinicians require patients to have a minimum UPDRS III score of 30/108 in the "off" state (18). The minimal degree of improvement required after a dopaminergic challenge to be considered a candidate for surgery is not well established. The Core Assessment Program for the Surgical Interventional Therapies in Parkinson's Disease (CAPSIT-PD) recommends a 33% improvement or greater before recommending surgery (19). We rarely offer surgery to patients who do not demonstrate at least a 30% improvement in the UPDRS III score. By performing these measures, one also derives information helpful in educating patients and their families about which symptoms are most likely to respond to surgery. Symptoms and signs resistant to levodopa will likely be resistant to surgical intervention, as well—with the notable exception of medication-resistant tremor. We also find that videotaping the patient's preoperative examination during the "off" and "on" UPDRS III assessments provides a useful visual record of baseline motor dysfunction, which can later be reviewed postoperatively to gauge treatment response.

3.5. Cognitive Status

A clear understanding of the patient's cognitive function is important when considering surgical candidacy. Dementia is common in patients with Parkinson's disease, with the prevalence increasing with advanced age and disease progression (20). Most clinicians do not offer surgery to patients with bona fide dementia, as this finding suggests more widespread disease that may be a marker for less robust motor response to surgery and because the presence of dementia produces practical obstacles to achieving optimal outcomes. Patients with dementia have difficulty tolerating and cooperating with the awake surgical procedures typically employed. Patients with dementia also have difficulty accurately observing and articulating their symptoms, making adjustment of deep brain stimulation parameters and medications more difficult. Finally, patients with preexisting dementia may experience a worsening of their cognitive status following surgery (21–23).

To screen for dementia, a Mini Mental Status Exam (MMSE) can be performed. It is generally accepted that a MMSE score of ≤ 24 is an indicator of poor surgical candidacy (18). Certainly, if a question exists about a patient's cognitive status, formal neuropsychological testing should be performed. In fact, many clinicians at experienced surgical centers evaluate all patients with a battery of neurocognitive tests preoperatively. Patients with Parkinson's disease can develop cognitive deficits in areas of executive functioning, visuospatial processing, attention and set shifting, and memory function. In the neurocognitive testing battery, it is important to include measures of general cognitive functioning, such as the Mattis Dementia Rating Scale (MDRS) ; measures of executive functioning and attention, such as verbal fluency tests, paced auditory serial addition tests, and the Wisconsin Card Sorting Test; measures of short- and long-term memory function; measures of visuospatial function; and measures of language function. In some instances, results from neuropsychological testing may reveal a pattern of dementia that is more compatible with Alzheimer's disease, diffuse Lewy body disease, or progressive supranuclear palsy, offering evidence against recommending surgery. Some clinicians exclude patients based on a MDRS total score of $\leq 120–130/144$ (18,19). We generally use a rejection criterion of a MDRS total score 2 or more standard deviations below the age-adjusted mean normal score or the criterion of 2 or more (out of 5) subtest scores that lie beyond 2 standard deviations.

3.6. Psychiatric Symptoms

Patients with Parkinson's disease are prone to depression, anxiety, and psychotic symptoms, including hallucinations and delusions. These symptoms can be a direct result of the disease process or exacerbated by medications used to control the symptoms of Parkinson's disease. Approximately 40% of Parkinson's disease patients suffer from depression. The literature is conflicting on the effect of surgical treatment on mood. Some studies suggest improvement in mood after surgery (24,25); however, a growing body of literature suggests, in some individuals, that depression and anxiety can worsen after surgery (26,27). Although there is no clear evidence that the presence of preexisting mood disorder increases the risk of postoperative disturbance in mood, it seems reasonable to assume that before proceeding with surgery, mood disorders should be effectively treated with medication. Furthermore, offering surgery to patients with severe preexisting depression or anxiety that does not adequately respond to pharmacological treatment may not be advisable. The Beck Depression Inventory (BDI) or the Montgomery and Asberg Depression Rating Scale (MADRS) can be used to assess depression. In our center, if a patient has a score of ≥18 on the BDI, then surgery is generally not recommended. The CAPSIT-PD recommends a score ranging from 7 to 19 on the MADRS as an exclusion criterion (19).

Parkinson's disease patients referred for surgery are also at greater risk for psychiatric symptoms, as they usually have relatively advanced disease and are being treated with moderate to high doses of medications that have the potential to cause psychiatric adverse effects. Patients with active hallucinations or delusions may be at increased risk for psychiatric complications after surgery. A wide range of psychiatric symptoms has been described following subthalamic nucleus deep brain stimulation surgery, including hallucinations, severe psychosis, mania, and impulsivity (25). Many times these symptoms occur in the immediate postoperative period, when patients are hospitalized, and are transient. Cases of persistent postoperative behavioral disturbance have been reported, though, and these may be more likely to occur in patients who are prone to these problems preoperatively (21). Thus, patients with active psychotic symptoms should not undergo surgical treatment (21,28). In many instances, reduction of antiparkinsonian medication or addition of an atypical antipsychotic agent will improve these symptoms, with the patient then able to proceed with surgery. Certainly, if a patient's psychotic symptoms are mild and clearly medication-induced, then surgical treatment may be beneficial, since following surgery, reduction in medication, and its associated adverse effects, is often possible.

3.7. Surgical Risk

Surgery is contraindicated by the presence of any medical condition that substantially increases its risk. The two most important risks of surgery are hemorrhagic stroke and, especially for deep brain stimulation surgery, device-related infection (29,30). In large surgical series, the risk of symptomatic hemorrhage complicating deep brain stimulation lead insertion is 1.5–3% per lead implant. The risk of a hemorrhage resulting in permanently increased morbidity is 0.5–1% per lead. This risk is increased in the setting of untreated hypertension, coagulopathy, or evidence on magnetic resonance imaging (MRI) of significant small vessel ischemic disease or extensive cerebral atrophy. Most clinicians require that a screening MRI of the brain be obtained, prior to making a final determination about surgical candidacy. The risk of serious infection of a newly implanted device, defined as an infection requiring reoperation to remove all or part of the implanted hardware, is 2–5% per device. Conditions that increase this risk, such as long-standing severe diabetes or need for chronic immunosuppression, are relative contraindications for device insertion. Such patients may be more appropriate candidates for unilateral pallidotomy.

3.8. Patient Expectations and Social Support

Candidates for surgery should demonstrate a clear understanding of the procedures entailed in their surgical treatment, potential risks of surgery, and realistic expectations about what can be achieved with surgery. Patients need to understand that currently available surgical treatments will not "cure" their disease or likely alter disease progression and that the goal of surgery is suppression of motor symptoms and optimization of motor function. Patients need to understand that the benefits of surgery will take time to accrue, particularly for treatment with deep brain stimulation, in which a number of visits may be required to optimize stimulator settings and concomitant medication. Patients and their families should be committed to working closely with the medical team in the postoperative management of their deep brain stimulation therapy, both in the early postoperative period and over time.

3.9. Multidisciplinary Consensus

An effective method for arriving at decisions regarding the surgical candidacy of patients is to collect the required data for each patient and then convene a conference in which these details are discussed by the multidisciplinary team. We find it extremely helpful for all team members to review together the medical history, motor testing scores, neurocognitive and psychiatric data, neuroimaging findings, and general clinical impressions (summarized in Table 4). This process allows a consensus decision to be reached on the suitability of each particular patient for surgical treatment and fosters a consistent and cohesive treatment approach.

4. ABLATIVE PROCEDURES vs. DEEP BRAIN STIMULATION

Surgical approaches to treat Parkinson's disease include destructive procedures, such as pallidotomy and thalamotomy, and the nonablative technique of deep brain stimulation. Deep brain stimulation is a nondestructive and reversible means of disrupting the abnormal function of neurons in brain structures affected by Parkinson's disease. It mimics to some extent

Table 4 Summary of Generally Accepted Criteria for Surgical Candidacy

Inclusion criteria	Exclusion criteria
Diagnosis of idiopathic Parkinson's disease	Serious surgical comorbidities
Disabling motor symptoms, including motor fluctuation or dyskinesia, despite optimized pharmacological treatment	Uncontrolled psychiatric illness, including anxiety and mood disorder (BDI >18)
Robust motor response (other than tremor) to levodopa (>30% improvement of UPDRS III score)	Dementia (MMSE $\leq$ 24, MDRS $\leq$ 120)
Clear understanding of risks and realistic expectations from surgery	Preoperative MRI with extensive white matter changes or severe cerebral atrophy

UPDRS III, Unified Parkinson's Disease Rating Scale, Part III (motor subscale); BDI, Beck Depression Inventory; MMSE, Mini Mental Status Examination; MDRS, Mattis Dementia Rating Scale; MRI, Magnetic Resonance Imaging.

the effect of a lesion in the target structure that is stimulated, although the exact mechanism by which this occurs remains unclear. The deep brain stimulation system consists of a four-contact lead placed into the brain that is connected to a programmable generator, implanted in the subclavicular region, via a wire tunneled under the scalp down to the chest. The stimulation parameters are programmed noninvasively to deliver the appropriate level of stimulation to the optimal anatomic region to maximize symptomatic benefit and minimize adverse effects. The benefits of deep brain stimulation compared to ablative surgery are its nondestructive nature, reversibility, and adjustability. In addition, when used bilaterally the technique does not generally produce the speech, swallowing, or cognitive complications commonly seen with ablative procedures (thalamotomy and pallidotomy); thus, deep brain stimulation is preferred for the provision of bilateral treatment (31–33). For patients in whom deep brain stimulation is not an appropriate option (e.g., patients who will be unable to adhere to follow-up requirements for stimulator programming), consideration can be given to treatment with a unilateral pallidotomy.

5. UNILATERAL vs. BILATERAL TREATMENT

The ability to safely provide bilateral treatment with deep brain stimulation has lead to this treatment being used bilaterally in the majority of Parkinson's disease patients who experience bilateral appendicular and/or axial motor symptoms. In moderately advanced patients with Parkinson's disease, bilateral treatment with subthalamic or pallidal deep brain stimulation provides incremental benefit over unilateral treatment and allows for a greater reduction in post-operative medication requirements (34,35). Unilateral deep brain stimulation used in patients with bilateral symptoms generally provides incomplete benefit and can result in more challenging postoperative management. Certainly, in patients with unilateral or strongly asymmetric motor symptoms, contralateral unilateral surgical intervention with deep brain stimulation is appropriate.

6. PREVIOUS SURGERY FOR PARKINSON'S DISEASE

In general, previous surgery does not exclude the possibility of additional surgical intervention. In a patient with a previous unilateral pallidotomy who continues to experience contralateral benefit but now requires treatment on the opposite side, pallidal deep brain stimulation on the opposite side of the brain can be used. Alternatively, if the benefits from the previous pallidotomy have waned, bilateral subthalamic nucleus deep brain stimulation can be employed with excellent benefit (36). Patients with a previous thalamotomy can also be successfully treated with bilateral subthalamic nucleus or globus pallidus deep brain stimulation.

7. AREAS OF CONTROVERSY

7.1. Earlier Intervention

The possibility of intervening earlier in the course of disease with surgical treatments has been proposed. There is speculation that subthalamic nucleus deep brain stimulation could potentially exert a neuroprotective effect. This hypothesis is based on indirect evidence implicating glutamate toxicity in Parkinson's disease and the possibility that deep brain stimulation of the subthalamic nucleus, by reducing glutaminergic outflow, could produce a neuroprotective effect (37). It remains to be proven, however, whether this hypothesis has merit. Others have suggested that reduction of medication or potential avoidance of medication exposure, often possible following surgery, could result in less neuronal toxicity, leading to a secondary neuroprotective effect. Today, there is no clear evidence that levodopa is neurotoxic in vivo (38). In fact, some studies suggest dopamine agonists may have a neuroprotective effect (39,40). These issues will need further study. At this time, there is no convincing evidence to recommend surgical intervention with deep brain stimulation based on its bestowing a neuroprotective effect. One of the most convincing arguments for earlier surgical intervention with deep brain stimulation therapy, though, is the promise of allowing patients with Parkinson's disease to enjoy a better quality of life by improved control of symptoms (41). A large clinical trial will be required to determine if treating milder patients with deep brain stimulation will have this desired effect in the context of an acceptable risk/benefit analysis.

7.2. Upper Age Limit

Whether there is an upper age limit above which surgery should no longer be offered is the topic of debate. Several previous studies have shown that patients older than 70 years benefit less from pallidotomy compared to younger patients (42). Similar findings of only modest motor improvement in older patients after subthalamic nucleus deep brain stimulation surgery have also been reported (16,43). Others have found an increased incidence of cognitive dysfunction in older patients after surgery (21). Older patients may tolerate surgery less well and may be more susceptible to transient postoperative confusion, especially after bilateral subthalamic nucleus deep brain stimulation surgery. We and others, however, have found no difference in postoperative outcomes in patients with advanced age, providing these patients are carefully selected and exhibit a robust response to a dopaminergic challenge (10,44,45). We typically do not exclude patients from surgery based on age alone. If older patients experience severe motor fluctuation, dyskinesia, a good response to levodopa, no signs of dementia or major psychiatric disturbance, and are in good general health, we will offer surgical treatment.

7.3. Surgical Brain Target Selection

The surgical treatment of choice today for most patients with Parkinson's disease is deep brain stimulation. The best location for stimulation, however, remains controversial. Both the subthalamic nucleus and globus pallidus internus have been studied extensively as target locations for deep brain stimulation, and both have been shown to treat the cardinal motor features of Parkinson's disease. To date, few rigorously conducted comparison studies have been completed to determine the relative merits and disadvantages of stimulation at each target and whether treatment at one target might, indeed, be superior to the other. Comparative studies to date and a meta-analysis of reports concerning deep brain stimulation of the subthalamic nucleus or of the globus pallidus have shown no statistically significant difference in the motor improvement provided by these treatments (46). A large-scale, multicenter, prospective randomized study sponsored by the Department of Veterans Affairs Cooperative Studies Program, the National Institute of Neurological Disease and Stroke, and Medtronic Neurological comparing bilateral subthalamic nucleus and globus pallidus deep brain stimulation is currently underway. The findings from this landmark study are expected to clarify numerous issues concerning the use of deep brain stimulation at the two targets.

In many centers, deep brain stimulation of the subthalamic nucleus is the default surgical treatment. Subthalamic nucleus stimulation may currently offer several advantages over pallidal stimulation. These include the larger scope of published experience with deep brain stimulation of the subthalamic nucleus, the greater familiarity that many neurosurgeons have in mapping and operating upon this target, and the suggestion from clinical practice that postoperative medication reduction is greater in patients treated at this target (47). Conversely, pallidal stimulation may offer some advantages over subthalamic stimulation. Some have suggested that globus pallidus deep brain stimulation provides a direct antidyskinetic effect on levodopa-induced dyskinesia, allowing medication levels to be maintained to help treat symptoms in a synergistic manner (7). Additionally, cognitive, mood, and behavior abnormalities may be less prevalent in patients treated with globus pallidus deep brain stimulation compared with those receiving subthalamic nucleus stimulation, though this remains to be proven (48).

Interventions at the thalamic target (specifically, the ventral intermediate nucleus of the thalamus), whether with deep brain stimulation or ablation, are effective in suppressing contralateral parkinsonian tremor but do not address other motor symptoms (49,50). In contrast, deep brain stimulation of either the subthalamic nucleus or of the globus pallidus can provide effective tremor control while simultaneously improving other parkinsonian motor symptoms, diminishing motor fluctuation, and suppressing dyskinesia. Thus, even in those patients with Parkinson's disease who predominantly manifest tremor as their main source of disability, basal ganglia targets seem to be preferable to the thalamic target in many of these instances.

8. FUTURE OF PARKINSON'S DISEASE SURGERY AND PATIENT SELECTION

The value of currently available surgical treatments for Parkinson's disease—particularly deep brain stimulation—is their ability to often dramatically suppress motor symptoms and provide patients with more consistent, high quality motor function. Patient selection for these procedures therefore heavily emphasizes patients with significant motor disability and focuses on those patients with relatively advanced disease in whom the risks of surgery can be justified by the benefits typically achieved. There is vital need to provide patients with therapies that do more than merely provide symptomatic benefit, however. Disease-modifying treatments that decelerate or halt disease progression, repair and restore degenerated neural circuits, and protect against the symptomatic declaration of disease in the first place are desperately needed. As these restorative and protective therapies, likely delivered using neurosurgical approaches, become available, selection criteria for their use will undoubtedly evolve. In the future, our therapies will be directed at those patients with new-onset or newly diagnosed Parkinson's disease and a mild level of symptomatology.

Thus, it seems likely that the field of surgical movement disorders will arrive at the point of being able to provide patients a spectrum of interventional therapies along the continuum of Parkinson's disease progression, with patient candidacy algorithms designed according to the efficacy and risk/benefit calculus at each stage of the disease.

REFERENCES

1. Volkmann J, Allert N, Voges J, Sturm V, Schnitzler A, Freund HJ. Long-term results of bilateral pallidal stimulation in Parkinson's disease. Ann Neurol 2004; 55(6):871–875.
2. Krause M, Fogel W, Mayer P, Kloss M, Tronnier V. Chronic inhibition of the subthalamic nucleus in Parkinson's disease. J Neurol Sci 2004; 219(1–2): 119–124.
3. Thobois S, Mertens P, Guenot M, Hermier M, Mollion H, Bouvard M, Chazot G, Broussolle E, Sindou M. Subthalamic nucleus stimulation in Parkinson's disease: clinical evaluation of 18 patients. J Neurol 2002; 249(5):529–534.
4. Loher TJ, Burgunder JM, Pohle T, Weber S, Sommerhalder R, Krauss JK. Long-term pallidal deep brain stimulation in patients with advanced Parkinson disease: 1-year follow-up study. J Neurosurg 2002; 96(5):844–853.
5. Simuni T, Jaggi JL, Mulholland H, Hurtig HI, Colcher A, Siderowf AD, Ravina B, Skolnick BE, Goldstein R, Stern MB, Baltuch GH. Bilateral stimulation of the subthalamic nucleus in patients with Parkinson disease: a study of efficacy and safety. J Neurosurg 2002; 96(4):666–672.
6. Pinter MM, Alesch F, Murg M, Seiwald M, Helscher RJ, Binder H. Deep brain stimulation of the subthalamic nucleus for control of extrapyramidal features in advanced idiopathic Parkinson's disease: one year follow-up. J Neural Transm 1999; 106(7/8):693–709.
7. Burchiel KJ, Anderson VC, Favre J, Hammerstad JP. Comparison of pallidal and subthalamic nucleus deep brain stimulation for advanced Parkinson's disease: results of a randomized, blinded pilot study. Neurosurgery 1999; 45(6):1375–1382; discussion 1382–1374.
8. Ghika J, Villemure JG, Fankhauser H, Favre J, Assal G, Ghika-Schmid F. Efficiency and safety of bilateral contemporaneous pallidal stimulation (deep brain stimulation) in levodopa-responsive patients with Parkinson's disease with severe motor fluctuations: a 2-year follow-up review. J Neurosurg 1998; 89(5):713–718.
9. Kumar R, Lozano AM, Kim YJ, Hutchison WD, Sime E, Halket E, Lang AE. Double-blind evaluation of subthalamic nucleus deep brain stimulation in advanced Parkinson's disease. Neurology 1998; 51(3):850–855.
10. Kleiner-Fisman G, Fisman DN, Sime E, Saint-Cyr JA, Lozano AM, Lang AE. Long-term follow up of bilateral deep brain stimulation of the subthalamic nucleus in patients with advanced Parkinson disease. J Neurosurg 2003; 99(3):489–495.
11. Tavella A, Bergamasco B, Bosticco E, Lanotte M, Perozzo P, Rizzone M, Torre E, Lopiano L. Deep brain stimulation of the subthalamic nucleus in Parkinson's disease: long-term follow-up. Neurol Sci 2002; 23(suppl 2):S111–S112.

12. Krack P, Batir A, Van Blercom N, Chabardes S, Fraix V, Ardouin C, Koudsie A, Limousin PD, Benazzouz A, LeBas JF, Benabid AL, Pollak P. Five-year follow-up of bilateral stimulation of the subthalamic nucleus in advanced Parkinson's disease. N Engl J Med 2003; 349(20):1925–1934.

13. Deep-Brain Stimulation for Parkinson's Disease Study Group. Deep-brain stimulation of the subthalamic nucleus or the pars interna of the globus pallidus in Parkinson's disease. N Engl J Med 2001; 345(13):956–963.

14. Goetz CG. Rating scale for dyskinesia in Parkinson's disease. Mov Disord 1999; 14(suppl 1):48–53.

15. Jenkinson C, Fitzpatrick R, Peto V. The Parkinson's Disease Questionnaire. User Manual for the PDQ-39, PDQ-8, and PDQ Summary Index. Oxford: Oxford Health Services Research Unit, 1998.

16. Charles PD, Van Blercom N, Krack P, Lee SL, Xie J, Besson G, Benabid AL, Pollak P. Predictors of effective bilateral subthalamic nucleus stimulation for PD. Neurology 2002; 59(6):932–934.

17. Fahn S, Elton RL. Members of the UPDRS development committee. Unified Parkinson's disease rating scale. In: Fahn S, Marsden CD, Calne CB, Goldstien M, eds. Recent Developments in Parkinson's Disease. Florham Park, NJ: MacMillan Healthcare Information, 1987:153–163.

18. Pollak P. Deep brain stimulation. Annual Course of the American Academy of Neurology, San Diego, CA, 2000.

19. Defer GL, Widner H, Marie RM, Remy P, Levivier M. Core assessment program for surgical interventional therapies in Parkinson's disease (CAPSIT-PD). Mov Disord 1999; 14(4):572–584.

20. Aarsland D, Andersen K, Larsen JP, Lolk A, Kragh-Sorensen P. Prevalence and characteristics of dementia in Parkinson disease: an 8-year prospective study. Arch Neurol 2003; 60(3):387–392.

21. Saint-Cyr JA, Trepanier LL, Kumar R, Lozano AM, Lang AE. Neuropsychological consequences of chronic bilateral stimulation of the subthalamic nucleus in Parkinson's disease. Brain 2000; 123(Pt 10):2091–2108.

22. Trepanier LL, Saint-Cyr JA, Lozano AM, Lang AE. Neuropsychological consequences of posteroventral pallidotomy for the treatment of Parkinson's disease. Neurology 1998; 51(1):207–215.

23. Scott R, Gregory R, Hines N, Carroll C, Hyman N, Papanasstasiou V, Leather C, Rowe J, Silburn P, Aziz T. Neuropsychological, neurological, and functional outcome following pallidotomy for Parkinson's disease. A consecutive series of eight simultaneous bilateral and twelve unilateral procedures. Brain 1998; 121(Pt 4):659–675.

24. Troster A, Fields J, Wilkinson S, Pahwa R, Koller W, Lyons K. Effect of motor improvement on quality of life following subthalamic stimulation is mediated by changes in depressive symptomatology. Stereotact Funct Neurosurg 2003; 80(1–4):43–47.

25. Funkiewiez A, Ardouin C, Caputo E, Krack P, Fraix V, Klinger H, Chabardes S, Foote K, Benabid AL, Pollak P. Long term effects of bilateral subthalamic nucleus stimulation on cognitive function, mood, and behaviour in Parkinson's disease. J Neurol Neurosurg Psychiatry 2004; 75(6):834–839.

26. Saint-Cyr JA, Trepanier LL. Neuropsychologic assessment of patients for movement disorder surgery. Mov Disord 2000; 15(5):771–783.

27. Doshi P, Chhaya N, Bhatt M. Depression leading to attempted suicide after bilateral subthalamic nucleus stimulation for Parkinson's disease. Mov Disord 2002; 17(5):1084–1085.

28. Lang AE, Widner H. Deep brain stimulation for Parkinson's disease: patient selection and evaluation. Mov Disord 2002; 17(suppl 3):S94–S101.

29. Hariz MI. Complications of deep brain stimulation surgery. Mov Disord 2002; 17(suppl 3):S162–S166.

30. Umemura A, Jaggi JL, Hurtig HI, Siderowf AD, Colcher A, Stern MB, Baltuch GH. Deep brain stimulation for movement disorders: morbidity and mortality in 109 patients. J Neurosurg 2003; 98:779–784.

31. Hallett M, Litvan I. Evaluation of surgery for Parkinson's disease: a report of the Therapeutics and Technology Assessment Subcommittee of the American Academy of Neurology. Neurology 1999; 53:1910–1921.

32. Hallett M, Litvan I. Scientific position paper of the Movement Disorder Society evaluation of surgery for Parkinson's disease. Mov Disord 2000; 15:436–438.

33. Starr P, Vitek J, Bakay R. Ablative surgery and deep brain stimulation for Parkinson's disease. Neurosurgery 1998; 43:989–1015.

34. Marks WJ Jr, Christine C, Clay H, Heath S, Aminoff M, Starr P. Unilateral chronic deep brain stimulation of the globus pallidus or subthalamic nucleus in patients with medically refractory Parkinson's disease: short-term results from a randomized trial. Neurology 2000; 54(suppl 3):A188–A189.

35. Marks WJ Jr, Christine C, Ostrem J, Starr P. A prospective, randomized trial of globus pallidus vs. subthalamic nucleus deep brain stimulation for Parkinson's disease. Mov Disord 2004; 19(suppl 9):S318–S319.

36. Mogilner AY, Sterio D, Rezai AR, Zonenshayn M, Kelly PJ, Beric A. Subthalamic nucleus stimulation in patients with a prior pallidotomy. J Neurosurg 2002; 96(4):660–665.

37. Benazzouz A, Piallat B, Pollak P, Benabid AL. Responses of substantia nigra pars reticulata and globus pallidus complex to high frequency stimulation of the subthalamic nucleus in rats: electrophysiological data. Neurosci Lett 1995; 189(2):77–80.

38. Fahn S, Parkinson's Study Group. Results of the ELLDOPA (earlier vs. later levodopa) study. Mov Disord 2002; 17(suppl 5):S13–S14.

39. Lida M, Miyazaki L, Tanaka K, Kabuto H, Iwata-Ichikawae, Ogawa N. Dopamine D2 receptor-mediated antioxidant and neuroprotective effect of ropinirole, a dopamine agonist. Brain Res 1999; 838:51–59.

40. Sawada H, Ibi M, Kihara T, Urushitani M, Akaike A, Kimura J, Shimohama S. Dopamine D2-type agonists protect mesencephalic neurons from glutamate neurotoxicity: mechanisms of neuroprotective treatment against oxidative stress. Ann Neurol 1998; 44(1):110–119.

41. Mesnage V, Houeto JL, Welter ML, Agid Y, Pidoux B, Dormont D, Cornu P. Parkinson's disease: neurosurgery at an earlier stage? J Neurol Neurosurg Psychiatry 2002; 73(6):778–779.

42. Van Horn G, Hassenbusch SJ, Zouridakis G, Mullani NA, Wilde MC, Papanicolaou AC. Pallidotomy: a comparison of responders and nonresponders. Neurosurgery 2001; 48(2):263–271; discussion 271–273.

43. Welter ML, Houeto JL, Tezenas du Montcel S, Mesnage V, Bonnet AM, Pillon B, Arnulf I, Pidoux B, Dormont D, Cornu P, Agid Y. Clinical predictive factors of subthalamic stimulation in Parkinson's disease. Brain 2002; 125:575–583.

44. Tavella A, Bergamasco B, Bosticco E, Lanotte M, Perozzo P, Rizzone M, Torre E, Lopiano L. Deep brain stimulation of the subthalamic nucleus in Parkinson's disease: long-term follow-up. Neurol Sci 2002; 23:S111–S112.

45. Ostrem J, Christine C, Starr P, Heath S, Marks WJ Jr. Effect of patient age on response to subthalamic nucleus or globus pallidus deep brain stimulation for Parkinson's disease: results from a prospective, randomized study. Neurology 2004; 62(suppl 5):A396.

46. Weaver FM, Follett K, Hur K, Stern M. A meta-analysis of studies of deep brain stimulation for persons with Parkinson's disease. VA HSR&D 2003 National Meeting, Washington, DC, Feb 13–15, 2003.

47. Follett KA. Comparision of pallidal and subthalamic deep brain stimulation for the treatment of levodopa-induced dyskinesias. Neurosurg Focus 2004; 17(1):14–19.

48. Vitek J. Deep brain stimulation for Parkinsons' disease. A critical re-evaluation of STN versus GPi DBS. Stereotact Funct Neurosurg 2002; 78:119–131.

49. Putzke J, Wharen RJ, Wszolek Z, Turk M, Strongosky A, Uitti R. Thalamic deep brain stimulation for tremor-predominant Parkinson's disease. Parkinsonism Relat Disord 2003; 10(2):81–88.

50. Kumar R, Lozano AM, Sime E, Lang AE. Long-term follow-up of thalamic deep brain stimulation for essential and parkinsonian tremor. Neurology 2003; 61(11):1601–1604.

51. Gelb DJ, Oliver E, Gilman S. Diagnostic criteria for Parkinson's disease. Arch Neurol 1999; 56(1):33–39.

3

Surgical Technique and Complication Avoidance

Joshua M. Rosenow

Department of Neurosurgery, Feinberg School of Medicine of Northwestern University, Chicago, Illinois, U.S.A.

Ali R. Rezai

Department of Neurosurgery, Cleveland Clinic Lerner College of Medicine, Cleveland, Ohio, U.S.A.

1. INTRODUCTION

The rapid rise in the number of patients undergoing subthalamic nucleus (STN) stimulation for Parkinson's disease is remarkable, given the traditional view that STN lesions cause disabling hemiballismus and the hypothesis that deep brain stimulation (DBS) produces a "functional lesion." However, human trials followed the demonstration that STN lesions could alleviate many of the symptoms observed in primate models of Parkinson's disease (1–3). The clinical benefits of chronic electrical stimulation of the STN were first reported by the Grenoble group in 1994 (4) and a lengthier paper in 1995 (5) describing the first three patients to have electrodes implanted chronically in the STN for the treatment of Parkinson's disease.

In this chapter, we present a practical methodology for implanting deep brain stimulating electrodes in the STN. While the techniques and preferences described here are ones our group has found work best (6,7), alternative successful styles do exist (8–11). Moreover, the advent of frameless techniques has added an extra dimension to the procedure. In general, the anatomic and physiologic considerations for the frame-based and frameless techniques are essentially the same. However, each frameless system has its own nuances regarding setup and alignment. This chapter will focus on the traditional frame-based procedure and will not delve into the multiple frameless systems available.

2. PATIENT SELECTION AND PREPARATION

Patients considered for surgery must not have any medical contraindications to anesthesia and surgery in general. Moreover, they should not have a history of a bleeding diathesis. Any anticoagulant medications, including aspirin, ticlopidine, clopidogrel, and all nonsteroidal anti-inflammatory drugs, should be discontinued at least 7–10 days preoperatively to ensure the return of normal blood clotting function. Other medications that may affect platelet function, such as valproic acid and high dose vitamin E, should also be discontinued.

In addition, patients should be willing and able, both physically and cognitively, to undergo an awake surgical procedure requiring several hours of immobilization in a stereotactic frame. Moreover, surgical candidates need to be able to remain attentive and cooperative under stressful conditions. Lastly, the patient and family must be willing and able to bear the responsibilities for maintaining a chronically implanted hardware system.

3. FRAME PLACEMENT

Patients are admitted the evening before surgery so that they may be optimized medically and obtain a portion of their preoperative imaging studies. By completing the magnetic resonance imaging (MRI) sequence preoperatively, patients do not need to spend time in the claustrophobic space of the MRI magnet while in the stereotactic frame. This also significantly improves efficiency by decreasing the amount of imaging time on the morning of surgery.

Most stereotactic head frames are compatible with the currently available surgical planning stations. We use the Leksell model G stereotactic head frame (Elekta, Stockholm, Sweden). It is easier to apply the frame with the patient sitting upright rather than supine. The frame should be positioned with the base parallel to the line between the anterior and posterior commissures (the AC–PC line), which may be approximated by the line extending from the lateral canthus to the tragus. Ear bars may be used to stabilize the frame during fixation, with padded ear plugs used to minimize discomfort. Alternatively, an assistant may be used to position the frame while the lead individual applies the pins.

The pins must be placed correctly to avoid damage to subcutaneous and intracranial structures. In patients with prior craniotomies, pin placement within the bone flap may cause the flap to fracture inwards and penetrate the brain. The anterior pins should be placed two fingerbreadths above the orbital rim, taking care to avoid the supraorbital nerve. Damaging the nerve may cause persistent pain and potentially even neuroma formation. Posteriorly, pins should be located so as to avoid penetration of the cerebral venous sinuses. The height of the base of the frame should allow prospective targets to lie comfortably within the frame's coordinate system, avoiding the extremes, which will mechanically hamper positioning the arc for targeting. In addition, since the pins create significant artifactual distortion of computed tomography (CT) imaging, they should be placed such that they do not distort the anterior commissure, the posterior commissure, or the STN.

Pins should have firm, direct purchase on the skull without scything at an extreme angle. Moreover, pin lengths should be chosen so that the frame and its posts do not contact the patient's nose, scalp, neck, or shoulders to avoid the risk of developing a pressure sore. Moreover, the blunt ends should not extend more than 5 mm from the external face of the stereotactic frame post so as not to interfere with placement of fiducial boxes for imaging. A spinal needle used to inject lidocaine may be inserted through the pin hole of the post to approximate the necessary pin length.

A generous amount of local anesthetic is infiltrated into the scalp and down to the periostium prior to fixing the pins. Given the length of the procedure, it is advantageous to use a long-acting mixture such as a 1:1 combination of 0.5% lidocaine with 1:200,000 epinephrine and 0.75% marcaine. Beginning the infiltration slowly, or adding one part sodium bicarbonate to nine parts anesthetic, ameliorates some of the burning sensation associated with these drugs. Sometimes administering a small amount of a short-acting benzodiazepine, such as midazolam, aids in reducing the patient's anxiety about frame placement and improves cooperation. The tips of the pins may be coated in antibiotic ointment prior to fixation.

Once applied, the pins should be tightened in opposing pairs to evenly distribute pressure on the skull. Pins should be hand tight and should not be over tightened. Over-tightening can result in frame distortion, which can create a source of targeting error. Intraoperative alteration in pin position will invalidate all stereotactic planning already completed. If the pins are set appropriately, it should be possible to gently shake the patient's head, gripping the frame, without causing pain. Pain results from pin slippage. If performed carefully, this maneuver can provide added assurance against intraoperative displacement.

4. TARGET PLANNING

4.1. Image Acquisition

While MRI has superior soft-tissue resolution, CT is less susceptible to the distortional artifacts produced by the inhomogeneities in the magnetic field and thus more accurately represents the actual position of intracerebral structures in space. Consequently, we rely on image fusion to allow us to capitalize on the respective advantages of each methodology. Our surgical planning utilizes several MRI sequences (1.5 T Siemens Magnetom Vision, Symphony, or Sonata) and one CT sequence (Siemens Emotion or Plus4). As previously stated, a volumetric T1-weighted axial MRI (MPRAGE) (TR 20, TE 6, Flip angle 30°, 256 field of view, 1 mm thick slices 256 × 256 matrix) is obtained on the day of surgery or up to several days preoperatively without the stereotactic frame in place. A coronal T2 sequence (TR 5000, TE 96, Flip angle 180°, 300 field of view, 2 mm thick slices 154 × 256 matrix) is performed from in front of the anterior commissure to behind the posterior commissure. The STN may be directly visualized on this sequence and it serves as an additional method for determining our initial target, as will be described below. A CT scan is then obtained with the patient, frame, and CT fiducial box secured to the table to ensure that the frame is parallel to the axis of scanning. The gantry angle must be kept at 0° in order to allow most planning software to construct a volumetric cranial model. The field of view is enlarged so that all of the fiducial rods are visible. Images are taken at 1–2 mm intervals from the base of the frame through the top of the fiducial set. While stereotactic surgery initially relied on contrast ventriculography to visualize the anterior and posterior commissures, the superb visualization of these structures on modern MRI machines renders this technique unnecessary.

4.2. Target and Trajectory

Targeting is performed using several methods. The T2-weighted MRI may be used for direct anatomical targeting of the STN. A defined stereotactic formula in combination with a stereotactic atlas indirectly targets the structure. Lastly, microelectrode recording (MER) locates the nucleus via neurophysiologic mapping.

After CT scanning the patient is transported to the operating room. The acquired images are uploaded into a planning station via the hospital intranet or from an optical disk. We utilize the Stealth Station Treon Plus (Medtronic Surgical Navigation Technologies, Colorado, U.S.A.). The CT scan serves as the reference examination against the multiple MRI exams. The CT and the MRI series are fused using automated image fusion software. The fused images are inspected to confirm that structures on each scan overlie each other. If this fusion is found to be unsatisfactory, corresponding points on each exam may be chosen for a manual point merge. Alternatively, the MRI may be fused to the CT scan using the point merge system.

The stereotactic coordinate system is then established by registering the fiducial rods. Ideally, this should be done on the CT images set to bone windows so that artifacts are reduced. The CT scan is utilized due to its more accurate spatial resolution. Once the rods are identified, the computer can then assign a triplanar set of Cartesian coordinates to any intracranial structure.

The commissures and at least one midline point are then identified and stored. Because stereotactic targeting formulas were all determined with the use of ventriculography, the posterior portion of the AC and the anterior portion of the PC should be selected to correspond with those regions visualized on a ventriculogram (Fig. 1). The computer then aligns the images to parallel the intercommissural line. If the Leksell frame is placed perfectly, both the AC and PC will have identical X- and Z-coordinates.

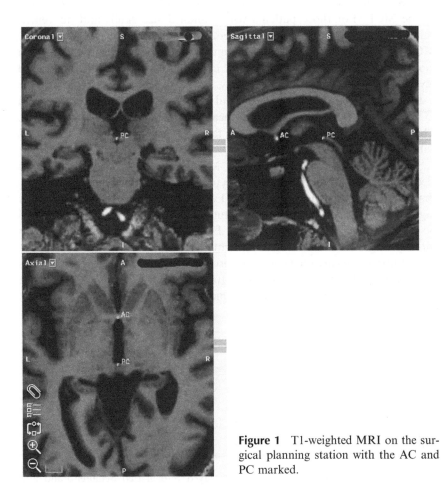

Figure 1 T1-weighted MRI on the surgical planning station with the AC and PC marked.

If redundancy in planning to minimize the chance of error is desired, we advocate a separate manual calculation of the location of the mid-commissural point (MCP). Most CT and MRI scanners provide enough image analysis functions to derive the displacement of AC and PC from frame center. These numbers can easily be transformed into stereotactic coordinates by adding or subtracting them from the $x = 100$, $y = 100$, and $z = 100$ (frame center). By convention, point displacement to the left, anterior, or inferior of frame center are added to 100, while displacement to the right, posterior, or superior of frame center are subtracted from 100. If no planning station is available, we recommend obtaining all imaging with the frame and performing separate AC/PC calculations on the CT and MRI consoles to provide redundancy.

Standard stereotactic formulas are used to locate the STN in relation to the MCP. For those patients with standard size skulls and no ventriculomegaly, we target 12.5–13 mm from the midline, 4 mm posterior to the MCP, and 5 mm below the intercommissural line. In older patients with more generous ventricles, the lateral coordinate may need to be shifted several tenths of a millimeter laterally. Some stereotactic systems provide a digitized version of the Schaltenbrand and Wahren Atlas that is morphed to conform to the patient's caudate head, thalamic height, and brainstem. This is then overlaid on the formulaic targets to confirm that the target lies within the STN.

Figure 2 shows a T1-weighted MRI with the overlayed atlas and electrode trajectories. A typical trajectory will pass through the anterior thalamus, the zona incerta/fields of Forel, the STN, and the substantial nigra pars reticulata (SNpr). The distinct electrical signatures of each will be used to determine the final target. Figure 3 demonstrates the ability to directly target the STN using T2-weighted MRI.

Entry points are then chosen to provide the ring and arc measurements for targeting. The trajectory taken to the target can be as important as the target itself. This should be approximately 1 cm anterior to the coronal

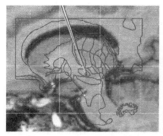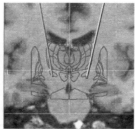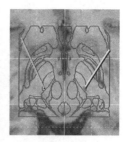

Figure 2 T1-weighted MRI with the overlayed reformatted Schaltenbrand and Wahren Atlas and bilateral electrode tracks.

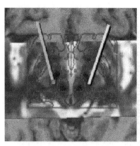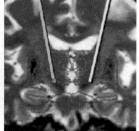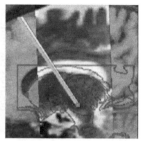

Figure 3 T2-weighted MRI with the overlayed reformatted Schaltenbrand and Wahren Atlas and bilateral electrode tracks. Direct targeting serves to confirm formula-derived coordinates.

suture so the sagittal angle of approach will result in the microelectrode traversing appropriate superficial structures. Similarly, the entry point should be between 2 and 3 cm from the midline in order to avoid the medial bridging veins and avoid a lateral tract in the internal capsule. In addition to the risk of damaging the internal capsule, lateral trajectories that do not pass through the thalamus and zona incerta provide limited MER data. The precise entry point may be refined on the planning console such that the trajectory passes through the crown of a gyrus rather than into a sulcus. This avoids inadvertently damaging sulcal or pial vessels which lie on the cortical surface. After selecting preliminary points, the images are then reformatted to the trajectory view, which provides three orthogonal planes positioned with respect to the trajectory rather than the patient's anatomy. The approach then may be traced at millimeter intervals to ensure that no deep sulci are transgressed and that the ventricular ependyma is not scythed. While many groups use a standard entry point for all patients and do not make the effort to intensively refine the trajectory in this manner (Table 1), we feel that this step attempts to minimize the risk of deep hemorrhage.

5. SURGICAL TECHNIQUE

A Foley catheter is placed. The patient's head in the frame is rigidly fixed to the operating table in a comfortable position anticipating a 4–6 hr procedure. The frame is set to the target's Cartesian coordinates and the Leksell arc is placed on the patient with the arc and ring settings for the entry point, which is marked on the skin. The head is then prepped and draped using sterile procedure. Prophylactic intravenous antibiotics are administered. Preliminary review of our infection data suggests that antibiotics should be administered approximately 45 min prior to the skin incision. Steroids and anticonvulsants are not routinely given. The patient is sedated with a short-acting agent such as propofol for this portion of the operation. Long-acting

Table 1 Clues as to whether the Trajectory is Too Posterior, Anterior, Medial, or Lateral when Targeting the Subthalamic Nucleus

	Too posterior	Too anterior	Too medial	Too lateral
Thalamus	Bottom of thalamus lower than anticipated; VOP encountered	Bottom of thalamus higher than anticipated	Bottom of thalamus lower than anticipated	Bottom of thalamus higher than anticipated
Zona incerta	Small width	Large width	Large width	Small width
STN neuronal activity	Sensori-motor driven neurons encountered	Sensori-motor driven neurons encountered	Few sensori-motor driven discharges	Sensori-motor driven neurons encountered
STN—height and width	Encountered lower than anticipated; small width	Encountered higher than anticipated; small width	Encountered lower than anticipated; small width	Encountered higher than anticipated; small width
STN—height and width after moving anteriorly	Encountered higher; larger width	Encountered lower; smaller width	No difference	No difference
STN—height and width after moving posteriorly	Encountered lower; smaller width	Encountered lower; larger width	No difference	No difference
STN—height and width after moving medially	No difference	No difference	Encountered lower	Encountered higher
STN—height and width after moving laterally	No difference	No difference	Encountered higher	Encountered lower
Distance between bottom of STN and top of SNR	Small	Large	Small	Large or SNR may not be encountered
Microstimulation effects	Paresthesias (except over the top of STN—see text)	Muscle contraction	Diplopia, eyelid closure	Muscle contraction

benzodiazepines are avoided due to their effect on the neurophysiology. Because the patient must be quickly returned to an awake and cooperative state when needed, the use of narcotics is limited as well. We usually perform bilateral electrode implantations in a single setting. Alternatively, staged procedures may be used.

The patient is draped such that the neurophysiology and anesthesia teams may observe the patient and interact with him or her but are isolated from the surgical team. After generous infiltration with local anesthetic, two incisions are made. Scalp incisions can be curvilinear to accommodate the burr hole cap, or may be made as parasagittal linear incisions that pass directly over the burr hole. For bilateral procedures, the preliminary steps (scalp opening and burr hole creation) are completed on the left side before moving the frame coordinates to the right side target and performing the entire procedure on that side. Once the first electrode is implanted, the frame is once again set to the left side target and microelectrode recording and lead placement is completed there. This serves the dual purpose of rapidly completing all the skull drilling (eliminating the need for heavy sedation) and reducing the number of frame movements. Burr holes are made with an air drill and self-stopping perforator exactly 14 mm in diameter in order to allow the use of the Medtronic silastic burr hole ring and cover, if desired. The dura is coagulated and then opened in a cruciate manner. The dural leaves are thoroughly coagulated to prevent oozing of blood into the burr hole. If the silastic ring is not used, and alternative burr hole ring such as the Navigus Stim-Loc (Image-Guided Neurologics, Inc., Melbourne, FL, U.S.A.) is then secured to the scalp with self-drilling screws.

The pia arachnoids are bipolar cauterized to obtain absolute hemostasis. A generous opening in the pia is then created with a #11 blade to allow passage of the cannula. It is important not to make this opening too small or the brain will be deformed as the cannula is passed, risking hemorrhage from cortical vessels and bridging veins. The cannula is inserted into the brain with a constant gentle rotating motion to gently push aside, rather than tear, any small vessels it encounters. We offset the cannula holder on the Leksell frame such that we provide for 15 mm of MER distance above our intended target. For example, the radius of the frame is 190 mm. We typically use a cannula 170 mm in length, which would typically stop 20 mm above our target. Therefore, we use a +5 mm offset. Fibrin glue is used to seal the hole during each track to prevent the egress of the cerebrospinal fluid and the entry of air. At this time, physiologic mapping is performed using MER.

6. MAPPING THE STN: CONFIRMING THE OPTIMAL TARGET

The strategy we use in attempting to locate the optimal target site varies based on the structure targeted, reflecting differences in the type of anatomical/

physiological information needed (12). In targeting STN, the goal of the initial microelectrode penetration, and that of any subsequent trajectories, is to find the optimal trajectory through STN. This is in contrast to targeting other regions such as the thalamus or globus pallidus, where the purpose of the initial penetration is to identify the anatomical boundaries of structures to be avoided. The criteria we use to define an optimal tract are:

1. At least 5 mm of sensori-motor STN (region of the STN whose neurons can be activated by passive movement).
2. No adverse effects during microstimulation, up to 90 µA.
3. Some improvement in symptoms, whether as a result of a "micro-subthalamotomy" effect or in response to microstimulation, although this is inconstant.

If the frame is well placed and the imaging adequate, this trajectory can be often be located with a single microelectrode penetration. When using the single-electrode approach, the entire trajectory must be studied in order to accurately anatomically localize the tract as well as to provide enough information to facilitate any potential correction of the target/trajectory on subsequent tracts. Clues are provided by the depth and width of the various structures traversed by the microelectrode. Our trajectory begins 15 mm above the image-guided target, which typically places the tip of our cannula in the reticular or anterior thalamus. From here our trajectory takes us through the zona incerta (ZI), fields of Forel, the STN, and into the substantia nigra pars reticulata (SNpr). Landmarks to be noted along the tract include the bottom of thalamus, the width of the ZI/fields of Forel, the height at which the STN is encountered, the amount of the STN traversed and the distance between the bottom of STN and the top of SNpr. Sensori-motor testing usually begins when neuronal activities characteristic of STN are encountered, and is performed at each location where a neuron is encountered provided it is at least 0.4 mm past the last neuronal recording site. The 0.4 mm criterion serves two purposes. First, it would be impractical to record at shorter intervals considering the time involved. Second, it helps to ensure that unique units are tested.

Structures are identified by their neuronal firing characteristics. Parameters include discharge frequency, discharge regularity, and neuronal density (as indicated in the number of different extracellular action potentials recognized in the recording at a single site or the distance traversed before an active site is encountered). Figure 4 shows a graphical representation of the firing characteristics of the different structures encountered along with a view of the operative setup. Note that distances are relative because there are many technical factors and individual idiosyncrasies influencing the lengths and depths of anatomical/physiological structures.

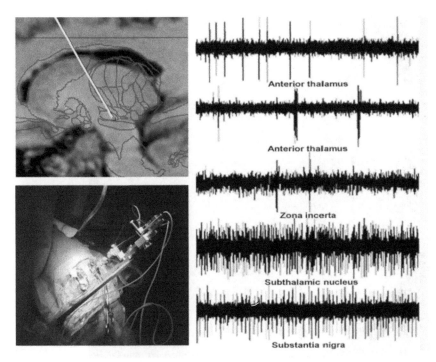

Figure 4 The microelectrode recording (MER) characteristics of the structures encountered during STN targeting. The small picture shows an intraoperative view of the MER setup.

7. SECURING THE ELECTRODE

After identifying an appropriate track and target, the fluoroscopy machine is draped and bought into the field. Crosshair targets are placed in the Leksell frame to serve as reference markers for both depth confirmation and parallax avoidance. The fluoroscope and/or operating table are adjusted such that the targets on the frame are aligned with one another. The picture should be rotated so that the cannula approaches the center of the targets from the upper left corner of the screen. The cannula should be clearly visible and not obstructed by the crosses on the target markers. The electrode (Model 3387, Medtronic Neurologic, Minneapolis, MN, U.S.A.) is then measured such that the distal edge of the distal contact (contact 0) will be at the ventral edge of the physiologically determined target (bottom of the STN). The electrode is either advanced via the microdrive or threaded by hand. If the electrode is advanced by hand, it is recommended that the microdrive be set so that the distance the electrode must travel freely beyond the cannula to the target is minimized. For some drive systems, this means retracting the drive only to the ventral target depth before exchanging the

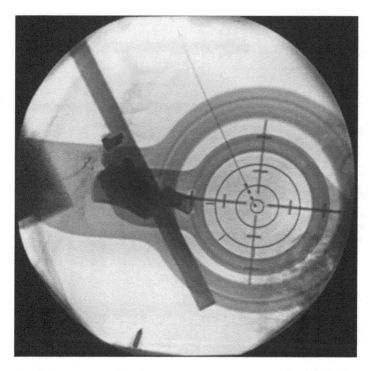

Figure 5 Fluoroscopic view of the macroelectrode at the target visualized with the targeting disks in place on the stereotactic frame.

microelectrode for the macroelectrode. Figure 5 depicts the fluoroscopic view of the electrode at target.

Macrostimulation is performed with the hand-held stimulator set at 130 Hz and 90 μsec pulse width. Bipolar stimulation is performed, first with contact 0 as negative and contact 3 as positive though gradually escalating voltages. At each level, the patient is assessed for both therapeutic effects and adverse side effects. Finger taps, fist opening/closing, and speech are assessed at each voltage setting. Worrisome effects include sustained paresthesias, dysarthria, forced gaze deviation, and muscle contractions. Most side effects are attributable to stimulation of the internal capsule. However, an electrode that is too deep in the midbrain may produce disconjugate eye deviation and some sensory changes from stimulation of the oculomotor nerve fibers or the medial lemniscus, respectively. The contacts may be varied to determine if a satisfactory combination exists. The results of macrostimulation are not intended to predict a patient's final outcome, but only to verify that an acceptable therapeutic window exists between effective stimulation and unacceptable side effects.

The Navigus Stim-Loc burr hole ring includes a disc that seats in the ring and rotates to grasp and secure the electrode. This device maintains a constant electrode position during microdrive removal. The electrode is then secured in the notch in the burr hole ring and the cover is placed. All steps are performed with fluoroscopic visualization. The position of the electrode at the termination of macrostimulation (final position) is saved on one of the screens of the dual screen fluoroscopy unit. The tip of the electrode is then monitored on fluoroscopy, shooting a new x-ray after each piece of the microdrive is removed to ensure that the electrode remains stable.

Other devices to secure the electrode are available. At present, these rings lack a fixation device that can be employed prior to removal of the microdrive and stylet. With these devices, the surgeon must vigilantly monitor the fluoroscopy as individual pieces of the microdrive are removed to ensure that the electrode does not stray from the correct position. Compensation is often required (e.g., pulling the electrode back by approximately 1 mm). Some surgeons prefer to use microplate systems or methyl methacrylate to secure electrodes. While these approaches avoid electrode displacement, they have been anecdotally associated with lead fracture.

Finally, the electrodes are connected to the extension wires, which are either externalized or buried. The use of the extender protects the exposed connection leads from moisture and allows the end of the lead to be easily palpated at the time of connection to the distal connector and the implantable pulse generator (IPG). It is critical not to overtighten the screws in the extender. This subtle error can induce curvature in the lead, which can increase the difficulty of removal at the time of IPG implantation. Finally, the wounds are copiously irrigated and the galea is reapproximated followed by closure of the skin. Attention to sterile technique throughout the procedure is critical, and the number of individuals passing in and out of the operating suite should be minimized to reduce the risk of hardware contamination.

8. ADVERSE EVENTS

If there is any intraoperative evidence of hemorrhage, such as bleeding from the cannula, gentle irrigation down the cannula is performed until the effluent is clear. We have had cases of active intraoperative hemorrhage where this has taken over 90 min, but it is crucial to continue as long as the patient is neurologically stable. Clinical hypervigilance is imperative. Any neurological deterioration such as the onset of lethargy or a new focal deficit is cause for immediately aborting the procedure and proceeding immediately to the CT scanner. If the patient cannot protect his or her airway, they should be intubated prior to leaving the operating room. Equipment to perform an emergent craniotomy should be readily available at all times.

We have generally left the stereotactic frame in place for emergent postoperative scans. In theory, the frame can facilitate the aspiration of deep hemorrhages that are inducing mass effect. However, we have never been forced to utilize the frame for such an aspiration.

Several events may provide clues to the presence of an occult intraoperative hemorrhage. As there are no active neurons within a hemorrhage cavity, a microelectrode that encounters or produces a hemorrhage along its track will record only silence. Therefore, unexpected electrical silence not attributable to problems with the electrode itself or its position (such as in the internal capsule) should raise the suspicion of an intraoperative hemorrhage. In addition, deviation of the electrode tip on fluoroscopy after placement not only signals the presence of the development of an intracranial hemorrhage, but also provides some information as to the magnitude of the problem. Reports quote the risk of intraoperative hemorrhage during DBS electrode implantation as ranging between 0.3% and 3.6% (9,13–15).

As with all implanted hardware systems, there is a certain risk of complications related to the hardware itself. In Koller et al.'s (16) series of 53 patients, the incidence of infection was 3.8% with a 1.9% malfunction rate. The Grenoble group's (9) large series of 197 patients contained three patients who experienced infections and five with scalp erosions leading to exposed hardware, for a total rate of 2.5%. The European Multicentre Study (13) yielded a rate of 2.7% and the North American trial reported 2.9%. Among the 143 patients in the multicenter prospective series of patients undergoing GPi or STN DBS (17), there were five leads that migrated, four infected leads, two broken leads, one scalp erosion, and one incidence of equipment malfunction. Of note, the manufacturer of the DBS equipment claims that the rate of lead migration is approximately 1%, lead fracture 0.5%, short circuit 1%, equipment failure 1.5%, infection 1.5%, and scalp erosion 2.5% (18). Overall, 25.3% of patients and 18.5% of electrodes included in the Toronto series (14) developed a complication of any type. Half of these involved infected leads or scalp erosions. Importantly, five of six infected electrodes that the group attempted to save with debridement and intravenous antibiotics eventually needed to be explanted anyway.

9. POSTOPERATIVE CARE

A CT scan is obtained soon after the operation to both assess electrode position and to rule out intracranial hemorrhage. AP and lateral skull x-rays are also performed (Fig. 6). Patients are observed in a monitored setting (either ICU or step-down unit) overnight and are mobilized on the morning of postoperative day one. The Foley catheter is usually removed in the recovery room or the next day. Antibiotics are given for 24 hr postoperatively. Most patients are discharged on postoperative day two. Patients undergo postoperative MRI scanning for the purposes of electrode position confirmation and functional imaging studies (Fig. 7). There have been recent

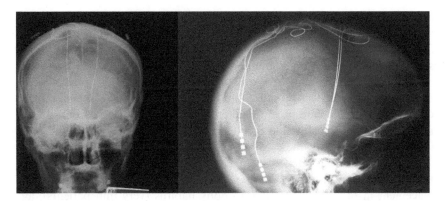

Figure 6 Postoperative AP and lateral skull x-rays demonstrating the implanted STN DB electrodes.

guidelines published regarding the safety of implanted neurostimulation systems in the MRI environment (19).

10. IPG IMPLANTATION

We prefer to perform implantation of the programmable pulse generators between 7 and 14 days after electrode placement. Alternatively, this may be done the same day as the electrode placement. The procedure is performed under general anesthesia. Once again, prophylactic antibiotics are

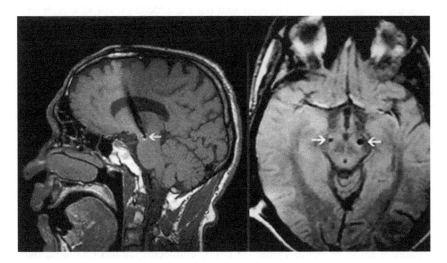

Figure 7 Postoperative axial and sagittal T1-weighted MRI scans showing the implanted STN DBS electrodes.

administered 45 min prior to skin incision. The head is thoroughly cleaned and prepped along with the neck and upper chest. One side is draped and implanted at a time, so two separate instrument tables are required to assure sterility and prevent cross-contamination.

The connector is palpated and a short linear incision is made adjacent to it. The connector is externalized and the boot removed. The connector is discarded. Extreme care must be taken during this step to prevent distraction of the lead, which could result in lead fracture, contact breakage, or insulation tears. All of these complications render the electrode useless.

A subcutaneous pocket is then created. The most common location for the IPG placement is infraclavicular. However, certain patients may require placement in other locations due to body habitus (very thin patients), age (pediatric patients), a history of prior surgery in the region, or vanity. In addition, certain activities such as hunting require the use of the chest to stabilize equipment. The IPG should be placed in a location that minimizes pressure and trauma to the unit. Anecdotal reports cite local trauma as an infection risk with other implanted hardware systems. Other locations include the subcostal area and the flank as well as the lumbar region and buttocks. All of these alternate sites require the use of a longer extension lead. The standard extension is 51 cm in length, but a 66 cm version is available.

The subcutaneous tunneling device is passed from the cranial incision to the pocket incision. Passing incisions are used as needed, but is should be remembered that the extension is passed from the generator pocket to the cranial incision. Once the tunnel is created, the proximal extension connector is placed in its carrier and brought cranially through the tunnel until it exits the cranial incision. The slim-line boot is placed on the electrode and the lead and connector are attached. Once again, excessive force on the screws should be avoided. The current equipment includes a torque wrench that is designed to prevent this. The boot is slid over the connector and secured with multiple ties. Some surgeons will smear a small amount of bone wax over the connector to prevent moisture from entering the connector and causing a short circuit. The other end of the extension is placed into the generator and the screws are tightened.

In the infraclavicular region, the subcutaneous pocket is developed over the pectoralis fascia. This should be sized so as to hold the IPG without leaving significant excess space that could become filled with seroma. Thin individuals may require the IPG placed below the fascia to ensure enough tissue coverage to prevent erosion. The generator is tacked down to the pectoralis fascia with two silk sutures to prevent migration and rotation. Any extra extension lead is coiled beneath the IPG. Gentle traction on the extension is used to remove any significant kinks or bends in the lead. The connector should be seated over the occipital region rather than in the neck, where the connector could become subjected to excessive torque, risking lead fracture. All incisions are thoroughly irrigated with dilute betadine solution and antibiotic-impregnated saline. A multilayer closure is performed.

REFERENCES

1. Aziz TZ, Peggs D, Agarwal E, et al. Subthalamic nucleotomy alleviates parkinsonism in the 1-methyl-4-phenyl-1,2,3,6-tetrahydropyridine (MPTP)-exposed primate. Br J Neurosurg 1992; 6:575–582.
2. Aziz TZ, Peggs D, Sambrook MA, et al. Lesion of the subthalamic nucleus for the alleviation of 1-methyl-4-phenyl-1,2,3,6-tetrahydropyridine (MPTP)-induced parkinsonism in the primate. Mov Disord 1991; 6:288–292.
3. Bergman H, Wichmann T, DeLong MR. Reversal of experimental parkinsonism by lesions of the subthalamic nucleus. Science 1990; 249:1436–1438.
4. Benabid AL, Pollak P, Gross C, et al. Acute and long-term effects of subthalamic nucleus stimulation in Parkinson's disease. Stereotact Funct Neurosurg 1994; 62:76–84.
5. Limousin P, Pollak P, Benazzouz A, et al. Effect of parkinsonian signs and symptoms of bilateral subthalamic nucleus stimulation. Lancet 1995; 345: 91–95.
6. Rezai A, Hutchison W, Lozano A. Chronic subthalamic nucleus stimulation for Parkinson's disease. Neurosurg Oper Atlas 1999; 8:196–207.
7. Sterio D, Zonenshayn M, Mogilner AY, et al. Neurophysiological refinement of subthalamic nucleus targeting. Neurosurgery 2002; 50:58–67; discussion 67–69.
8. Ashby P, Kim YJ, Kumar R, et al. Neurophysiological effects of stimulation through electrodes in the human subthalamic nucleus. Brain 1999; 122: 1919–1931.
9. Benabid AL, Benazzouz A, Hoffmann D, et al. Long-term electrical inhibition of deep brain targets in movement disorders. Mov Disord 1998; 13:119–125.
10. Pollak P, Krack P, Fraix V, et al. Intraoperative micro- and macrostimulation of the subthalamic nucleus in Parkinson's disease. Mov Disord 2002; 17: S155–S161.
11. Zonenshayn M, Rezai AR, Mogilner AY, et al. Comparison of anatomic and neurophysiological methods for subthalamic nucleus targeting. Neurosurgery 2000; 47:282–292; discussion 292–294.
12. Loddenkemper T, Pan A, Neme S, et al. Deep brain stimulation in epilepsy. J Clin Neurophysiol 2001; 18:514–532.
13. Limousin P, Speelman JD, Gielen F, et al. Multicentre European study of thalamic stimulation in parkinsonian and essential tremor. J Neurol Neurosurg Psychiatry 1999; 66:289–296.
14. Oh MY, Abosch A, Kim SH, et al. Long-term hardware-related complications of deep brain stimulation. Neurosurgery 2002; 50:1268–1274.
15. Schuurman PR, Bosch DA, Bossuyt PM, et al. A comparison of continuous thalamic stimulation and thalamotomy for suppression of severe tremor. N Engl J Med 2000; 342:461–468.
16. Koller W, Pahwa R, Busenbark K, et al. High-frequency unilateral thalamic stimulation in the treatment of essential and parkinsonian tremor. Ann Neurol 1997; 42:292–299.

17. Bilateral deep brain stimulation (DBS) of the subthalamic nucleus (STN) or the globus pallidus interna (GPi) for treatment of advanced Parkinson's disease. Tecnologica MAP Suppl 2001; 1–8.
18. Medtronic I. Deep Brain Stimulation 3387/89 Lead Kit: Implant Manual. Minneapolis, MN: Medtronic, Inc., 2002.
19. Rezai AR, Finelli D, Nyenhuis JA, et al. Neurostimulation systems for deep brain stimulation: in vitro evaluation of magnetic resonance imaging-related heating at 1.5 tesla. J Magn Reson Imaging 2002; 15:241–250.

4

Surgical Results

Jean-Guy Villemure

*Neurosurgery Service, Centre Hospitalier Universitaire Vaudois,
Lausanne, Switzerland*

Joseph Ghika and François Vingerhoets

*Neurology Service, Centre Hospitalier Universitaire Vaudois,
Lausanne, Switzerland*

1. INTRODUCTION

The expected results following the surgical treatment of Parkinson's disease
(PD) must take into account many variables: selection criteria, anatomical target, targeting methodology, surgical methodology, and methods of evaluating
results.

Some of these issues are addressed in other chapters of this book. Selection
of patients and indications are the crucial steps in ascertaining a correct diagnosis, confirming the likelihood of clinical benefit, and estimating potential complications or side effects. There have been many anatomical structures targeted over
the past five decades for the treatment of PD, and results have varied according
to these targets. Furthermore, the surgical methodology utilized (i.e., lesioning
or stimulating) has also led to different results. This latter issue, namely surgical
technique, is addressed in other sections of this book. However, for the same
target, the surgical methodology employed will not only influence the results
on PD symptoms or signs, but also those on the type, severity, and frequency
of adverse events.

In this chapter, we will focus on the results obtained with respect to specific targets (thalamus, pallidum, subthalamus) and the methodology (lesion, stimulation) used.

2. THALAMUS

2.1. Thalamotomy

The ventralis intermedius (VIM) nucleus of the thalamus has been one of the earliest stereotactic targets for the treatment of PD, with results being predominantly, not to say exclusively, on tremor. Many series report initial control of tremor in up to 90% of patients, with the effect fading gradually in some 10–20%. The results at 3 months postoperation are usually permanent and thus very satisfactory in most patients (70–80%) (1–4). Rigidity appears to be improved as well, with lesions located slightly more anteriorly (ventralis oralis posterior, or VOP), and few reports outline some benefits on L-dopa-induced dyskinesia obtained with such a target (4,5). Bilateral lesions have been associated with adverse events in over 30% of patients, a reason why contralateral surgery was carried out at varying intervals from the first surgery to decrease the complications (6–11).

2.1.1. Complications/Side Effects

The anatomical location of the lesion within the thalamus, unilaterality, or bilaterality, as well as its size are responsible for most of the side effects encountered with thalamotomy. These manifest as dysarthria, paresthesia, ataxia of gait, dystonia, limb weakness, and cognitive decline (2,4,8,10,11). Dysarthria, ataxia, and cognitive decline occur more frequently in bilateral lesions, at a frequency reaching 50% in some series (12). Hemorrhagic complications are relatively rare, occurring in less than 2% of cases.

2.2. VIM-Deep Brain Stimulation

The introduction of chronic thalamic stimulation by Benabid et al. (13) has confirmed the efficacy of the methodology. This allows to obtain the benefits of lesional surgery with a decrease in side effects of bilateral surgeries. However, the lack of efficacy of the thalamic target on the other symptoms of PD, namely rigidity, bradykinesia, and dyskinesia, has been clearly demonstrated (4,13–24). A randomized prospective study comparing thalamotomy and VIM-deep brain stimulation (DBS) confirmed the superiority of stimulation over thalamotomy for control of tremor, in addition to greater improvement in activities of daily living (ADL) in the DBS group (4). Other studies comparing thalamotomy and VIM-DBS have also been reported (24,25). The long lasting effect of VIM-DBS for tremor-dominant PD has been demonstrated (17,26–28). Similar to the results obtained with thalamotomy, VIM-DBS is effective only against tremor and does not influence the other clinical features of PD to any significant degree.

2.2.1. Complications/Side Effects

The same side effects that are encountered with thalamotomy are also seen with unilateral and bilateral VIM-DBS, but they can be modulated, to a great extent, with adjustments of the stimulation parameters (29). The literature reports dysarthria (10%) (18,19), ataxia (5%) (14), limb weakness (5%) (24), paresthesiae (10–20%) (18,24), and dystonia (5%) (22,24) as the side effects. Complications related to hardware are inherent to this type of surgery and have been reported to occur in 4% to as high as 20–25% of patients (14,30,31). There appears to be a higher number of occurrences of hardware and functional complications reported in the literature. However, such complications have not been encountered at such a high rate in our experience. They are to some extent operator dependent. Infection occurs in 2–3.5%, while hemorrhage has been rare at this site (<1%) (4,31,32).

2.3. Summary—Thalamic Target

- VIM is an excellent target to control tremor.
- Thalamotomy and thalamic stimulation are both effective in controlling tremor.
- Other symptoms of PD are not really modified.
- There are no significant benefits on bradykinesia and axial signs.
- Anteriorly (VOP) placed target may moderately improve rigidity as well.
- Anteriorly (VOP) placed target may moderately improve drug-induced dyskinesia.
- Functional complications are in part due to size and location of target (motor, sensory).
- Dysarthria is frequent (10%), and occurs in 30–50% of patients after bilateral surgeries.
- Cognitive deficits are more frequent with bilateral surgeries, and represent a contraindication to bilateral lesioning.
- Functional complications are less frequent, and can be modulated with stimulation techniques.
- DBS hardware complications vary in incidence between 4% and 25%.

3. PALLIDUM

The pars interna of the globus pallidus (GPi), being a major relay in the basal ganglia circuit, became a surgical target for the treatment of PD 50 years ago. Following Hassler's introduction of the thalamic target and the excellent results obtained on tremor, the pallidum target (33) faced competition due to the advent of effective antiparkinsonian drugs, and was reintroduced only in the early 1990s (34), when motor complications of these treatments became a major burden. Surgical methodologies consisting of either lesion or stimulation, either unilateral or bilateral, have been applied to the GPi.

3.1. Pallidotomy

Between the mid- and late 1990s, many clinical reports confirmed the benefits of pallidotomy for PD. The early results obtained with pallidotomy, either unilateral (34–38) or bilateral (40–43), confirmed that GPi was mainly effective on dyskinesia with improvements in PD signs being insufficient to allow drug reduction. One study concerning 40 patients—with follow-up longer than 52 months in 20 patients—confirmed the longest benefit in patients presenting a very asymmetric involvement and who were treated for their worse side (44–46). Few other long-term follow-up reports confirm benefits for all cardinal signs, with a fading effect starting within 2 years following surgery (44,47–51). Some long-term effects remain in less than 50% of the population. No clear predictive factors responsible for long-term effects have been identified.

Staged bilateral pallidotomy, done in a high proportion of patients who have undergone unilateral surgery, confirms the lack of efficacy of unilateral surgery. This strategy, most frequently done at a point later in time from the original surgery (34,51,52) to decrease complications, or contemporaneous pallidotomies (51,53,54), has not introduced any convincing arguments in support of its superiority on the duration of efficacy, but as expected, the benefits have been bilateral.

3.1.1. Complications/Side Effects

Most series of pallidotomy report complications when the surgery is bilateral. These are characterized by transient paresis (35), corticobulbar syndrome (12,54,55), visual field defect (34,56), cognitive deficit of various amplitude (12,40,54,57–59), delayed ischemic stroke (60), hemorrhage (53), abscess (53) and mood changes (38,54). These have been either transient or permanent. They relate to the proximity of the target to the internal capsule, to the optic tract, and to the cortico-bulbar fibers. The site and size of the lesions are correlated with the type and severity of the complications. Hemorrhagic complications have occurred in 1–3% (61).

3.2. Pallidal Stimulation

Bilateral chronic stimulation of the GPi for PD was first reported by Siegfried and Lippitz (62). Most reports concern bilateral stimulation, and few reports address the results obtained in unilateral stimulation (63). The results expected were similar to those obtained with pallidotomy, with the added inherent flexibility provided by the stimulation technique, thus decreasing the rate of permanent complications. Reports with short- and long-term follow-up of patients with bilateral pallidal stimulation, most frequently carried out contemporaneously, confirmed the results obtained with lesional methodology with regards to the benefits and duration. Benefits on the motor function fade gradually during the first and second postoperative years while the improvement in dyskinesias is maintained (54,65–77).

3.2.1. Complications/Side Effects

Complications, in the motor or cognitive sphere, encountered with GPi-DBS are much less frequent than with pallidotomy, and are reversible to some degree with adjustments of stimulation parameters (59,66,68,77,78). Complications related to stimulation hardware are inherent to this methodology (12,30,31). In the DBS for PD study group (DBSPDSG) report, the incidence of hardware complications within the first 6 months is of the order of 9% (74). Hemorrhagic complications appear to be higher at that target for DBS and were found to be as high as 6.7% per lead in one series (32) and at 10% in the DBSPDSG report (74).

3.3. Summary—Pallidal Target

- Pallidotomy and pallidal stimulation are effective in improving all features of PD but mainly contralateral drug-induced dyskinesias.
- Improvement is observed contralateral to surgery, with no significant sustained effect on ipsilateral motor function or dyskinesia.
- There is improvement in the Unified Parkinson's Disease Rating Scale (UPDRS) motor scores in the "off" period. This improvement is seen preferentially in the tremor, rather than in the rigidity, and bradykinesia.
- This improvement is insufficient to allow drug reduction.
- Medication cannot be reduced significantly, if at all.
- There is no significant effect on axial signs, i.e., on postural instability and gait.
- Functional complications are related to size and site of lesion, or site and intensity of stimulation, as well as to the bilaterality.
- Functional complications are less frequent with DBS, and their severity is modifiable with adjustment of stimulation parameters.
- Occurrences of hemorrhagic complications with DBS are high, and the highest of all targets for PD.

4. SUBTHALAMIC NUCLEUS

4.1. Subthalamotomy

Lesions of the subthalamic nucleus (STN) have been associated with hemiballism, and surgeons have been reluctant to lesion this nucleus to treat advanced PD (79). There are, however, many reports, some dating as far as 1963, of STN lesioning in PD (80). Few reports of subthalamotomy describe hemiballism as a complication, even when present transiently (81) or permanently (82). Benefits resulting from subthalamotomy have been noted on motor function, with follow-up as long as 24 months, with unilateral subthalamotomy for unilateral predominating symptoms (80,81,84,85), but long-term motor and cognitive assessments in bilateral cases are lacking. Although hemiballism is a proven complication of subthalamotomy, its incidence and long-lasting presence have not been clearly demonstrated (86,87).

4.2. STN-DBS

Chronic stimulation of the STN, either unilaterally but most frequently bilaterally, has been carried out for more than 10 years (88). Its introduction and efficacy have been such that it has become the target and technique of choice for the surgical treatment of PD in most centers. Many reports have demonstrated that motor functions improve significantly (50% UPDRS-motor) apart from improvements in ADL (50%), and the possibility of reducing medication allows for a major improvement in dyskinesia scores (89–104). While most series refer to short-term follow-up, Krack et al.'s group reported on 5-year long-term outcomes in 49 consecutive patients treated with bilateral STN-DBS (105). All parkinsonian signs except speech improved with treatment, and this improvement has been sustained over the baseline data for the whole period of 5 years. Worsening of akinesia, speech, and gait were observed over the years, and interpreted as possibly reflecting the progression of the disease. Similar interpretation was given for some patients who developed progressive dementia, considering that stimulation had no documented effect of cognitive functions (106–109). Mood changes characterized by hypomania or depression have been observed in the early post-operative phase. No direct effect of stimulation on mood could be clearly documented (105).

In our series of 50 consecutive patients treated with bilateral STN-DBS with a median follow-up of 18 months, we observed improvement of all features of PD, i.e., UPDRS-motor, 58%; fluctuations, 78%; and dyskinesia, 95%. Twenty-two patients remained off drugs after surgery, while medication was reduced by 55% in the others.

Bilateral STN-DBS has also proved effective following failure of pallidotomy and bilateral pallidal stimulation (78,110–112).

4.2.1. Complications/Side Effects

In a consecutive series of 50 bilateral STN-DBS, we encountered the following adverse events. Frame displacement was noted in a patient with severe tremor, leading to the misplacement of electrodes, which required replacement, with the patient being drug-free since then. Two patients required repositioning of one electrode, based on lack of positive response during trial stimulation period, and magnetic resonance imaging (MRI) confirmation of medial placement. One patient was clearly documented as having suffered a peroperative air embolism without consequences. One patient presented a panic attack characterized by hyperventilation and lack of cooperation at the time of skin incision, which led to abortion of surgery. The patient was successfully implanted 7 days later under general anesthesia, and has remained drugfree. One patient presented a seizure as the dura was being opened by electrocoagulation, which prompted us to stop surgery and reschedule it. There were two connector wounds dehiscence treated by local revision without having to remove the electrodes. One patient presented bilateral infection at the stimulator site, manifesting 3 months after placement, and requiring removal of generators and extension cables, which were reimplanted 3 and 5 months later. Six patients presented transient or prolonged cognitive problems or confusional states.

The rate of hemorrhage has been shown to be of the order of 2–2.5% per lead (32,105), and is 3% in the DBSPDSG (74), for the STN target. We have documented on routine post-operative MRI a small thalamic hemorrhage in 1 of 80 consecutive patients who underwent bilateral STN-DBS; in most of our patients, one-track microelectrode recording was obtained.

Stimulation hardware complications in STN-DBS have been the subject of some reports and are observed to occur in as low as 4% to as high as 20–25% of patients (12,30,31). We did not encounter more than 6% incidence of hardware complications in our initial series.

Many authors report cognitive (114), behavioral (113,115,116), and psychiatric (105,108) mood changes associated with STN-DBS. (115,117–120). Axial signs, advanced age, and cognitive deficits are clearly identified as unfavorable factors (88,102,121).

4.3. Summary—Subthalamic Nucleus

- Subthalamotomy and chronic bilateral STN-DBS improve all motor features of PD.
- STN-DBS allows marked reduction, and even cessation, of antiparkinsonian medication.
- Dyskinesia is markedly improved.
- The beneficial effects of STN-DBS are sustained for at least 5 years.
- Worsening of motor and cognitive functions may occur with time, and seems to reflect the evolution of the disease.
- STN-DBS has proven to be effective, following failure of bilateral pallidotomy.
- The current status of subthalamotomy does not allow comparison with STN-DBS as to long-term outcome and complications.

- With STN-DBS, age and cognitive functions are predictive factors of outcome.
- STN-DBS may be complicated with serious transient or permanent cognitive problems.
- More mood changes are observed with STN-DBS than at other targets.
- According to reports, stimulation hardware complications occur in 4–25% of cases.

5. PREOPERATIVE PHYSIOLOGICAL DEFINITION OF THE TARGET

There is continuous debate concerning the indications for recordings in movement disorder surgery. There are three possible scenarios: microelectrode "guided" target definition, microelectrode "assisted" target definition, or no use of recording. In the first instance, there is a need for multiple microelectrode trajectories that determine, on the basis of neural noise and single cell recordings, the best anatomical definition of the target. In the "assisted" use of recordings, the anatomical definition of the target is determined, in its rostro-caudal extent, without looking for further refinement within the nucleus. Finally, microrecording may not be used at all. However, most teams use either micro- or macrostimulation for determining the positive and negative effects of a specific target's stimulation. Some have reported the superiority of the information obtained from the stimulation as compared to the microrecordings (123). The usefulness of a preoperative physiological definition of the target is confirmed by the results obtained, and by taking into account, the benefits and side effects of the technique. There are no randomized studies on this topic; however, there are many reports that comment on the benefits and complications (89–104,124–126,128).

Discrepancies between anatomical, radiological localization, and stereotactic targeting using microelectrodes have been reported (100,122,127,128). Some explanations may account for these minimal, but important differences, including inherent mechanical aspects such as frame fixation, stereotactic device rigidity, and isocentric accuracy, cerebrospinal fluid (CSF) drainage related to the size of dural opening, and length of surgery, which may allow brain shift, rigidity, and perfect axis of instrumentation reaching the target, etc. All these may contribute to the discrepancies reported, and in these instances microrecording may allow preoperative correction to the physiological target. However, it is assumed that the physiological microrecording-based STN target identification would provide the best clinical response, but this has never clearly been proven. Taking into account some reports that describe the beneficial effect of DBS, aimed at the STN, but where the effective plot is outside the nucleus, the necessity of operating within the STN nucleus is being questioned. This has raised the importance of the role played by adjacent anatomical structures in the benefits thus obtained (128,129). It has also been our experience that the effective stimulation contact proved to be outside the STN in some 20% of cases; in slightly more than half of these, the clinical outcome has been very favorable. However, most patients whose stimulated contacts are within the STN boundaries have a good clinical outcome. Nevertheless, the technique of microrecording provides an additional physiological indicator to place the permanent lesion or electrode at a target, which may be considered ideal. When combined with per-operative stimulation, it appears to increase the likelihood for a good outcome. We have used microrecording "assisted" STN targeting (126), combined with macrostimulation to determine electrode placement within the STN (92,102).

Possible benefits of microrecording are, however, to be weighted against the adverse events related to the use of such a technique. Microrecordings add some time to surgery, and this will vary according to the number of trajectories and extent of recordings done—from 20 to 30 minutes per trajectory. We will not discuss microrecording hardware problems that may interfere with interpretation of data and are inherent to the technique. Excluding the time necessary to carry microrecording, the only other issues related to recording are the risks of hemorrhage and infection. The latter is difficult to assess and its incidence must be extremely low.

The potential hemorrhagic complications related to additional brain penetration should be compared with the benefits of microrecordings, and this issue represents the core of the debate. Incidence of hemorrhage reported in the literature has to take into account targets, techniques, and whether the hemorrhage is symptomatic or not. Not all reports are explicit about the latter. The analysis by Starr, based on 357 implants (32), of the incidence of hemorrhage in DBS surgery for PD, essential tremor, or dystonia is illustrative. All patients underwent imaging within 24 hours of surgery. There was an overall incidence of 3.1% hemorrhage per lead, with 1.4% that were symptomatic. The following two observations were made: the target had a significant effect on the rate of hemorrhage (2.5% STN, 6.7% pallidum, 0% VIM), and there was no correlation with the number of microelectrode recording trajectories (average 2.6). This latter observation is not in accordance with the observations made by the DBSPDSG (74), who reported that the "increased numbers of microelectrode passes were associated with an increased risk of intracranial bleeding." That study, however, confirmed the higher hemorrhagic rate at the pallidum (10%) as compared with the STN (3%). In our experience with STN-DBS and one track microrecording, the incidence of hemorrhage per lead, as documented by MRI routinely done the day after surgery, has been less than 1%.

The technique of microelectrode guided or assisted STN targeting is being challenged by the emerging evidence of MRI accuracy for such targeting (130–132) with reports of comparable clinical outcome (133).

6. CONCLUSIONS

The main surgical targets have historically been, and remain, the VIM nucleus of the thalamus, the postero-infero-lateral portion of the globus pallidus internus (GPi), and subthalamic nucleus. While the thalamic target has been successful in controlling parkinsonian tremor, it has had little, if any, impact on bradykinesia, rigidity, and dyskinesia. This had been the target of choice over a 40-year period, until Laitinen re-emphasized the benefits obtained with the GPi target in improving the motor fluctuations encountered in akineto-rigid patients suffering from drug-induced dyskinesias. The pallidal target has not, however, allowed patients to benefit from a lower medication dosage, and many series have confirmed its non-lasting efficacy in controlling symptoms. The definition of the role of the STN in the pathophysiology of PD and the surgical results obtained with surgery at this target have led most teams to consider at this time, the STN as the ideal target for the surgical treatment of PD.

While similar benefits on motor functions are obtained with lesion or stimulation at these targets, results obtained with these methodologies have confirmed the superiority of the stimulation technique in terms of overall benefits and reduction of complications or side effects. In that respect, comparative data concerning lesion and stimulation of the STN are too scarce to allow a statement, but STN-DBS provides excellent results with low morbidity.

At this point in time, it is obvious that, on the one hand, the stimulation technique has replaced the lesional approach, and on the other hand, the STN has turned out to be the best target for the treatment of PD. There remain considerations for targeting the thalamus in long-standing, stable dominant parkinsonian tremor, but there are really no reasons not to target the STN. Additionally, one could also find a reason to perform a thalamic lesion in a unilateral long-standing non–dominant parkinsonian tremor, in order to avoid the cost of the stimulation equipment. In our opinion, there are no more indications for pallidal surgery in PD.

The microrecordings during STN-DBS surgery, combined with clinical observations resulting from stimulation, are excellent tools for determining the final electrode position. It does not seem that an effective stimulation requires refined positioning of the electrode within the STN. There are indications that some structures in the neighborhood of the STN may also be responsible for clinical improvement with DBS. However, stimulating within the STN has been demonstrated to be effective. While it is assumed that the greater number of brain penetrations with electrodes should be associated with a greater risk of hemorrhage, there are conflicting reports related to the issue. There is emerging evidence that further refinement in MRI-based targeting provides an accuracy comparable to the preoperative physiological localization techniques. More clinical studies are necessary before MRI-based targeting and surgery under anesthesia can be recommended as standard practice.

In our opinion, STN-DBS represents, at present, the surgical treatment of choice for advanced PD.

REFERENCES

1. Brophy BP, Kimber TJ, Thompson PD. Thalamotomy for Parkinsonian tremor. Stereotact Funct Neurosurg 1997; 69:1–4.
2. Schuurman PR, Bosch A, Bossuyt PMM, Bonsel GJ, van Someren EJW, de Bie RMA, Merkus MP, Speelman JD. A comparison of continuous thalamic stimulation and thalamotomy for suppression of severe tremor. N Engl J Med 2000; 342:461–468.
3. Linhares MN, Tasker RR. Microelectrode-guided thalamotomy for Parkinson's disease. Neurosurgery 2000; 46(2):390–395.
4. Siegfried J, Blond S. The Neurosurgical Treatment of Parkinson's Disease. Baltimore, MD: Williams and Wilkins, 1997:66–72.
5. Narabayashi H, Yokosch F, Nakajima Y. Levodopa induced dyskinesia and thalamotomy. J Neurol Neurosurg Psychiatry 1984; 47:831–839.
6. Kelly PJ, Gillingham FJ. The long-term results of stereotaxic surgery and L-dopa therapy in patients with Parkinson's disease: a 10-year follow-up study. J Neurosurg 1980; 53:332–337.
7. Nagaseki Y, Shibazaki T, Hirai T, Kawashima Y, Hirato M, Wada H, Miyazaki M, Ohye C. Long-term follow-up results of selective VIM-thalamotomy. J Neurosurg 1986; 65:296–302.
8. Wester K, Hauglie-Hanssen E. Stereotaxic thalamotomy—experiences from the levodopa era. J Neurol Neurosurg Psychiatry 1990; 53:427–430.
9. Fox MW, Ahlskog JE, Kelly PJ. Stereotactic ventrolateralis thalamotomy for medically refractory tremor in post-levodopa era Parkinson's disease patients. J Neurosurg 1991; 75:723–730.
10. Jankovic J, Cardoso F, Grossman RG, Hamilton WJ. Outcome after stereotactic thalamotomy for parkinsonian, essential, and other types of tremor. Neurosurgery 1995; 37:680–686.
11. Tasker RR. Thalamotomy for Parkinson's disease and other types of tremor. II. The outcome of thalamotomy for tremor. Gildenberg PL, Tasker RR, eds. Textbook of Stereotactic and Functional Neurosurgery. New York: McGraw-Hill, 1998:1179–1198.
12. Hariz MI. Complications of movement disorder surgery and how to avoid them. Prog Neurol Surg 2000; 15:246–265.
13. Benabid AL, Pollak P, Louveau A, Henry S, de Rougemont J. Combined (thalamotomy and stimulation) stereotactic surgery of the VIM thalamic nucleus for bilateral Parkinson's disease. Appl Neurophysiol 1987; 50:344–346.
14. Benabid AL, Pollak P, Gervason C, Hoffmann D, Gao DM, Hommel M, Perret JE, de Rougemont J. Long-term suppression of tremor by chronic stimulation of the ventral intermediate thalamic nucleus. Lancet 1991; 337: 403–406.

15. Blond S, Caparros-Lefebvre D, Parker F, Assaker R, Petit H, Guieu JD, Christiaens JL. Control of tremor and involuntary movement disorders by chronic stereotactic stimulation of the ventral intermediate thalamic nucleus. J Neurosurg 1992; 77:62–68.

16. Benabid AL, Pollak P, Seigneuret E, Hoffmann D, Gay E, Perret J. Chronic VIM thalamic stimulation in Parkinson's disease, essential tremor and extrapyramidal dyskinesias. Acta Neurochir Suppl (Wien) 1993; 58:39–44.

17. Benabid AL, Pollak P, Gao D. Chronic electrical stimulation of the ventralis intermedius nucleus of the thalamus as a treatment of movement disorders. J Neurosurg 1996; 84:203–214.

18. Alesch F, Pinter MM, Helscher RJ, Fertl L, Benabid AL, Koos WT. Stimulation of the ventral intermediate thalamic nucleus in tremor dominated Parkinson's disease and essential tremor. Acta Neurochir (Wien) 1995; 136:75–81.

19. Ondo W, Jankovic J, Schwartz K, Almaguer M, Simpson RK. Unilateral thalamic deep brain stimulation for refractory essential tremor and Parkinson's disease tremor. Neurology 1998; 51:1063–1069.

20. Hariz GM, Bergenheim AT, Hariz MI, Lindberg M. Assessment of ability/disability in patients treated with chronic thalamic stimulation for tremor. Mov Disord 1998; 13:78–83.

21. Limousin P, Speelman JD, Gielen F, Janssens M. Multicentre European study of thalamic stimulation in parkinsonian and essential tremor. J Neurol Neurosurg Psychiatry 1999; 66:289–296.

22. Pollak P, Benabid AL, Gervason CL, Hoffmann D, Seigneuret E, Perret J. Long-term effects of chronic stimulation of the ventral intermediate thalamic nucleus in different types of tremor. Adv Neurol 1993; 60:408–413.

23. Speelman JD, Schuurman PR, de Bie RMA, Bosch DA. Thalamic surgery and tremor. Mov Disord 1998; 113(suppl 3):103–106.

24. Koller W, Pahwa R, Busenbark K, et al. High-frequency unilateral thalamic stimulation in the treatment of essential and parkinsonian tremor. Ann Neurol 1997; 42:292–299.

25. Tasker RR, Munz M, Junn FS, et al. Deep brain stimulation and thalamotomy for tremor compared. Acta Neurochir Suppl (Wien) 1997; 68:49–53.

26. Krauss JK, Simpson RK Jr, Ondo WG, Pohle T, Burgunder JM, Jankovic J. Concepts and methods in chronic thalamic stimulation for treatment of tremor: technique and application. Neurosurgery 2001; 48(3):535–541.

27. Putzke JD, Wharen RE, Wszolek ZK, Turk MF, Strongosky AJ, Uitti RJ. Thalamic depp brain stimulation for tremor-predominant Parkinson's disease. Parkinsonism Relat Disord 2003; 10:81–88.

28. Rehncrona S, Johnels B, Widner H, Tomqvist AL, Hariz M, Sydow O. Long-term efficacy of thalamic deep brain stimulation for tremor: double-blind assessments. Mov Disord 2003; 18:163–170.

29. Hariz MI. Complications of deep brain stimulation surgery. Mov Disord 17, S3, 202, S162–S166.

30. Joint C, Nardi D, Parkin S, Gregory R, Aziz T. Hardware related problems of deep brain stimulation. Mov Disord 2002; 17:S175–S180.

31. Lyons KE, Wilkinson SB, Overman J, Pahwa R. Surgical and hardware complications of subthalamic stimulation: a series of 160 procedures. Neurology 2004; 63(4):612–616.

32. Binder DK, Rau G, Starr PA. Hemorrhagic complications of microelectrode-guided deep brain stimulation. Stereotact Funct Neurosurg 2003; 80:28–31.

33. Svennilson E, Torvik A, Lowe R, Leksell L. Treatment of parkinsonism by stereotactic thermolesions in the pallidal region. A clinical evaluation of 81 cases. Acta Psychiatr Neurol Scand 1960; 35:358–377.

34. Laitinen LV, Bergenheim AT, Hariz MI. Leksell's posteroventral pallidotomy in the treatment of parkinson's disease. J Neurosurg 1992; 76:53–61.

35. Lozano AM, Lang AE, Galvez-Jimenez N, Miyasaki J, Duff J, Hutchinson WD, Dostrovsky JO. Effect of GPi pallidotomy on motor function in Parkinson's disease. Lancet 1995; 346:1383–1387.

36. Baron MS, Vitek JL, Bakay RA, Green J, Kaneoke Y, Hashimoto T, Turner RS, Woodard JL, Cole SA, McDonald WM, DeLong MR. Treatment of advanced Parkinson's disease by posterior GPi pallidotomy: 1-year results of a pilot study. Ann Neurol 1996; 40:355–366.

37. Uitti RJ, Wharen RE Jr, Turk MF, Lucas JA, Finton MJ, Graff-Radford NR, Boylan KB, Goerss SJ, Kall BA, Adler CH, Caviness JN, Atkinson EJ. Unilateral pallidotomy for Parkinson's disease: comparison of outcome in younger versus elderly patients. Neurology 1997; 49:1072–1077.

38. Lang AE, Lozano AM, Montgomery E, Duff J, Tasker R, Hutchinson W. Posteroventral medial pallidotomy in advanced Parkinson's disease. N Engl J Med 1997; 337:1036–1042.

39. Samii A, Turnbull IM, Kishore A, Schulzer M, Mak E, Yardley S, Calne DB. Reassessment of unilateral pallidotomy in Parkinson's disease: a 2-year follow-up study. Brain 1999; 122:417–425.

40. Galvez-Jimenez N, Lozano AM, Duff J, Trepanier L, Saint-Cyr JA, Lang AE. Bilateral pallidotomy: pronounced amelioration of incapacitating levodopa-induced dyskinesias but accompanying cognitive decline. Mov Disord 1996; 11(suppl 1):242.

41. Kishore A, Turnbull IM, Snow BJ, de la Fuente-Fernandez R, Schulzer M, Mak E, Yardley S, Calne DB. Efficacy, stability and predictors of outcome of pallidotomy for Parkinson's disease: six-month follow-up with additional 1-year observations. Brain 1997; 120:729–737.

42. Shannon KM, Penn RD, Kroin JS, Adler CH, Janko KA, York M, Cox SJ. Stereotactic pallidotomy for the treatment of Parkinson's disease: efficacy and adverse effects at 6 months in 26 patients. Neurology 1998; 50:434–438.

43. Samuel M, Caputo E, Brooks DJ, et al. A study of medial pallidotomy for Parkinson's disease: clinical outcome, MRI location and complications. Brain 1998; 121:59–75.

44. Fazzini E, Dogali M, Sterio D, Eidelberg D, Beric A. Stereotactic pallidotomy for Parkinson's disease: a long-term follow-up of unilateral pallidotomy. Neurology 1997; 48:1273–1277.

45. Gross RE, Lombardi WJ, Lang AE, Duff J, Hutchison WD, Saint-Cyr JA, Tasker RR, Lozano AM. Relationship of lesion location to clinical outcome

following microelectrode-guided pallidotomy for Parkinson's disease. Brain 1999; 122:405–416.

46. Fine J, Duff J, Chen R, Hutchison W, Lozano A, Lang AE. Long-term follow-up of unilateral pallidotomy in advanced Parkinson's disease. N Engl J Med 2000; 342:1708–1714.

47. Lai EC, Jankovic J, Krauss JK, Ondo WG, Grossman RG. Long-term efficacy of posteroventral pallidotomy in the treatment of Parkinson's disease. Neurology 2000; 55(8):1218–1222.

48. Alkhani A, Lozano AM. Pallidotomy for Parkinson disease: a review of contemporary literature. J Neurosurg 2001; 94:43–49.

49. Valldeoriola F, Martinez-Rodriguez J, Tolosa E, Rumia J, Alegret M, Pilleri M, Ferrer E. Four year follow-up study after unilateral pallidotomy in advanced Parkinson's disease. J Neurol 2002; 249:1671–1677.

50. de Bie RM, Schuurman PR, Esselink RA, Bosch DA, Speelman JD. Bilateral pallidotomy in Parkinson's disease: a retrospective study. Mov Disord 2002; 17:533–538.

51. Hariz MI, Bergenheim AT. A 10-year follow-up review of patients who underwent Leksell's posteroventral pallidotomy for Parkinson disease. J Neurosurg 2001; 94:552–558.

52. Kim R, Alterman R, Kelly PJ, Fazzini E, Eidelberg D, Beric A, Sterio D. Efficacy of bilateral pallidotomy. Neurosurg Focus 1997; 2(3):e8.

53. Iacono RP, Shima F, Lonser RR, Kuniyoshi S, Maeda G, Yamada S. The results, indications and physiology of posteroventral pallidotomy for patients with Parkinson's disease. Neurosurgery 1995; 36:1118–1127.

54. Ghika J, Ghika-Schmid F, Fankhauser H, Assal G, Vingerhoets F, Albanese A, Bogousslavsky J, Favre J. Bilateral contemporaneous posteroventral pallidotomy for the treatment of Parkinson's disease: neuropsychological and neurological side effects: report of four cases and review of the literature. J Neurosurg 1999; 91: 313–321.

55. Merello M, Starkstein S, Nouzeilles MI, Kuzis G, Leiguarda R. Bilateral pallidotomy for treatment of Parkinson's disease induced corticobulbar syndrome and psychic akinesia avoidable by globus pallidus lesion with contralateral stimulation. J Neurol Neurosurg Psychiatry 2001; 71:611–614.

56. Laitinen LV, Hariz MI. Movement Disorders. Youmans JR, ed. Neurological Surgery. 4th ed. Philadelphia, PA: W.B. Saunders, 1996:3575–3609.

57. Hua Z, Guodong G, Qinchuan L, Yaqun Z, Qinfen W, Xuelian W. Analysis of complications of radiofrequency pallidotomy. Neurosurgery 2003; 52: 89–101.

58. Trepanier LL, Saint-Cyr JA, Lozano AM, Lang AI. Neuropsychological consequences of posteroventral pallidotomy for the treatment of Parkinson's disease. Neurology 1998; 51:207–215.

59. Ardouin C, Pillon B, Peiffer E, Bejjani P, Limousin P, Damier P, Arnulf I, Benabid AL, Agid Y, Pollak P. Bilateral subthalamic or pallidal stimulation for Parkinson's disease affects neither memory nor executive functions: a consecutive series of 62 patients. Ann Neurol 1999; 46(2):217–223.

60. Hariz MI, DeSalles AAF. The side effects and complications of posteroventral pallidotomy. Acta Neurochir Suppl 1997; 68:42–48.

61. Higouchi Y, Iacono RP. Surgical complications in patients with Parkinson's disease after posteroventral pallidotomy. Neurosurgery 2003; 52:558–571.
62. Siegfried J, Lippitz B. Chronic electrical stimulation of the VL-VPL complex and of the pallidum in the treatment of movement disorders: personal experience since 1982. Stereotact Funct Neurosurg 1994; 62:71–75.
63. Visser-Vandewalle V, van der Linden C, Temel Y, Nieman F, Celik H, Beuls E. Long-term motor effect of unilateral pallidal stimulation in 26 patients with advanced Parkinson disease. J Neurosurg 2003; 99(4):701–707.
64. Iacono RP, Lonser RR, Mandybur G, Yamada S. Stimulation of the globus pallidus in Parkinson's disease. Br J Neurosurg 1995; 9(4):505–510.
65. Gross C, Rougier A, Guehl D, Boraud T, Julien J, Bioulac B. High-frequency stimulation of the globus pallidus internalis in Parkinson's disease: a study of seven cases. J Neurosurg 1997; 87(4):491–498.
66. Pahwa R, Wilkinson S, Smith D, Lyons K, Miyawaki E, Koller WC. High-frequency stimulation of the globus pallidus for the treatment of Parkinson's disease. Neurology 1997; 49:249–253.
67. Bejjani B, Damier P, Arnulf I, Bonnet AM, Vidailhet M, Dormont D, Pidoux B, Cornu P, Marsault C, Agid Y. Pallidal stimulation for Parkinson's disease. Two targets? Neurology 1997; 49(6):1564–1569.
68. Ghika J, Villemure JG, Fankhauser H, Favre J, Assal G, Ghika-Schmid F. Efficiency and safety of bilateral contemporaneous pallidal stimualtion in levo-dopa responsive patients with parkinson's disease with severe motor fluctuations: a 2-year follow-up review. J Neurosurg 1998; 89:713–718.
69. Kumar R, Lozano AM, Montgomery E, Lang AE. Pallidotomy and deep brain stimulation of the pallidum and subthalamic nucleus in advanced Parkinson's disease. Mov Disord 1998; 13(suppl 1):73–82.
70. Krack P, Pollak P, Limousin P, Hoffmann D, Xie J, Benazzouz A, Benabid AL. Opposite motor effects of pallidal stimulation in Parkinson's disease. Ann Neurol 1998; 43(2):180–192.
71. Gálvez-Jiménez N, Lozano A, Tasker R, Duff J, Hutchison W, Lang AE. Pallidal stimulation in Parkinson's disease patients with a prior unilateral pallidotomy. Can J Neurol Sci 1998; 25:300–305.
72. Burchiel KJ, Anderson VC, Favre J, Hammerstad JP. Comparison of pallidal and subthalamic nucleus deep brain stimulation for advanced Parkinson's disease: results of a randomized, blinded pilot study. Neurosurgery 1999; 45: 1375–1382.
73. Volkmann J, Sturm V, Weiss P, Kappler J, Voges J, Koulousakis A, Lehrke R, Hefter H, Freund HJ. Bilateral high-frequency stimulation of the internal globus pallidus in advanced Parkinson's disease. Ann Neurol 1998; 44:953–961.
74. The Deep-brain stimulation of the subthalamic nucleus or pars interna of the globus pallidus in Parkinson's disease. N Engl J Med 2001; 345:956–993.
75. Durif F, Lemaire JJ, Debilly B, Dordain G. Long-term follow-up of globus pallidus chronic stimulation in advanced Parkinson's disease. Mov Disord 2002; 17:803–807.
76. Loher TJ, Burgunder JM, Pohle T, Weber S, Sommerhalder R, Krauss JK. Long-term pallidal deep brain stimulation in patients with advanced Parkinson disease: 1-year follow-up study. J Neurosurg 2002; 96(5):844–853.

77. Volkmann J, Albert N, Voges J, Sturm V, Schnitzler A, Freund HJ. Long-term results of bilateral pallidal stimulation in Parkinson's disease. Ann Neurol 2004; 55:871–875.
78. Volkmann J, Allert N, Voges J, Weiss PH, Freund HJ, Sturm V. Safety and efficacy of pallidal or subthalamic nucleus stimulation in advanced PD. Neurology 2001; 56(4):548–551.
79. Guridi J, Obeso JA. The subthalamic nucleus, hemiballismus and Parkinson's disease: reappraisal of a neurosurgical dogma. Brain 2001; 124(Pt 1):5–19.
80. Andy OJ, Jurko MF, Sias FR. Subthalamotomy in treatment of parkinsonian tremor. J Neurosurg 1963; 20:860–870.
81. Su PC, Tseng HM, Liu HM, Yen RF, Liou HH. Treatment of advanced Parkinson's disease by subthalamotomy: one-year results. Mov Disord 2003; 18(5):531–538.
82. Chen CC, Lee ST, Wu T, Chen CJ, Huang CC, Lu CS. Hemiballism after subthalamotomy in patients with Parkinson's disease: report of 2 cases. Mov Disord 2002; 17(6):1367–1371.
83. Gill SS, Heywood P. Bilateral dorsolateral subthalamotomy for advanced Parkinson's disease. Lancet 1997; 350(9086):1224.
84. Alvarez L, Macias R, Guridi J, Lopez G, Alvarez E, Maragoto C, Teijeiro J, Torres A, Pavon N, Rodriguez-Oroz MC, Ochoa L, Hetherington H, Juncos J, DeLong MR, Obeso JA. Dorsal subthalamotomy for Parkinson's disease. Mov Disord 2001; 16(1):72–78.
85. Patel NK, Heywood P, O'Sullivan K, McCarter R, Love S, Gill SS. Unilateral subthalamotomy in the treatment of Parkinson's disease. Brain 2003; 126(Pt 5): 1136–1145.
86. Klostermann W, Vieregge P, Kompf D. Apraxia of eyelid opening after bilateral stereotaxic subthalamotomy. J Neuroophthalmol 1997; 17(2):122–123.
87. Tseng HM, Su PC, Liu HM. Persistent hemiballism after subthalamotomy: the size of the lesion matters more than the location. Mov Disord 2003; 18(10): 1209–1211.
88. Benabid AL, Krack PP, Benazzouz A, Limousin P, Koudsie A, Pollak P. Deep brain stimulation of the subthalamic nucleus for Parkinson's disease: methodologic aspects and clinical criteria. Neurology 2000; 55(12 suppl 6): S40–S44.
89. Krack P, Limousin P, Benabid AL, Pollak P. Chronic stimulation of subthalamic nucleus improves levodopa-induced dyskinesias in Parkinson's disease. Lancet 1997; 350:1676(letter).
90. Kumar R, Lozano AM, Kim YJ, Hutchison WD, Sime E, Halket E, Lang AE. Double-blind evaluation of subthalamic nucleus deep brain stimulation in advanced Parkinson's disease. Neurology 1998; 51:850–855.
91. Limousin P, Krack P, Pollak P, Benazzouz A, Ardouin C, Hoffmann D, Benabid AL. Electrical stimulation of the subthalamic nucleus in advanced Parkinson's disease. N Engl J Med 1998; 339:1105–1111.
92. Vingerhoets FJ, Villemure JG, Temperli P, Pollo C, Pralong E, Ghika J. Subthalamic DBS replaces levodopa in Parkinson's disease: two-year follow-up. Neurology 2002; 58(3):396–401.

93. Simuni T, Jaggi JL, Mulholland H, Hurtig HI, Colcher A, Siderowf AD, Ravina B, Skolnick BE, Goldstein R, Stern MB, Baltuch GH. Bilateral stimulation of the subthalamic nucleus in patients with Parkinson disease: a study of efficacy and safety. J Neurosurg 2002; 96(4):666–672.

94. Herzog J, Volkmann J, Krack P, Kopper F, Potter M, Lorenz D, Steinbach M, Klebe S, Hamel W, Schrader B, Weinert D, Muller D, Mehdorn HM, Deuschl G. Two-year follow-up of subthalamic deep brain stimulation in Parkinson's disease. Mov Disord 2003; 18(11):1332–1337.

95. Jarraya B, Bonnet AM, Duyckaerts C, Houeto JL, Cornu P, Hauw JJ, Agid Y. Parkinson's disease, subthalamic stimulation, and selection of candidates: a pathological study. Mov Disord 2003; 18(12):1517–1520.

96. Patel NK, Plaha P, O'Sullivan K, McCarter R, Heywood P, Gill SS. MRI directed bilateral stimulation of the subthalamic nucleus in patients with Parkinson's disease. J Neurol Neurosurg Psychiatry 2003; 74(12):1631–1637.

97. Kleiner-Fisman G, Fisman DN, Sime E, Saint-Cyr JA, Lozano AM, Lang AE. Long-term follow up of bilateral deep brain stimulation of the subthalamic nucleus in patients with advanced Parkinson disease. J Neurosurg 2003; 99(3): 489–495.

98. Rousseaux M, Krystkowiak P, Kozlowski O, Ozsancak C, Blond S, Destee A. Effects of subthalamic nucleus stimulation on parkinsonian dysarthria and speech intelligibility. J Neurol 2004; 251(3):327–334.

99. Krause M, Fogel W, Mayer P, Kloss M, Tronnier V. Chronic inhibition of the subthalamic nucleus in Parkinson's disease. J Neurol Sci 2004; 219(1–2):119–124.

100. Jaggi JL, Umemura A, Hurtig HI, Siderowf AD, Colcher A, Stern MB, Baltuch GH. Bilateral stimulation of the subthalamic nucleus in Parkinson's disease: surgical efficacy and prediction of outcome. Stereotact Funct Neurosurg 2004; 82(2–3):104–114.

101. Rodriguez-Oroz MC, Zamarbide I, Guridi J, Palmero MR, Obeso JA. Efficacy of deep brain stimulation of the subthalamic nucleus in Parkinson's disease 4 years after surgery: double blind and open label evaluation. J Neurol Neurosurg Psychiatry 2004; 75(10):1382–1385.

102. Russmann H, Ghika J, Villemure JG, Robert B, Bogousslavsky J, Burkhard PR, Vingerhoets FJ. Subthalamic nucleus deep brain stimulation in Parkinson disease patients over age 70 years. Neurology 2004; 63(10):1952–1954.

103. Thobois S, Mertens P, Guenot M, Hermier M, Mollion H, Bouvard M, Chazot G, Broussolle E, Sindou M. Subthalamic nucleus stimulation in Parkinson's disease: clinical evaluation of 18 patients. J Neurol 2002; 249(5):529–534.

104. Tavella A, Bergamasco B, Bosticco E, Lanotte M, Perozzo P, Rizzone M, Torre E, Lopiano L. Deep brain stimulation of the subthalamic nucleus in Parkinson's disease: long-term follow-up. Neurol Sci 2002; 23(suppl 2):S111–S112.

105. Krack P, Batir A, Van Blercom N, Chabardes S, Fraix V, Ardouin C, Koudsie A, Limousin PD, Benazzouz A, LeBas JF, Benabid AL, Pollak P. Five-year follow-up of bilateral stimulation of the subthalamic nucleus in advanced Parkinson's disease. N Engl J Med 2003; 349(20):1925–1934.

106. Pillon B, Ardouin C, Damier P, Krack P, Houeto JL, Klinger H, Bonnet AM, Pollak P, Benabid AL, Agid Y. Neuropsychological changes between "off"

and "on" STN or GPi stimulation in Parkinson's disease. Neurology 2000; 55:411–418.

107. Jahanshahi M, Ardouin CM, Brown RG, Rothwell JC, Obeso J, Albanese A, Rodriguez-Oroz MC, Moro E, Benabid AL, Pollak P, Limousin-Dowsey P. The impact of deep brain stimulation on executive function in Parkinson's disease. Brain 2000; 123:1142–1154.

108. Houeto JL, Mesnage V, Mallet L, Pillon B, Gargiulo M, du Moncel ST, Bonnet AM, Pidoux B, Dormont D, Cornu P, Agid Y. Behavioural disorders, Parkinson's disease and subthalamic stimulation. J Neurol Neurosurg Psychiatry 2002; 72:701–707.

109. Funkiewiez A, Ardouin C, Caputo E, Krack P, Fraix V, Klinger H, Chabardes S, Foote K, Benabid AL, Pollak P. Long term effects of bilateral subthalamic nucleus stimulation on cognitive function, mood, and behaviour in Parkinson's disease. J Neurol Neurosurg Psychiatry 2004; 75(6):834–839.

110. Villemure JG, Vingerhoets F, Temperli P, Pollo C, Ghika J. Effect of bilateral subthalamic deep brain stimulation (STN-DBS) after bilateral contemporaneous pallidal DBS (Gpi-DBS) in Parkinson's disease (PD). Neurology 2000; 54(suppl 3):A186.

111. Houeto JL, Bejjani PB, Damier P, Staedler C, Bonnet AM, Pidoux B, Dormont D, Cornu P, Agid Y. Failure of long-term pallidal stimulation corrected by subthalamic stimulation in PD. Neurology 2000; 55(5):728–730.

112. Mogilner AY, Sterio D, Rezai AR, Zonenshayn M, Kelly PJ, Beric A. Subthalamic nucleus stimulation in patients with a prior pallidotomy. J Neurosurg 2002; 96(4):660–665.

113. Morrison CE, Borod JC, Perrine K, Beric A, Brin MF, Rezai A, Kelly P, Sterio D, Germano I, Weisz D, Olanow CW. Neuropsychological functioning following bilateral subthalamic nucleus stimulation in Parkinson's disease. Arch Clin Neuropsychol 2004; 19(2):165–181.

114. Pahwa R, Wilkinson SB, Overman J, Lyons KE. Bilateral subthalamic stimulation in patients with Parkinson disease: long-term follow up. J Neurosurg 2003; 99:71–77.

115. Romito LM, Raja M, Daniele A, Contarino MF, Bentivoglio AR, Barbier A, Scerrati M, Albanese A. Transient mania with hypersexuality after surgery for high frequency stimulation of the subthalamic nucleus in Parkinson's disease. Mov Disord 2002; 17:1371–1374.

116. Woods SP, Fields JA, Troster AI. Neuropsychological sequelae of subthalamic nucleus deep brain stimulation in Parkinson's disease: a critical review. Neuropsychol Rev 2002; 12(2):111–126.

117. Berney A, Vingerhoets F, Perrin A, Guex P, Villemure JG, Burkhard PR, Benkelfat C, Ghika J. Effect on mood of subthalamic DBS for Parkinson's disease: a consecutive series of 24 patients. Neurology 2002; 59:1427–1429.

118. Doshi PK, Chhaya N, Bhatt MH. Depression leading to attempted suicide after bilateral subthalamic nucleus stimulation for Parkinson's disease. Mov Disord 2002; 17:1084–1085.

119. Funkiewiez A, Ardouin C, Krack P, Fraix V, Van Blercom N, Xie J, Moro E, Benabid AL, Pollak P. Acute psychotropic effects of bilateral subthalamic

nucleus stimulation and levodopa in Parkinson's disease. Mov Disord 2003; 18:524–530.

120. Herzog J, Reiff J, Krack P, Witt K, Schrader B, Muller D, Deuschl G. Manic episode with psychotic symptoms induced by subthalamic nucleus stimulation in a patient with Parkinson's disease. Mov Disord 2003; 18(11):1382–1384.

121. Welter ML, Houeto JL, Tezenas du Montcel S, Mesnage V, Bonnet AM, Pillon B, Arnulf I, Pidoux B, Dormont D, Cornu P, Agid Y. Clinical predictive factors of subthalamic stimulation in Parkinson's disease. Brain 2002; 125(3):575–583.

122. Zonenshayn M, Rezai AR, Mogilner AY, Beric A, Sterio D, Kelly PJ. Comparison of anatomic and neurophysiological methods for subthalamic nucleus targeting. Neurosurgery 2000; 47:282–292.

123. Houeto JL, Welter ML, Bejjani PB, Tezenas du Montcel S, Bonnet AM, Mesnage V, Navarro S, Pidoux B, Dormont D, Cornu P, Agid Y. Subthalamic stimulation in Parkinson disease: intraoperative predictive factors. Arch Neurol 2003; 60(5):690–694.

124. Benazzouz A, Breit S, Koudsie A, Pollack P, Krack P, Benabid AL. Intraoperative microrecordings of the subthalamic nucleus in Parkinson's disease. Mov Disord 2002; 17(suppl3):S145–S149.

125. Molinuevo JL, Valldeoriola F, Valls-Sole J. Usefulness of neurophysiologic techniques in stereotactic subthalamic nucleus stimulation in advanced Parkinson's disease. Clin Neurophysiol 2003; 114:1793–1799.

126. Pralong E, Ghika J, Temperli P, Pollo C, Vingerhoets F, Villemure JG. Electrophysiological localization of the subthalamic nucleus in parkinsonian patients. Neurosci Lett 2002; 325:144–146.

127. Guridi J, Rodriguez-Oroz MC, Ramos E, Linazasoro G, Obeso JA. Discrepancy between imaging and neurophysiology in deep brain stimulation of medial pallidum and subthalamic nucleus in Parkinson's disease. Neurologia 2002; 17:183–192.

128. Lanotte MM, Rizzone M, Bergamasco B, Faccani G, Melcarne A, Lopiano L. Deep brain stimulation of the subthalamic nucleus: anatomical, neurophysiological, and outcome correlations with the effects of stimulation. J Neurol Neurosurg Psychiatry 2002; 72(1):53–58.

129. Caire F, Derost P, Coste J, Durif F, Frenoux E, Lemaire JJ. Deep brain stimulation for Parkinson's disease: anatomical location of effective contacts in the subthalamic area. Acta Neurochir 2004; 146(8):869.

130. Andrade-Souza YM, Schwalb JM, Hamani C, Eltahawy H, Saint-Cyr J, Lozano AM. Comparison of three methods of targeting the subthalamic nucleus for chronic stimulation in Parkinson disease. Acta Neurochir 2004; 146(8):869.

131. Vayssiere N, Fertit HE, Cif L, Hemm S, Coubes P. Quality control procedure for stereotactic magnetic resonance imaging during neurosurgery of movement disorders. Acta Neurochir 2004; 146(8):881.

132. Vayssiere N, Charif M, Garrigues G, Cif L, Touchon J, Coubes P. Treatment of Parkinson's disease by deep brain stimulation: evaluation of an MRI-based surgery under general anesthesia. Acta Neurochir 2004; 146(8):905.

133. Zrinzo L, Blomstedt P, Dowsey-Limousin P, Hariz M. Accuracy of stereotactic targeting in deep brain stimulation. Acta Neurochir 2004; 146(8):909.

5

Novel Surgical Strategies: Motor Cortex Stimulation, Transplantation, Gene Therapy, Stem Cells, and CNS Drug Delivery

Jason M. Schwalb and Andres M. Lozano

Division of Neurosurgery, Toronto Western Hospital, University of Toronto and University Health Network, Toronto, Ontario, Canada

1. INTRODUCTION

Deep brain stimulation (DBS) and lesional stereotactic surgery are well-established treatments for Parkinson's disease (PD). This chapter will discuss the limitations of current strategies and potential novel therapies in the treatment of PD. These include attempts to replace dopaminergic neurons, prevention of ongoing loss of dopaminergic neurons, and direct infusion of pharmacologic agents. However, before discussing novel therapies, some of the lessons learned in previous clinical trials for adrenal chromaffin and human fetal mesencephalic transplants will be examined. Ethical issues raised by these studies will also be examined.

2. LIMITATIONS OF CURRENT THERAPY

As discussed in the previous chapter by Villemure, Ghika, and Vingerhoets, DBS is a highly effective treatment for medically refractory PD. DBS reduces dopamine-related dyskinesias and improves motor function when not taking dopaminergic drugs (1–3). When DBS of the subthalamic nucleus

(STN) is performed, dopamine dosage can be significantly decreased (1,2,4,5). In short, DBS reduces fluctuations in functions related to levodopa dosing and bioavailability.

Performing lesions and placing DBS systems seem to be equally effective, at least when using the nucleus ventralis intermedialis (Vim) thalami as a target (6). However, there is a much higher risk of serious complications with lesional techniques (6–8), especially if performed bilaterally (9–12).

There are several limitations to DBS and lesional techniques that have spurred researchers to investigate alternative surgical therapies. DBS does not confer benefits above a patient's best condition "on" medication. There is little or no effect on autonomic dysfunction or depression associated with PD. Akinesia, speech, postural stability, freezing of gait, and cognitive function worsen between the first and the fifth year after surgery (13). It is also unknown whether DBS alters the natural history of PD.

In addition, there are significant risks and costs related to DBS and long-term hardware implantation. There is a risk of intraparenchymal bleeding associated with targeting deep structures. Late hardware complications include DBS electrode fracture, extension wire failure, lead migration, erosion, infection, foreign body reaction, pulse generator malfunction, and pain over the pulse generator (14–21). Rates of these complications vary from center to center, from 2.7% to 50% of patients.

3. MOTOR CORTEX STIMULATION

As early as 1979, it was reported that electrical stimulation of the primary motor cortex can reduce rigidity and tremor in patients with PD (22). Some neurosurgeons who placed chronic motor cortex stimulators in patients with poststroke pain also noted reductions in rigidity and tremor (23–25). On the basis of these observations, a group from Turin, Italy, performed chronic motor cortex stimulation (MCS) in five patients with PD (26–28). Although the electrode was placed over the area of the motor cortex involved in movement of the face and arm of the opposite side, these patients were reported to have significant improvement in their ambulation and other bilateral symptoms. Although the core assessment program for surgical interventional therapies (CAPSIT) was not used for evaluation (29), the Turin group reported improvements in drug-induced dyskinesia, focal dystonia, tremor, gait, and speech. One of their patients had a significant reduction in levodopa medication needed to control her symptoms.

There are several other reasons to believe that MCS might be effective in the treatment of PD. Patients with tremor from PD have electrical oscillations in their motor cortices that correlate with their tremors, as detected by electroencephalography (EEG) or magnetoencephalography (MEG) and electromyography (EMG) (30,31). These oscillations precede the physical tremor in PD, indicating that the primary motor cortex is involved in the generation of the tremor (31). Positron emission tomography (PET) and functional magnetic resonance imaging have demonstrated disturbances in the activity of premotor and motor cortices in PD that improve in response to effective medical and surgical therapy (32–36). However, some of the changes associated with PD may be due to pronounced disruption of connections between the basal ganglia and the motor cortex, so that therapies directed at the basal ganglia may not have an effect (37). Experiments on monkeys made parkinsonian with the drug N-methyl-4-phenyl-1,2,3,6-tetrahydropyridine (MPTP) suggest that some of their rigidity and akinesia may be caused by excessive synchrony of the neurons in the motor cortex which causes persistent contraction of muscles with opposing actions (37). In addition, unilateral MCS improved motor performance in three baboons made parkinsonian with MPTP (38).

Techniques of directly altering the function of these cortical areas have been applied in a limited fashion with some promising results. Transcranial magnetic stimulation (TMS), wherein a magnetic stimulus is given through the skull to induce a current and transient activation and/or inactivation of the cortical brain area underneath, can reset the tremors of patients with PD (39). There have also been transient improvements in bradykinesia and gait dysfunction in patients with PD [reviewed in (40,41)]. TMS causes an acute release of dopamine in the striatum in humans and macaques, which may be responsible for some of the benefits seen with TMS in patients with PD (42,43). There is some evidence that TMS may induce effects in a similar way to chronic electrical stimulation (44).

MCS has several possible advantages over lesional and DBS techniques. It is a less complex operation, involving techniques that are more commonly practiced by neurosurgeons. Electrophysiologic localization of the motor cortex does not require the same degree of complexity as localization of the Vim, globus pallidus pars interna (GPi), or STN, and is therefore less expensive and time consuming. There may be bilateral effects from a unilateral electrode (26–28). Placing the electrode on the surface of the brain does not violate the brain, so there should be a lower risk of intraparechymal hemorrhage. It may be less likely that DBS of deep structures will result in unwanted side effects from current spread to adjacent structures, such as paresthesias, dizziness, dysarthria, depression, gait disorders, and visual disturbances (1,6,7,45–49). Therefore, this technique may be useful in patients at risk for DBS, e.g., those with multiple vascular lesions in the brain, cognitive or psychiatric problems, or advanced age.

4. HISTORY OF TRANSPLANTATION

The hallmark of PD is the loss of dopaminergic neurons in the substantia nigra pars compacta (SNc) (50,51). The hope has been that replacement of lost dopaminergic neurons will reverse the symptoms of the disease. This avenue of research has been aided by the use of animal models of PD, namely the use of the neurotoxins MPTP in mice and nonhuman primates and 6-hydroxydopamine (6-OHDA) in rats, which cause an acute loss of dopaminergic neurons.

The first attempt at replacement of dopaminergic neurons in humans with PD was with adrenal chromaffin cells, which are derived embryologically from the neural crest. Dopaminergic cells were harvested from the adrenal glands of patients and then placed into their postcommissural putamina, the site enervated by the SNc that is involved in appendicular motor function. This method avoided any issues of immunosuppression, since autotransplants were used. Unfortunately, very few of the cells survived the transplantation process and there was little clear, sustained benefit in the patients treated (52–54). Part of the problem may have been that these cells were also affected by the patients' disease process.

After this experience, it was hoped that cells derived from the substantia nigra of 6–9-week-old human fetuses could be used. On the basis of multiple open label studies suggesting benefit [reviewed in (55)], the National Institutes of Health (NIH) funded two randomized trials of fetal nigral transplantation (56,57). In both studies, the patients and evaluating neurologists were blinded to whether the patient was given the transplant or underwent trepanation alone.

There are many lessons for subsequent trial design to be learned by evaluating these trials closely (Table 1). In the study by Freed and colleagues (56), tissue from two embryos per side was transplanted into the postcommissural putamina of the patients in the therapy arm of the trial via a transfrontal approach. Tissue was transplanted up to 4 weeks after it had been obtained. No immunosuppression was given. There were no changes in global rating scales. There were no improvements of Unified PD Rating Scale (UPDRS) scores when "on" medication. UPDRS motor subscores "off" medication decreased 18% at 12 months in the transplantation group and remained stable in the sham-surgery group ($p = 0.04$ using the general estimating equation). Preoperative response to levodopa challenge was predictive of a positive response (58,59). In comparison, in open label studies, bilateral STN DBS improved "off" medication UPDRS motor subscores by 56% at 12 months (3).

Olanow and colleagues transplanted tissue from either one or four embryos per side into the postcommissural putamina of patients in the therapy arms of the trial via an approach from Kocher's point (57). Tissue was transplanted within 2 days of being obtained. All patients, including those in the sham-surgery group, were immunosuppressed with cyclosporine from 2 weeks prior to the procedure to 6 months afterwards. There were significant improvements in UPDRS motor subscores at 6 and 9 months after surgery, but not afterwards. The only significant treatment effect at 24

Table 1 Differences in Study Design of the Randomized Trials of Fetal Nigral Transplantation

Trial	Number of embryos	Time from harvest to transplantation	Approach	Immunosuppression	Length of follow-up
Freed et al. (2001)	2 per side	Within 4 weeks	Transfrontal through forehead	No	12 months
Olanow et al. (2003)	1 or 4 per side	Within 2 days	Via Kocher's point	Yes, 2 weeks preop to 6 months postop	24 months

months was in patients with less severe motor scores (UPDRS <49) who received transplants from four donors per side. These patients improved by 1.5 ± 4.2 points, compared to a 21.4 ± 4.3 decrement in the group that underwent trepanation alone. These findings suggest that therapies may be more likely to be helpful in less advanced disease and that 12 month follow-up may be insufficient for subsequent trials.

[18]F-fluorodopa (FDOPA) PET scanning and postmortem examination revealed viable dopaminergic neurons in both trials (Fig. 1). However, this did not correlate with clinical benefit.

Of concern, patients who received transplants in both trials had increased risk of postoperative confusion, hallucinations, or increases in psychosis compared to the sham-surgery groups. In addition, in both studies, 15–56% of those who received transplants developed dystonia and dyskinesia more than a year after surgery that could not be controlled by eliminating levodopa therapy. Some of these patients required STN or pallidal DBS to control their dyskinesias (58). In the trial by Freed and colleagues, but not the trial by Olanow et al., all of these subjects had initial clinical improvement as measured by UPDRS. Their average UPDRS "on" and "off" motor subscores were better preoperatively than patients who did

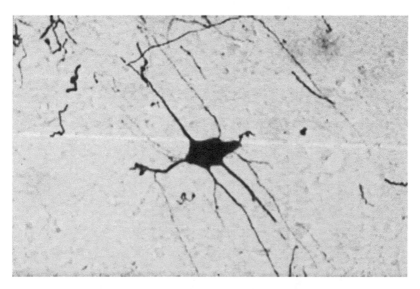

Figure 1 Human fetal dopamine neuron in putamen of Parkinson's patient dying 8 years after cell transplantation. The cell is immunostained for tyrosine hydroxylase and has multiple neuronal processes growing out from the cell body. Other staining methods used on other transplanted cells in the same patient revealed neuromelanin pigment particles typical of mature substantia nigra dopamine neurons (magnification ×400). *Source*: From Ref. 188. Copyright 2002 National Academy of Sciences, U.S.A.

not develop dyskinesias (60). This complication was probably not the result of absolute overproduction of dopamine, since PET scans did not demonstrate FDOPA uptake that was higher than in normal patients without PD (60). Regional imbalance and partial, but inadequate, graft survival have been proposed as possible causes of this complication (57,60).

All in all, these trials indicate that fetal nigral transplantation is not a viable clinical therapy at the present time. There was no benefit over best condition "on" medication. Apart from the ethical and political issues inherent in using fetal tissue, the therapy, under the different protocols used in these two randomized trials, was not as effective as bilateral STN DBS. However, valuable lessons can be learned from these trials: (a) immunosuppression may not be necessary for the survival of some types of grafts; (b) improvement in dopamine delivery into the postcommissural putamen, as measured by PET, does not necessarily correlate with clinical improvement; (c) the patients who are most likely to gain benefit from transplantation may be those who are younger with less advanced disease. It may be "too late" to transplant patients with more advanced disease.

5. ETHICS OF SHAM SURGERY

There was much controversy before the fetal transplant trials regarding the use of sham surgery as a control (61–63), which has continued (64–67). Much of the justification for using sham surgery was based upon drug trials on patients with early stage PD, which demonstrated a significant placebo effect (68,69). There is also increased endogenous dopamine release and decreased activity of subthalamic nucleus neurons in response to placebo, in patients with advanced PD who are usually considered eligible for DBS or transplantation (70–73).

Of concern, there were some "nonserious" adverse effects reported in the sham surgery arm of the trial by Freed and colleagues, including increased "off" time, freezing, dyskinesias, depression, constipation, headaches, and worsened "on" states (56). It is unclear whether these changes were transient or not, or whether this reflects variablity of the disease over time that would have been seen if the control group had not undergone sham surgery.

The controlled, randomized trials demonstrate that the natural history of advanced PD is quite variable. There are few data about the natural history of advanced PD [reviewed in (74)]. There is significant fluctuation in UPDRS motor "off" scores if evaluating patients more frequently than every 4 or 6 months. Patients who enter trials with fairly good scores (<49) have significant worsening at 24 months, while those with higher scores, and therefore worse disease, tend to remain fairly stable (57). Patients in the control arm of the trial by Freed and colleagues had fairly stable disease over time, while those in the study by Olanow et al. had significant deterioration over the 2 years of the study.

Freed and colleagues (58), among others, have maintained that double-blind designs with sham surgery are necessary, since previous open label studies of fetal transplantation gave positive results. However, except for one study that included 22 patients (75), the open label studies cited were too small, containing 10 patients or less (76–87). It is unclear why previous trials did not reveal off-period dyskinesias, even when the patients were followed for 2 years (75).

At this point, it is unclear how significant and long-lasting the placebo effect is in patients receiving sham surgery, and therefore how necessary sham surgery controls are. The side effects reported in the sham surgery groups are concerning. It is doubtful that this gap in our knowledge will change unless a trial is performed with three groups: a treatment group, a sham-surgery group, and a third group that receives medical therapy alone but would have met inclusion criteria with similarly advanced PD.

6. FUTURE DIRECTIONS IN IMPLANTING DOPAMINERGIC NEURONS

In spite of the fact that delivering dopamine into the postcommisural putamen does not necessarily improve PD symptoms, several groups are working on cell-based strategies to do just this, several of which were initiated before the results of the fetal transplantation trials were known. Autotransplants of carotid body cell aggregates (88), porcine fetal tissue xenografts (89), and human retinal pigment epithelial cell transplants with gelatin microcarriers (90) have been performed in open label studies. These patients had modest improvements in "off" UPDRS scores. "On" state UPDRS III subscore changes have not been reported.

Human retinal pigment epithelial cell transplantation has proceeded to a Phase II, NIH-funded trial which started in December 2002 (91). These cells produce levodopa and may, therefore, act as constant levodopa infusion minipumps. They may also produce dopamine (90). This trial is expected to randomize 68 patients to either postcommissural placement of these cells with gelatin microcarriers (Spheramine®) or sham surgery. The investigators plan to follow the patients for 5 years.

Additional experimental work has focused on developing stem cell lines that can be induced to differentiate into neurons. This technology could supply large amounts of homogenous material for transplantation that could be more stably transported than primary fetal cultures. Murine neuronal stem cells, isolated before the embryonic stage of dopaminergic differentiation, can be propagated in culture, differentiate into dopaminergic neurons, survive intrastriatal transplantation, and induce functional recovery in animal models (92–97). Cells from earlier stages of embryonic rodent development, i.e., embryonic stem (ES) cells, can also differentiate into dopaminergic neurons in vitro (98–100) and in vivo (101). Human and nonhuman primate ES cells can be induced to differentiate into dopaminergic neurons as well (102–104). Unfortunately, some of the human embryonic stem cell lines that are eligible for NIH funding may be contaminated with murine cells (105).

Clonal cell lines, such as the C17.2 line, which is immortalized with the oncogene v-myc, can also express dopaminergic markers after transplantation (106). The ability to form dopaminergic neurons is significantly affected by host conditions and location. For example, C17.2 cells are more likely to form dopaminergic neurons when transplanted into damaged brain (107). This is also true of endogenous stem cells (see following text) (108).

Adult bone marrow stromal cells are being explored as an alternative source of dopaminergic neurons that avoid ethical and political concerns about using human embryonic tissue. It is possible to transplant these cells autologously, without a theoretical need for immunosuppression. These cells can be greatly expanded in culture without losing their ability to differentiate into different cell types (109). Although these cells are thought to be of mesodermal origin, they are also capable of differentiating into astrocytes, neurons, and oligodendrocytes, both in vitro and in vivo (110–117). They can be induced to differentiate in vitro into neurons with dopaminergic markers (118). In addition, marrow stromal cells have powerful effects on adjacent cells, promoting the outgrowth of neurites from hippocampal slices and reducing cell damage in an ischemia model (119).

However, many of the in vivo experiments demonstrating stem cell plasticity have been called into question because of fusion with host cells, especially in the case of bone marrow stromal cells (120–124). Subsequent characterization of the grafted cells can be misinterpreted due to markers expressed by the host tissue. Prior experiments that did not check for polyploidy have been called into question. There are no clear data on the stability of these chimeras and whether or not they may be oncogenic. However, there is good evidence, when polyploidy was looked for, that bone marrow stromal cells can differentiate into neurons in vivo and can be detected up to 6 years after transplantation (125). It is clear that stem cells can be differentiated into neurons in vitro and can cause functional recovery in animal models of PD.

It should be noted that some stem cells can enter the central nervous system and differentiate into neurons when administered intravenously (126–129). To date, these experimental models have been performed for conditions where there is breakdown of the blood–brain barrier, such as glioblastomas, trauma, and multiple sclerosis. One study has shown that marrow stromal cells can enter into the brains of MPTP-lesioned mice, but it is unknown whether these cells differentiated into neurons (130). It has been shown that cells used in bone marrow transplants can differentiate into hippocampal and cortical neurons in humans (125,131).

Other strategies include cografting with human Sertoli cells to prevent rejection. Sertoli cells provide local immunoprotection to cografted cells, including those from xenogeneic sources. Sertoli cells, which are found in the testes, normally provide local immunologic protection to developing germ cells (132,133). They may also directly encourage cell survival of dopaminergic neurons (134,135).

7. INDUCTION OF ENDOGENOUS STEM CELLS

In 1998, Eriksson and colleagues demonstrated that ongoing neurogenesis takes place in specific areas of the adult human brain, especially the hippocampus (136). Since then, some groups have worked on inducing endogenous stem cells in adult animals to differentiate into functional dopaminergic neurons. Although most neuronal stem cells reside in the subventricular zone, there are some indications that stem cells in the adult substantia nigra can be induced to differentiate into neurons under the appropriate conditions (108). Infusion of TGF-α into the striata of 6-OHDA lesioned rats induces proliferation, migration, and differentiation of endogenous stem cells, along with functional recovery (137).

8. TROPHIC FACTORS RATHER THAN DOPAMINERGIC NEURONS—GDNF THERAPY

While many groups have been working on replacing dopaminergic neurons, others have been pursuing strategies of preventing further loss of dopaminergic neurons with trophic factors. Glial cell line–derived neurotrophic factor (GDNF) is a member of the TGF-β superfamily that was isolated due to its ability to promote the survival and morphological differentiation of dopaminergic neurons in embryonic midbrain cultures and increase high-affinity dopamine uptake (138). Since its description in 1993, 1479 articles have been published in English on GDNF, of which 170 are reviews, as ascertained by searching PubMed (139). GDNF not only protects dopaminergic neurons from injury, but also induces axonal sprouting and regeneration when delivered into the cerebral ventricles, striatum, or substantia nigra of both rodents and nonhuman primates that have had neurotoxins administered prior to GDNF infusion [reviewed in (140)]. GDNF also causes increased dopamine turnover and release in the striatum and leads to functional recovery in animal models.

On this basis, a multicenter, randomized, double-blinded trial was initiated in which recombinant GDNF was injected monthly into the cerebral ventricles of PD patients via a subcutaneous filtered access port (141). "On" and "off" total and motor UPDRS scores were not improved by

GDNF at any of the doses tested. In addition, intrathecal GDNF caused adverse effects, such as nausea, anorexia, vomiting, weight loss, and paresthesias, often described as electric shocks (Lhermitte's sign). An autopsy of one of the study patients, who had many of these adverse side effects, revealed increased tyrosine hydroxylase immunoreactivity in the nucleus basalis and substantia innominata, but not in the striatum or substantia nigra (142).

It was hypothesized that GDNF was not getting to the target structures with intrathecal administration, whereas it had in studies involving animals with smaller brains. Therefore, Gill and colleagues continuously infused recombinant GDNF into the postcommissural putamina of five patients with PD (143). Their results were remarkable. This was the first study that showed improvement in UPDRS scores in the "on" state, suggesting functional regeneration. In addition, there were improvements in autonomic and sexual symptoms, as well as olfaction, which had not been seen in the fetal transplant trials or with DBS.

On the basis of this open label trial, a Phase 2 multicenter, double-blinded, randomized crossover trial was initiated in which 34 patients received either recombinant GDNF or saline. Unfortunately, there was no clinical difference between the GDNF group and the placebo group at 6 months [Amgen press release on June 28, 2004 (144)], in spite of improvements on F-DOPA PET studies (145). In addition, four of the patients developed antibodies to GDNF and GDNF at high doses was found to cause cerebellar degeneration in two nonhuman primates (145,146). As a result, the therapy was discontinued in the study patients and the trial was halted.

It is unclear why the results of the open label pilot study and the multicenter trial are different. Could the placebo effect in the open label study have been that strong? Other issues to consider are the different dosages and different catheter sizes used in these studies (146).

At this point, the fate of further GDNF trials is unclear. However, there are other trophic factors, which support dopaminergic survival and regeneration in animal models, that are candidates for human therapy, the GDNF homologs neurturin (147) and artemin (148), basic fibroblast growth factor (bFGF) (149), and brain derived neurotrophic factor (BDNF) (150,151).

9. GENE THERAPY FOR PARKINSON'S DISEASE

Another possible strategy is to modulate the ability of human cells to produce therapeutic molecules they do not normally produce. By inducing cells to produce neurotrophins, e.g., the complications associated with pumps and the cost of recombinant proteins could be avoided. Similarly, host cells could be induced to express dopamine without the need to transplant dopaminergic neurons. This strategy has been used in animal studies by introducing RNA or

DNA into cells with a variety of techniques, direct transfer of naked nucleic acids, liposomal transfer, and packaging in replication-deficient viruses. These methods differ in their stability of expression over time, the size of the construct that can be packaged, and immunogenicity. The most long-lasting transduction method is with lentiviruses, which use reverse transcriptase to integrate the gene of interest into the host DNA. The other main virus that has been investigated for gene therapy for PD is adeno-associated virus (AAV) (152). AAV can induce gene expression for at least 15 months in nonhuman primates and is not as immunogenic as adenovirus (153).

Several of these strategies are moving toward clinical trials. Initial animal studies showed improvement in parkinsonian symptoms by transducing neurons to express tyrosine hydroxylase (TH), the rate-limiting enzymatic step in dopamine synthesis (154). A subsequent study has shown that introducing genes for GTP-cyclohydrolase I, which synthesizes the TH cofactor tetrahydrobiopterin, and aromatic acid decarboxylase (AADC) along with TH can improve dopamine production and behavioral outcome (155). In this study, confocal microscopy has been used to show that striatal neurons can change their phenotypes and produce dopamine. Oxford Biomedica has proposed a clinical trial using this vector (156). Other studies have used different combinations of these genes (157–160). However, such trials may encounter similar problems to those seen with fetal transplantation, in that there is no regulation of gene expression and dopamine production other than the number of virions injected. Patients receiving this therapy could similarly develop "off" dyskinesias. Due to this concern, Avigen has proposed a trial of AADC gene therapy in the human striatum with an AAV vector (161). This would potentially increase responsiveness to levodopa therapy with effective regulation of dopamine production, since dopamine could not be synthesized without exogenous levodopa (157). In addition, Ceregene has proposed a trial with the GDNF homolog neurturin (162).

There is one active gene therapy trial in humans for PD, which takes advantage of the ability to change neuronal phenotype. Single injections of lidocaine or muscimol, a $GABA_A$ receptor agonist, into the thalamus arrest tremor (163–165). Single injections into the STN or GPi also reverse parkinsonian symptoms (166,167). On this basis, Luo and colleagues transfected STN neurons with two isoforms of the enzyme glutamic acid decarboxylase (GAD-65 and GAD-67), which synthesize GABA, using AAV vectors (168). This construct changed the phenotype of these glutamatergic projection neurons into GABAergic projection neurons, leading to increased GABA in the substantia nigra pars reticulata (Fig. 2). In addition, dopaminergic neurons were protected from injury with 6-OHDA. This group has initiated a open label trial in humans of stereotactic gene therapy using this construct at Weill Cornell Medical Center (169,170).

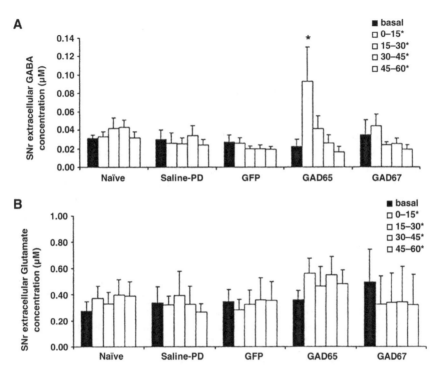

Figure 2 Increase in GABA, but not glutamate, concentrations in the SNr after electrical stimulation of the STN in transduced animals. Surprisingly, there was no increase in glutamate concentrations in the nontransduced animals. Sequential mean (A) GABA and (B) glutamate concentrations after electrical stimulation, as determined by microdialysis in 15 minute epochs, were pooled ($n = 4$ rats for each of the five groups). Groups were unlesioned control rats and parkinsonian rats transduced with saline, GFP, GAD65, or GAD67. Error bars represent SEMs. Asterisk, $p \leq 0.05$, repeated measures ANOVA. *Source*: From Ref. 168.

As with all medical therapies, there are risks associated with gene therapy. There is concern about recombination with wild-type virus, leading to a replication-competent virus that could cause disease. An immune response in one child to an adenoviral vector at the University of Pennsylvania led to his death (171,172). In a successful trial of gene therapy for children with X-linked severe combined immunodeficiency (SCID), 2 of the 11 children developed leukemia due to integration of the therapeutic gene into the host genome near a proto-oncogene (173,174).

Safety can be improved by inserting controls into the constructs. Overactive gene expression can be controlled by inserting a tetracycline-responsive element (175,176). When doxycycline, a tetracycline homolog that crosses the blood–brain barrier, is given orally, gene transcription is shut down or turned on. Similar gene switches using steroids, rapamycin, or ecdysone can also be used (175,177).

10. GENETIC MANIPULATION OF STEM CELLS

Stem cell therapy can be combined with gene therapy ex vivo to improve safety and efficacy and to produce large numbers of dopaminergic neurons. Neuronal stem cells can be transfected to produce GDNF (178). Bone marrow stromal cells transfected with GDNF provide a greater functional recovery than untransfected cells when injected intravenously into MPTP-lesioned mice (130). Neuronal stem cells can be immortalized and made to overexpress the nuclear receptor Nurr1, an important protein in the development of dopaminergic neurons (179). When exposed to fibroblast growth factor-8 (FGF-8) and sonic hedgehog signals, this cell line generates large numbers of dopaminergic cells. Murine ES cells that constitutively express Bcl-XL, an antiapoptotic protein of Bcl-2 family, form dopaminergic neurons, are more resistant to MPTP injury, and induce greater behavioral recovery in animal models than nontransfected cells (180).

Dezawa and colleagues recently showed that marrow stromal cells transduced with the Notch intracellular domain via lipofection can be induced to form almost pure neuronal cultures when exposed to a specific cocktail of trophic factors (181). Forty-one percent of these near-pure neuronal cultures were dopaminergic, whereas previous efforts produced cultures with 30% dopaminergic neurons with admixed glial cells (118). Dezawa and colleagues transplanted these neurons into the striata of 6-OHDA lesioned rats and demonstrated behavioral improvement of parkinsonian symptoms (181).

When patients in the randomized fetal mesencephalic transplantation trials developed "off" period dyskinesias, nothing could be done to modulate the transplanted cells. Many of these patients underwent DBS to control their dyskinesias (58). However, future cell transplantation protocols could have better built-in safety characteristics. Suicide genes like the herpes simplex virus thymidine kinase can be inserted into cells to be used in transplantation (182). If the cells become oncogenic, gancyclovir can be administered to the patient to selectively kill those cells that are dividing. Proliferation and differentiation of cells can also be controlled by using a tetracycline-responsive element to control the expression of inserted genes (175,176, 183,184).

11. CONCLUSIONS

There are many promising therapies for PD that are in various stages of development, which may supplement or replace DBS. These include cellular transplants, gene therapy, neurotrophic factors, motor cortex stimulation, and combined therapies. However, there are lessons to be learned from previous trials about the pitfalls likely to be encountered in clinical trials, as well as in our thinking about PD. For example, from the clinical trials of fetal mesencephalic tissue and GDNF, it is now clear that increased dopamine delivery to the putamen does not necessarily produce clinical improvement. This fact forces us to reassess our assumption that PD is primarily a disease of the substantia nigra, especially in the patients with advanced disease that is refractory to levodopa therapy. Autopsy data reveal involvement of the dorsal motor nucleus of the vagus nerve and the intermediate reticular zone in earliest stages of PD, before there is involvement of the substantia nigra [reviewed in (185)]. Patients with late-stage PD also have widespread disease in the temporal mesocortex and neocortex (185). We may need to develop animal models that resemble advanced, idiopathic PD more closely in order to develop effective therapies (186,187).

ADDITIONAL RESOURCES

The NIH publishes information on the Internet on clinical trials that it is funding at http://clinicaltrials.gov/ct/gui/ and http://www.ninds.nih.gov/parkinsonsweb/.

REFERENCES

1. Deep-brain stimulation of the subthalamic nucleus or the pars interna of the globus pallidus in Parkinson's disease. N Engl J Med 2001; 345:956–963.
2. Limousin P, Krack P, Pollak P, Benazzouz A, Ardouin C, Hoffmann D, Benabid AL. Electrical stimulation of the subthalamic nucleus in advanced Parkinson's disease. N Engl J Med 1998; 339:1105–1111.
3. Hamani C, Richter E, Schwalb JM, Lozano AM. Bilateral subthalamic nucleus stimulation for Parkinson's disease: a systematic review of the clinical literature. Neurosurgery, 2005; 56(6): 1313–1324.
4. Moro E, Scerrati M, Romito LM, Roselli R, Tonali P, Albanese A. Chronic subthalamic nucleus stimulation reduces medication requirements in Parkinson's disease. Neurology 1999; 53:85–90.
5. Katayama Y, Kasai M, Oshima H, Fukaya C, Yamamoto T, Ogawa K, Mizutani T. Subthalamic nucleus stimulation for Parkinson disease: benefits observed in levodopa-intolerant patients. J Neurosurg 2001; 95:213–221.
6. Schuurman PR, Bosch DA, Bossuyt PM, Bonsel GJ, van Someren EJ, de Bie RM, Merkus MP, Speelman JD. A comparison of continuous thalamic stimulation and thalamotomy for suppression of severe tremor. N Engl J Med 2000; 342:461–468.
7. Benabid AL, Pollak P, Gao D, Hoffmann D, Limousin P, Gay E, Payen I, Benazzouz A. Chronic electrical stimulation of the ventralis intermedius nucleus of the thalamus as a treatment of movement disorders. J Neurosurg 1996; 84:203–214.

8. Tasker RR. Deep brain stimulation is perferable to thalamotomy for tremor suppression. Surg Neurol 1998; 49:145–153; discussion 153–154.
9. Kelly PJ, Gillingham FJ. The long-term results of stereotaxic surgery and L-dopa therapy in patients with Parkinson's disease. A 10-year follow-up study. J Neurosurg 1980; 53:332–337.
10. Mohadjer M, Goerke H, Milios E, Etou A, Mundinger F. Long-term results of stereotaxy in the treatment of essential tremor. Stereotact Funct Neurosurg 1990; 54–55:125–129.
11. Burchiel KJ. Thalamotomy for movement disorders. Neurosurg Clin N Am 1995; 6:55–71.
12. Matsumoto K, Shichijo F, Fukami T. Long-term follow-up review of cases of Parkinson's disease after unilateral or bilateral thalamotomy. J Neurosurg 1984; 60:1033–1044.
13. Krack P, Batir A, Van Blercom N, Chabardes S, Fraix V, Ardouin C, Koudsie A, Limousin PD, Benazzouz A, LeBas JF, Benabid AL, Pollak P. Five-year follow-up of bilateral stimulation of the subthalamic nucleus in advanced Parkinson's disease. N Engl J Med 2003; 349:1925–1934.
14. Oh MY, Abosch A, Kim SH, Lang AE, Lozano AM. Long-term hardware-related complications of deep brain stimulation. Neurosurgery 2002; 50:1268–1274; discussion 1274–1276.
15. Merello M, Cammarota A, Leiguarda R, Pikielny R. Delayed intracerebral electrode infection after bilateral STN implantation for Parkinson's disease. Case report. Mov Disord 2001; 16:168–170.
16. Umemura A, Jaggi JL, Hurtig HI, Siderowf AD, Colcher A, Stern MB, Baltuch GH. Deep brain stimulation for movement disorders: morbidity and mortality in 109 patients. J Neurosurg 2003; 98:779–784.
17. Hamel W, Schrader B, Weinert D, Herzog J, Muller D, Deuschl G, Volkmann J, Mehdorn HM. Technical complication in deep brain stimulation. Zentralbl Neurochir 2002; 63:124–127.
18. Schwalb JM, Riina HA, Skolnick B, Jaggi JL, Simuni T, Baltuch GH. Revision of deep brain stimulator for tremor. Technical note. J Neurosurg 2001; 94:1010–1012.
19. Hariz MI. Complications of deep brain stimulation surgery. Mov Disord 2002; 17(suppl 3):S162–S166.
20. Beric A, Kelly PJ, Rezai A, Sterio D, Mogilner A, Zonenshayn M, Kopell B. Complications of deep brain stimulation surgery. Stereotact Funct Neurosurg 2001; 77:73–78.
21. Joint C, Nandi D, Parkin S, Gregory R, Aziz T. Hardware-related problems of deep brain stimulation. Mov Disord 2002; 17(suppl 3):S175–S180.
22. Woolsey CN, Erickson TC, Gilson WE. Localization in somatic sensory and motor areas of human cerebral cortex as determined by direct recording of evoked potentials and electrical stimulation. J Neurosurg 1979; 51:476–506.
23. Garcia-Larrea L, Peyron R, Mertens P, Gregoire MC, Lavenne F, Le Bars D, Convers P, Mauguiere F, Sindou M, Laurent B. Electrical stimulation of motor cortex for pain control: a combined PET-scan and electrophysiological study. Pain 1999; 83:259–273.

24. Katayama Y, Fukaya C, Yamamoto T. Control of poststroke involuntary and voluntary movement disorders with deep brain or epidural cortical stimulation. Stereotact Funct Neurosurg 1997; 69:73–79.

25. Nguyen JP, Pollin B, Feve A, Geny C, Cesaro P. Improvement of action tremor by chronic cortical stimulation. Mov Disord 1998; 13:84–88.

26. Canavero S, Bonicalzi V, Paolotti R, Castellano G, Greco-Crasto S, Rizzo L, Davini O, Maina R. Therapeutic extradural cortical stimulation for movement disorders: a review. Neurol Res 2003; 25:118–122.

27. Canavero S, Paolotti R, Bonicalzi V, Castellano G, Greco-Crasto S, Rizzo L, Davini O, Zenga F, Ragazzi P. Extradural motor cortex stimulation for advanced Parkinson disease. Report of two cases. J Neurosurg 2002; 97: 1208–1211.

28. Pagni CA, Zeme S, Zenga F. Further experience with extradural motor cortex stimulation for treatment of advanced Parkinson's disease. Report of 3 new cases. J Neurosurg Sci 2003; 47:189–193.

29. Defer GL, Widner H, Marie RM, Remy P, Levivier M. Core assessment program for surgical interventional therapies in Parkinson's disease (CAPSIT-PD). Mov Disord 1999; 14:572–584.

30. Hellwig B, Haussler S, Schelter B, Lauk M, Guschlbauer B, Timmer J, Lucking CH. Tremor-correlated cortical activity in essential tremor. Lancet 2001; 357:519–523.

31. Timmermann L, Gross J, Dirks M, Volkmann J, Freund HJ, Schnitzler A. The cerebral oscillatory network of parkinsonian resting tremor. Brain 2003; 126: 199–212.

32. Davis KD, Taub E, Houle S, Lang AE, Dostrovsky JO, Tasker RR, Lozano AM. Globus pallidus stimulation activates the cortical motor system during alleviation of parkinsonian symptoms. Nat Med 1997; 3:671–674.

33. Ceballos-Baumann AO, Boecker H, Bartenstein P, von Falkenhayn I, Riescher H, Conrad B, Moringlane JR, Alesch F. A positron emission tomographic study of subthalamic nucleus stimulation in Parkinson disease: enhanced movement-related activity of motor-association cortex and decreased motor cortex resting activity. Arch Neurol 1999; 56:997–1003.

34. Thobois S, Dominey P, Fraix V, Mertens P, Guenot M, Zimmer L, Pollak P, Benabid AL, Broussolle E. Effects of subthalamic nucleus stimulation on actual and imagined movement in Parkinson's disease: a PET study. J Neurol 2002; 249:1689–1698.

35. Hesselmann V, Sorger B, Girnus R, Lasek K, Maarouf M, Wedekind C, Bunke J, Schulte O, Krug B, Lackner K, Sturm V. Intraoperative functional MRI as a new approach to monitor deep brain stimulation in Parkinson's disease. Eur Radiol 2003.

36. Brooks DJ, Samuel M. The effects of surgical treatment of Parkinson's disease on brain function: PET findings. Neurology 2000; 55:S52–59.

37. Goldberg JA, Boraud T, Maraton S, Haber SN, Vaadia E, Bergman H. Enhanced synchrony among primary motor cortex neurons in the 1-methyl-4-phenyl-1,2,3,6-tetrahydropyridine primate model of Parkinson's disease. J Neurosci 2002; 22:4639–4653.

38. Drouot X, Oshino S, Lefaucheur J-P, L. B, Conde F, Keravel Y, Peschanski M, Hantraye P, Palfi S. Electrical neuromodulation of motor cortex facilitates locomotor activity in a primate model of Parkinson disease. Society for Neuroscience, Orlando, FL, November 2–7, 2002.

39. Britton TC, Thompson PD, Day BL, Rothwell JC, Findley LJ, Marsden CD. Modulation of postural wrist tremors by magnetic stimulation of the motor cortex in patients with Parkinson's disease or essential tremor and in normal subjects mimicking tremor. Ann Neurol 1993; 33:473–479.

40. Wassermann EM, Lisanby SH. Therapeutic application of repetitive transcranial magnetic stimulation: a review. Clin Neurophysiol 2001; 112:1367–1377.

41. Cantello R, Tarletti R, Civardi C. Transcranial magnetic stimulation and Parkinson's disease. Brain Res Rev 2002; 38:309–327.

42. Strafella AP, Paus T, Fraraccio M, Dagher A. Striatal dopamine release induced by repetitive transcranial magnetic stimulation of the human motor cortex. Brain 2003; 126:2609–2615.

43. Ohnishi T, Hayashi T, Okabe S, Nonaka I, Matsuda H, Iida H, Imabayashi E, Watabe H, Miyake Y, Ogawa M, Teramoto N, Ohta Y, Ejima N, Sawada T, Ugawa Y. Endogenous dopamine release induced by repetitive transcranial magnetic stimulation over the primary motor cortex: an [11C]raclopride positron emission tomography study in anesthetized macaque monkeys. Biol Psychiatry 2004; 55:484–489.

44. Canavero S, Bonicalzi V, Dotta M, Vighetti S, Asteggiano G, Cocito D. Transcranial magnetic cortical stimulation relieves central pain. Stereotact Funct Neurosurg 2002; 78:192–196.

45. Siegfried J, Lippitz B. Bilateral chronic electrostimulation of ventroposterolateral pallidum: a new therapeutic approach for alleviating all parkinsonian symptoms. Neurosurgery 1994; 35:1126–1129; discussion 1129–1130.

46. Pahwa R, Wilkinson S, Smith D, Lyons K, Miyawaki E, Koller WC. High-frequency stimulation of the globus pallidus for the treatment of Parkinson's disease. Neurology 1997; 49:249–253.

47. Bryant JA, De Salles A, Cabatan C, Frysinger R, Behnke E, Bronstein J. The impact of thalamic stimulation on activities of daily living for essential tremor. Surg Neurol 2003; 59:479–484; discussion 484–475.

48. Limousin P, Speelman JD, Gielen F, Janssens M. Multicentre European study of thalamic stimulation in parkinsonian and essential tremor. J Neurol Neurosurg Psychiatry 1999; 66:289–296.

49. Koller WC, Lyons KE, Wilkinson SB, Troster AI, Pahwa R. Long-term safety and efficacy of unilateral deep brain stimulation of the thalamus in essential tremor. Mov Disord 2001; 16:464–468.

50. Lang AE, Lozano AM. Parkinson's disease. Second of two parts. N Engl J Med 1998; 339:1130–1143.

51. Lang AE, Lozano AM. Parkinson's disease. First of two parts. N Engl J Med 1998; 339:1044–1053.

52. Velasco F, Velasco M, Rodriguez Cuevas H, Jurado J, Olvera J, Jimenez F. Autologous adrenal medullary transplants in advanced Parkinson's disease with particular attention to the selective improvement in symptoms. Stereotact Funct Neurosurg 1991; 57:195–212.

53. Ahlskog JE, Kelly PJ, van Heerden JA, Stoddard SL, Tyce GM, Windebank AJ, Bailey PA, Bell GN, Blexrud MD, Carmichael SW. Adrenal medullary transplantation into the brain for treatment of Parkinson's disease: clinical outcome and neurochemical studies. Mayo Clin Proc 1990; 65:305–328.

54. Goetz CG, Stebbins GT, Klawans HL, Koller WC, Grossman RG, Bakay RA, Penn RD. United Parkinson Foundation Neurotransplantation Registry on adrenal medullary transplants: presurgical, and 1- and 2-year follow-up. Neurology 1991; 41:1719–1722.

55. Hallett M, Litvan I. Scientific position paper of the Movement Disorder Society evaluation of surgery for Parkinson's disease. Task Force on Surgery for Parkinson's Disease of the American Academy of Neurology Therapeutic and Technology Assessment Committee. Mov Disord 2000; 15:436–438.

56. Freed CR, Greene PE, Breeze RE, Tsai WY, DuMouchel W, Kao R, Dillon S, Winfield H, Culver S, Trojanowski JQ, Eidelberg D, Fahn S. Transplantation of embryonic dopamine neurons for severe Parkinson's disease. N Engl J Med 2001; 344:710–719.

57. Olanow CW, Goetz CG, Kordower JH, Stoessl AJ, Sossi V, Brin MF, Shannon KM, Nauert GM, Perl DP, Godbold J, Freeman TB. A double-blind controlled trial of bilateral fetal nigral transplantation in Parkinson's disease. Ann Neurol 2003; 54:403–414.

58. Freed CR, Leehey MA, Zawada M, Bjugstad K, Thompson L, Breeze RE. Do patients with Parkinson's disease benefit from embryonic dopamine cell transplantation? J Neurol 2003; 250(suppl 3):III44–III46.

59. Freed CR, Breeze RE, Fahn S, Eidelberg D. Preoperative response to levodopa is the best predictor of transplant outcome. Ann Neurol 2004; 55:896; author reply 896–897.

60. Ma Y, Feigin A, Dhawan V, Fukuda M, Shi Q, Greene P, Breeze R, Fahn S, Freed C, Eidelberg D. Dyskinesia after fetal cell transplantation for parkinsonism: a PET study. Ann Neurol 2002; 52:628–634.

61. Cohen J. New fight over fetal tissue grafts. Science 1994; 263:600–601.

62. Cohen P. Focus: is it ethical for surgeons to cut patients open and sew them up without doing anything? New Sci 1999; 163:18–19.

63. Freeman TB, Vawter DE, Leaverton PE, Godbold JH, Hauser RA, Goetz CG, Olanow CW. Use of placebo surgery in controlled trials of a cellular-based therapy for Parkinson's disease. N Engl J Med 1999; 341:988–992.

64. London AJ, Kadane JB. Placebos that harm: sham surgery controls in clinical trials. Stat Methods Med Res 2002; 11:413–427.

65. Weijer C. I need a placebo like I need a hole in the head. J Law Med Ethics 2002; 30:69–72.

66. Miller FG. Sham surgery: an ethical analysis. Sci Eng Ethics 2004; 10:157–166.

67. Boer GJ, Widner H. Clinical neurotransplantation: core assessment protocol rather than sham surgery as control. Brain Res Bull 2002; 58:547–553.

68. Goetz CG, Janko K, Blasucci L, Jaglin JA. Impact of placebo assignment in clinical trials of Parkinson's disease. Mov Disord 2003; 18:1146–1149.

69. Shetty N, Friedman JH, Kieburtz K, Marshall FJ, Oakes D. The placebo response in Parkinson's disease. Parkinson Study Group. Clin Neuropharmacol 1999; 22:207–212.

70. de la Fuente-Fernandez R, Ruth TJ, Sossi V, Schulzer M, Calne DB, Stoessl AJ. Expectation and dopamine release: mechanism of the placebo effect in Parkinson's disease. Science 2001; 293:1164–1166.

71. de la Fuente-Fernandez R, Schulzer M, Stoessl AJ. The placebo effect in neurological disorders. Lancet Neurol 2002; 1:85–91.

72. de la Fuente-Fernandez R. Uncovering the hidden placebo effect in deep-brain stimulation for Parkinson's disease. Parkinsonism Relat Disord 2004; 10: 125–127.

73. Benedetti F, Colloca L, Torre E, Lanotte M, Melcarne A, Pesare M, Bergamasco B, Lopiano L. Placebo-responsive Parkinson patients show decreased activity in single neurons of subthalamic nucleus. Nat Neurosci 2004; 7:587–588.

74. Poewe WH, Wenning GK. The natural history of Parkinson's disease. Ann Neurol 1998; 44:S1–S9.

75. Kopyov OV, Jacques D, Lieberman A, Duma CM, Rogers RL. Clinical study of fetal mesencephalic intracerebral transplants for the treatment of Parkinson's disease. Cell Transplant 1996; 5:327–337.

76. Freed CR, Breeze RE, Rosenberg NL, Schneck SA, Wells TH, Barrett JN, Grafton ST, Mazziotta JC, Eidelberg D, Rottenberg DA. Therapeutic effects of human fetal dopamine cells transplanted in a patient with Parkinson's disease. Prog Brain Res 1990; 82:715–721.

77. Lindvall O, Brundin P, Widner H, Rehncrona S, Gustavii B, Frackowiak R, Leenders KL, Sawle G, Rothwell JC, Marsden CD, et al. Grafts of fetal dopamine neurons survive and improve motor function in Parkinson's disease. Science 1990; 247:574–577.

78. Freed CR, Breeze RE, Rosenberg NL, Schneck SA, Kriek E, Qi JX, Lone T, Zhang YB, Snyder JA, Wells TH, et al. Survival of implanted fetal dopamine cells and neurologic improvement 12 to 46 months after transplantation for Parkinson's disease. N Engl J Med 1992; 327:1549–1555.

79. Spencer DD, Robbins RJ, Naftolin F, Marek KL, Vollmer T, Leranth C, Roth RH, Price LH, Gjedde A, Bunney BS, et al. Unilateral transplantation of human fetal mesencephalic tissue into the caudate nucleus of patients with Parkinson's disease. N Engl J Med 1992; 327:1541–1548.

80. Widner H, Tetrud J, Rehncrona S, Snow B, Brundin P, Gustavii B, Bjorklund A, Lindvall O, Langston JW. Bilateral fetal mesencephalic grafting in two patients with parkinsonism induced by 1-methyl-4-phenyl-1,2,3,6-tetrahydropyridine (MPTP). N Engl J Med 1992; 327:1556–1563.

81. Freeman TB, Olanow CW, Hauser RA, Nauert GM, Smith DA, Borlongan CV, Sanberg PR, Holt DA, Kordower JH, Vingerhoets FJ, et al. Bilateral fetal nigral transplantation into the postcommissural putamen in Parkinson's disease. Ann Neurol 1995; 38:379–388.

82. Peschanski M, Defer G, N'Guyen JP, Ricolfi F, Monfort JC, Remy P, Geny C, Samson Y, Hantraye P, Jeny R, et al. Bilateral motor improvement and alteration of L-dopa effect in two patients with Parkinson's disease following intrastriatal transplantation of foetal ventral mesencephalon. Brain 1994; 117 (Pt3):487–499.

83. Defer GL, Geny C, Ricolfi F, Fenelon G, Monfort JC, Remy P, Villafane G, Jeny R, Samson Y, Keravel Y, Gaston A, Degos JD, Peschanski M, Cesaro P,

Nguyen JP. Long-term outcome of unilaterally transplanted parkinsonian patients. I. Clinical approach. Brain 1996; 119(Pt1):41–50.

84. Wenning GK, Odin P, Morrish P, Rehncrona S, Widner H, Brundin P, Rothwell JC, Brown R, Gustavii B, Hagell P, Jahanshahi M, Sawle G, Bjorklund A, Brooks DJ, Marsden CD, Quinn NP, Lindvall O. Short- and long-term survival and function of unilateral intrastriatal dopaminergic grafts in Parkinson's disease. Ann Neurol 1997; 42:95–107.

85. Hauser RA, Freeman TB, Snow BJ, Nauert M, Gauger L, Kordower JH, Olanow CW. Long-term evaluation of bilateral fetal nigral transplantation in Parkinson disease. Arch Neurol 1999; 56:179–187.

86. Levivier M, Dethy S, Rodesch F, Peschanski M, Vandesteene A, David P, Wikler D, Goldman S, Claes T, Biver F, Liesnard C, Goldman M, Hildebrand J, Brotchi J. Intracerebral transplantation of fetal ventral mesencephalon for patients with advanced Parkinson's disease. Methodology and 6-month to 1-year follow-up in 3 patients. Stereotact Funct Neurosurg 1997; 69:99–111.

87. Lopez-Lozano JJ, Bravo G, Brera B, Millan I, Dargallo J, Salmean J, Uria J, Insausti J. Long-term improvement in patients with severe Parkinson's disease after implantation of fetal ventral mesencephalic tissue in a cavity of the caudate nucleus: 5-year follow up in 10 patients. Clinica Puerta de Hierro Neural Transplantation Group. J Neurosurg 1997; 86:931–942.

88. Arjona V, Minguez-Castellanos A, Montoro RJ, Ortega A, Escamilla F, Toledo-Aral JJ, Pardal R, Mendez-Ferrer S, Martin JM, Perez M, Katati MJ, Valencia E, Garcia T, Lopez-Barneo J. Autotransplantation of human carotid body cell aggregates for treatment of Parkinson's disease. Neurosurgery 2003; 53:321–328; discussion 328–330.

89. Fink JS, Schumacher JM, Ellias SL, Palmer EP, Saint-Hilaire M, Shannon K, Penn R, Starr P, VanHorne C, Kott HS, Dempsey PK, Fischman AJ, Raineri R, Manhart C, Dinsmore J, Isacson O. Porcine xenografts in Parkinson's disease and Huntington's disease patients: preliminary results. Cell Transplant 2000; 9:273–278.

90. Bakay RA, Raiser CD, Stover NP, Subramanian T, Cornfeldt ML, Schweikert AW, Allen RC, Watts R. Implantation of spheramine in advanced Parkinson's disease (PD). Front Biosci 2004; 9:592–602.

91. http://clinicaltrials.gov/ct/gui/show/NCT00059007?order=27 (accessed November 4, 2004).

92. Studer L, Tabar V, McKay RD. Transplantation of expanded mesencephalic precursors leads to recovery in parkinsonian rats. Nat Neurosci 1998; 1:290–295.

93. Studer L, Csete M, Lee SH, Kabbani N, Walikonis J, Wold B, McKay R. Enhanced proliferation, survival, and dopaminergic differentiation of CNS precursors in lowered oxygen. J Neurosci 2000; 20:7377–7383.

94. Storch A, Paul G, Csete M, Boehm BO, Carvey PM, Kupsch A, Schwarz J. Long-term proliferation and dopaminergic differentiation of human mesencephalic neural precursor cells. Exp Neurol 2001; 170:317–325.

95. Stull ND, Iacovitti L. Sonic hedgehog and FGF8: inadequate signals for the differentiation of a dopamine phenotype in mouse and human neurons in culture. Exp Neurol 2001; 169:36–43.

96. Yan J, Studer L, McKay RD. Ascorbic acid increases the yield of dopaminergic neurons derived from basic fibroblast growth factor expanded mesencephalic precursors. J Neurochem 2001; 76:307–311.

97. Kim JH, Auerbach JM, Rodriguez-Gomez JA, Velasco I, Gavin D, Lumelsky N, Lee SH, Nguyen J, Sanchez-Pernaute R, Bankiewicz K, McKay R. Dopamine neurons derived from embryonic stem cells function in an animal model of Parkinson's disease. Nature 2002; 418:50–56.

98. Barberi T, Klivenyi P, Calingasan NY, Lee H, Kawamata H, Loonam K, Perrier AL, Bruses J, Rubio ME, Topf N, Tabar V, Harrison NL, Beal MF, Moore MA, Studer L. Neural subtype specification of fertilization and nuclear transfer embryonic stem cells and application in parkinsonian mice. Nat Biotechnol 2003; 21:1200–1207.

99. Kawasaki H, Mizuseki K, Nishikawa S, Kaneko S, Kuwana Y, Nakanishi S, Nishikawa SI, Sasai Y. Induction of midbrain dopaminergic neurons from ES cells by stromal cell-derived inducing activity. Neuron 2000; 28:31–40.

100. Lee SH, Lumelsky N, Studer L, Auerbach JM, McKay RD. Efficient generation of midbrain and hindbrain neurons from mouse embryonic stem cells. Nat Biotechnol 2000; 18:675–679.

101. Bjorklund LM, Sanchez-Pernaute R, Chung S, Andersson T, Chen IY, McNaught KS, Brownell AL, Jenkins BG, Wahlestedt C, Kim KS, Isacson O. Embryonic stem cells develop into functional dopaminergic neurons after transplantation in a Parkinson rat model. Proc Natl Acad Sci USA 2002; 99:2344–2349.

102. Park S, Lee KS, Lee YJ, Shin HA, Cho HY, Wang KC, Kim YS, Lee HT, Chung KS, Kim EY, Lim J. Generation of dopaminergic neurons in vitro from human embryonic stem cells treated with neurotrophic factors. Neurosci Lett 2004; 359:99–103.

103. Perrier AL, Tabar V, Barberi T, Rubio ME, Bruses J, Topf N, Harrison NL, Studer L. Derivation of midbrain dopamine neurons from human embryonic stem cells. Proc Natl Acad Sci USA 2004; 101:12543–12548.

104. Kawasaki H, Suemori H, Mizuseki K, Watanabe K, Urano F, Ichinose H, Haruta M, Takahashi M, Yoshikawa K, Nishikawa S, Nakatsuji N, Sasai Y. Generation of dopaminergic neurons and pigmented epithelia from primate ES cells by stromal cell-derived inducing activity. Proc Natl Acad Sci USA 2002; 99:1580–1585.

105. Bjorklund A, Dunnett SB, Brundin P, Stoessl AJ, Freed CR, Breeze RE, Levivier M, Peschanski M, Studer L, Barker R. Neural transplantation for the treatment of Parkinson's disease. Lancet Neurol 2003; 2:437–445.

106. Yang M, Stull ND, Berk MA, Snyder EY, Iacovitti L. Neural stem cells spontaneously express dopaminergic traits after transplantation into the intact or 6-hydroxydopamine-lesioned rat. Exp Neurol 2002; 177:50–60.

107. Yang M, Donaldson AE, Jiang Y, Iacovitti L. Factors influencing the differentiation of dopaminergic traits in transplanted neural stem cells. Cell Mol Neurobiol 2003; 23:851–864.

108. Lie DC, Dziewczapolski G, Willhoite AR, Kaspar BK, Shults CW, Gage FH. The adult substantia nigra contains progenitor cells with neurogenic potential. J Neurosci 2002; 22:6639–6649.

109. Prockop DJ, Azizi SA, Colter D, Digirolamo C, Kopen G, Phinney DG. Potential use of stem cells from bone marrow to repair the extracellular matrix and the central nervous system. Biochem Soc Trans 2000; 28:341–345.

110. Kopen GC, Prockop DJ, Phinney DG. Marrow stromal cells migrate throughout forebrain and cerebellum, and they differentiate into astrocytes after injection into neonatal mouse brains. Proc Natl Acad Sci USA 1999; 96: 10711–10716.

111. Mezey E, Chandross KJ, Harta G, Maki RA, McKercher SR. Turning blood into brain: cells bearing neuronal antigens generated in vivo from bone marrow. Science 2000; 290:1779–1782.

112. Sanchez-Ramos J, Song S, Cardozo-Pelaez F, Hazzi C, Stedeford T, Willing A, Freeman TB, Saporta S, Janssen W, Patel N, Cooper DR, Sanberg PR. Adult bone marrow stromal cells differentiate into neural cells in vitro. Exp Neurol 2000; 164:247–256.

113. Deng W, Obrocka M, Fischer I, Prockop DJ. In vitro differentiation of human marrow stromal cells into early progenitors of neural cells by conditions that increase intracellular cyclic AMP. Biochem Biophys Res Commun 2001; 282:148–152.

114. Kohyama J, Abe H, Shimazaki T, Koizumi A, Nakashima K, Gojo S, Taga T, Okano H, Hata J, Umezawa A. Brain from bone: efficient "meta-differentiation" of marrow stroma-derived mature osteoblasts to neurons with Noggin or a demethylating agent. Differentiation 2001; 68:235–244.

115. Song S, Sanchez-Ramos J. Preparation of neural progenitors from bone marrow and umbilical cord blood. Methods Mol Biol 2002; 198:79–88.

116. Suzuki H, Taguchi T, Tanaka H, Kataoka H, Li Z, Muramatsu K, Gondo T, Kawai S. Neurospheres induced from bone marrow stromal cells are multipotent for differentiation into neuron, astrocyte, and oligodendrocyte phenotypes. Biochem Biophys Res Commun 2004; 322:918–922.

117. Jin K, Mao XO, Batteur S, Sun Y, Greenberg DA. Induction of neuronal markers in bone marrow cells: differential effects of growth factors and patterns of intracellular expression. Exp Neurol 2003; 184:78–89.

118. Jiang Y, Jahagirdar BN, Reinhardt RL, Schwartz RE, Keene CD, Ortiz-Gonzalez XR, Reyes M, Lenvik T, Lund T, Blackstad M, Du J, Aldrich S, Lisberg A, Low WC, Largaespada DA, Verfaillie CM. Pluripotency of mesenchymal stem cells derived from adult marrow. Nature 2002; 418:41–49.

119. Zhong C, Qin Z, Zhong CJ, Wang Y, Shen XY. Neuroprotective effects of bone marrow stromal cells on rat organotypic hippocampal slice culture model of cerebral ischemia. Neurosci Lett 2003; 342:93–96.

120. Ying QL, Nichols J, Evans EP, Smith AG. Changing potency by spontaneous fusion. Nature 2002; 416:545–548.

121. Terada N, Hamazaki T, Oka M, Hoki M, Mastalerz DM, Nakano Y, Meyer EM, Morel L, Petersen BE, Scott EW. Bone marrow cells adopt the phenotype of other cells by spontaneous cell fusion. Nature 2002; 416:542–545.

122. Spees JL, Olson SD, Ylostalo J, Lynch PJ, Smith J, Perry A, Peister A, Wang MY, Prockop DJ. Differentiation, cell fusion, and nuclear fusion during ex vivo repair of epithelium by human adult stem cells from bone marrow stroma. Proc Natl Acad Sci USA 2003; 100:2397–2402.

123. Wang X, Willenbring H, Akkari Y, Torimaru Y, Foster M, Al-Dhalimy M, Lagasse E, Finegold M, Olson S, Grompe M. Cell fusion is the principal source of bone-marrow-derived hepatocytes. Nature 2003; 422:897–901.
124. Vassilopoulos G, Wang PR, Russell DW. Transplanted bone marrow regenerates liver by cell fusion. Nature 2003; 422:901–904.
125. Cogle CR, Yachnis AT, Laywell ED, Zander DS, Wingard JR, Steindler DA, Scott EW. Bone marrow transdifferentiation in brain after transplantation: a retrospective study. Lancet 2004; 363:1432–1437.
126. Pluchino S, Quattrini A, Brambilla E, Gritti A, Salani G, Dina G, Galli R, Del Carro U, Amadio S, Bergami A, Furlan R, Comi G, Vescovi AL, Martino G. Injection of adult neurospheres induces recovery in a chronic model of multiple sclerosis. Nature 2003; 422:688–694.
127. Fujiwara Y, Tanaka N, Ishida O, Fujimoto Y, Murakami T, Kajihara H, Yasunaga Y, Ochi M. Intravenously injected neural progenitor cells of transgenic rats can migrate to the injured spinal cord and differentiate into neurons, astrocytes and oligodendrocytes. Neurosci Lett 2004; 366:287–291.
128. Tang Y, Shah K, Messerli SM, Snyder E, Breakefield X, Weissleder R. In vivo tracking of neural progenitor cell migration to glioblastomas. Hum Gene Ther 2003; 14:1247–1254.
129. Chu K, Kim M, Park KI, Jeong SW, Park HK, Jung KH, Lee ST, Kang L, Lee K, Park DK, Kim SU, Roh JK. Human neural stem cells improve sensorimotor deficits in the adult rat brain with experimental focal ischemia. Brain Res 2004; 1016:145–153.
130. Park KW, Eglitis MA, Mouradian MM. Protection of nigral neurons by GDNF-engineered marrow cell transplantation. Neurosci Res 2001; 40:315–323.
131. Mezey E, Key S, Vogelsang G, Szalayova I, Lange GD, Crain B. Transplanted bone marrow generates new neurons in human brains. Proc Natl Acad Sci USA 2003; 100:1364–1369.
132. Emerich DF, Hemendinger R, Halberstadt CR. The testicular-derived Sertoli cell: cellular immunoscience to enable transplantation. Cell Transplant 2003; 12:335–349.
133. Sanberg PR, Borlongan CV, Saporta S, Cameron DF. Testis-derived Sertoli cells survive and provide localized immunoprotection for xenografts in rat brain. Nat Biotechnol 1996; 14:1692–1695.
134. Othberg AI, Willing AE, Cameron DF, Anton A, Saporta S, Freeman TB, Sanberg PR. Trophic effect of porcine Sertoli cells on rat and human ventral mesencephalic cells and hNT neurons in vitro. Cell Transplant 1998; 7: 157–164.
135. Sanberg PR, Borlongan CV, Othberg AI, Saporta S, Freeman TB, Cameron DF. Testis-derived Sertoli cells have a trophic effect on dopamine neurons and alleviate hemiparkinsonism in rats. Nat Med 1997; 3:1129–1132.
136. Eriksson PS, Perfilieva E, Bjork-Eriksson T, Alborn AM, Nordborg C, Peterson DA, Gage FH. Neurogenesis in the adult human hippocampus. Nat Med 1998; 4:1313–1317.
137. Fallon J, Reid S, Kinyamu R, Opole I, Opole R, Baratta J, Korc M, Endo TL, Duong A, Nguyen G, Karkehabadhi M, Twardzik D, Patel S, Loughlin S. In vivo induction of massive proliferation, directed migration, and differentiation

of neural cells in the adult mammalian brain. Proc Natl Acad Sci USA 2000; 97:14686–14691.

138. Lin LF, Doherty DH, Lile JD, Bektesh S, Collins F. GDNF: a glial cell line-derived neurotrophic factor for midbrain dopaminergic neurons. Science 1993; 260:1130–1132.

139. http://www.ncbi.nlm.nih.gov/entrez/query.fcgi (accessed October 7, 2004).

140. Kirik D, Georgievska B, Bjorklund A. Localized striatal delivery of GDNF as a treatment for Parkinson disease. Nat Neurosci 2004; 7:105–110.

141. Nutt JG, Burchiel KJ, Comella CL, Jankovic J, Lang AE, Laws ER Jr. Lozano AM, Penn RD, Simpson RK Jr. Stacy M, Wooten GF. Randomized, double-blind trial of glial cell line-derived neurotrophic factor (GDNF) in PD. Neurology 2003; 60:69–73.

142. Kordower JH, Palfi S, Chen EY, Ma SY, Sendera T, Cochran EJ, Mufson EJ, Penn R, Goetz CG, Comella CD. Clinicopathological findings following intra-ventricular glial-derived neurotrophic factor treatment in a patient with Parkinson's disease. Ann Neurol 1999; 46:419–424.

143. Gill SS, Patel NK, Hotton GR, O'Sullivan K, McCarter R, Bunnage M, Brooks DJ, Svendsen CN, Heywood P. Direct brain infusion of glial cell line-derived neurotrophic factor in Parkinson disease. Nat Med 2003; 9:589–595.

144. http://www.amgen.com/news/viewPR.jsp?id=585632 (accessed November 4, 2004).

145. Gill SS, Heywood P, Lozano AM, Lang AE, Moro E, Penn R, Dalvi A, Burchiel KJ, Nutt J, Kelly PJ, Hutchinson M, Elias WJ, Wooten F, Turner DA, Scott BL, Patel N, Laws ER Jr. Matcham J, Coffey R, Traub M. Bilateral intraputaminal infusion of liatermin (glial cell line-derived neurotrophic factor; r-metHuGDNF) in subjects with advanced Parkinson's disease. Congress of Neurological Surgeons, San Francisco, CA, October 16–21, 2004.

146. http://www.nature.com/news/2004/041004/pf/041004-6_pf.html (accessed October 7, 2004).

147. Horger BA, Nishimura MC, Armanini MP, Wang LC, Poulsen KT, Rosenblad C, Kirik D, Moffat B, Simmons L, Johnson E Jr. Milbrandt J, Rosenthal A, Bjorklund A, Vandlen RA, Hynes MA, Phillips HS. Neurturin exerts potent actions on survival and function of midbrain dopaminergic neurons. J Neurosci 1998; 18:4929–4937.

148. Rosenblad C, Gronborg M, Hansen C, Blom N, Meyer M, Johansen J, Dago L, Kirik D, Patel UA, Lundberg C, Trono D, Bjorklund A, Johansen TE. In vivo protection of nigral dopamine neurons by lentiviral gene transfer of the novel GDNF-family member neublastin/artemin. Mol Cell Neurosci 2000; 15: 199–214.

149. Fontan A, Rojo A, Sanchez Pernaute R, Hernandez I, Lopez I, Castilla C, Sanchez Albisua J, Perez Higueras A, Al-Rashid I, Rabano A, Gonzalo I, Angeles Mena M, Cools A, Eshuis S, Maguire P, Pruim J, Leenders K, Garcia de Yebenes J. Effects of fibroblast growth factor and glial-derived neuro-trophic factor on akinesia, F-DOPA uptake and dopamine cells in parkinso-nian primates. Parkinsonism Relat Disord 2002; 8:311–323.

150. Takeda M. [Intrathecal infusion of brain-derived neurotrophic factor protects nigral dopaminergic neurons from degenerative changes in 1-methyl-4-phenyl-

1,2,3,6-tetrahydropyridine-induced monkey parkinsonian model]. Hokkaido Igaku Zasshi 1995; 70:829–838.

151. Klein RL, Lewis MH, Muzyczka N, Meyer EM. Prevention of 6-hydroxydopamine-induced rotational behavior by BDNF somatic gene transfer. Brain Res 1999; 847:314–320.

152. Gao GP, Alvira MR, Wang L, Calcedo R, Johnston J, Wilson JM. Novel adeno-associated viruses from rhesus monkeys as vectors for human gene therapy. Proc Natl Acad Sci USA 2002; 99:11854–11859.

153. Schimmenti S, Boesen J, Claassen EA, Valerio D, Einerhand MP. Long-term genetic modification of rhesus monkey hematopoietic cells following transplantation of adenoassociated virus vector-transduced CD34+ cells. Hum Gene Ther 1998; 9:2727–2734.

154. Kaplitt MG, Leone P, Samulski RJ, Xiao X, Pfaff DW, O'Malley KL, During MJ. Long-term gene expression and phenotypic correction using adeno-associated virus vectors in the mammalian brain. Nat Genet 1994; 8:148–154.

155. Azzouz M, Martin-Rendon E, Barber RD, Mitrophanous KA, Carter EE, Rohll JB, Kingsman SM, Kingsman AJ, Mazarakis ND. Multicistronic lentiviral vector-mediated striatal gene transfer of aromatic L-amino acid decarboxylase, tyrosine hydroxylase, and GTP cyclohydrolase I induces sustained transgene expression, dopamine production, and functional improvement in a rat model of Parkinson's disease. J Neurosci 2002; 22: 10302–10312.

156. http://www.biomedica.co.uk/prosavin.htm (accessed November 4, 2004).

157. Leff SE, Spratt SK, Snyder RO, Mandel RJ. Long-term restoration of striatal L-aromatic amino acid decarboxylase activity using recombinant adenoassociated viral vector gene transfer in a rodent model of Parkinson's disease. Neuroscience 1999; 92:185–196.

158. Mandel RJ, Rendahl KG, Spratt SK, Snyder RO, Cohen LK, Leff SE. Characterization of intrastriatal recombinant adeno-associated virus-mediated gene transfer of human tyrosine hydroxylase and human GTP-cyclohydrolase I in a rat model of Parkinson's disease. J Neurosci 1998; 18:4271–4284.

159. During MJ, Samulski RJ, Elsworth JD, Kaplitt MG, Leone P, Xiao X, Li J, Freese A, Taylor JR, Roth RH, Sladek JR Jr. O'Malley KL, Redmond DE Jr. In vivo expression of therapeutic human genes for dopamine production in the caudates of MPTP-treated monkeys using an AAV vector. Gene Ther 1998; 5:820–827.

160. Ozawa K, Fan DS, Shen Y, Muramatsu S, Fujimoto K, Ikeguchi K, Ogawa M, Urabe M, Kume A, Nakano I. Gene therapy of Parkinson's disease using adeno-associated virus (AAV) vectors. J Neural Transm Suppl 2000:181–191.

161. http://www.avigen.com/product/clinical_trials.htm (accessed November 4, 2004).

162. http://www.ceregene.com/f-sci-park.html (accessed November 4, 2004).

163. Pahapill PA, Levy R, Dostrovsky JO, Davis KD, Rezai AR, Tasker RR, Lozano AM. Tremor arrest with thalamic microinjections of muscimol in patients with essential tremor. Ann Neurol 1999; 46:249–252.

164. Parrent AG, Tasker RR, Dostrovsky JO. Tremor reduction by microinjection of lidocaine during stereotactic surgery. Acta Neurochir Suppl (Wien) 1993; 58:45–47.

165. Dostrovsky JO, Sher GD, Davis KD, Parrent AG, Hutchison WD, Tasker RR. Microinjection of lidocaine into human thalamus: a useful tool in stereotactic surgery. Stereotact Funct Neurosurg 1993; 60:168–174.

166. Levy R, Lang AE, Dostrovsky JO, Pahapill P, Romas J, Saint-Cyr J, Hutchison WD, Lozano AM. Lidocaine and muscimol microinjections in sub-thalamic nucleus reverse Parkinsonian symptoms. Brain 2001; 124:2105–2118.

167. Penn RD, Kroin JS, Reinkensmeyer A, Corcos DM. Injection of GABA-agonist into globus pallidus in patient with Parkinson's disease. Lancet 1998; 351:340–341.

168. Luo J, Kaplitt MG, Fitzsimons HL, Zuzga DS, Liu Y, Oshinsky ML, During MJ. Subthalamic GAD gene therapy in a Parkinson's disease rat model. Science 2002; 298:425–429.

169. Oransky I. Gene therapy trial for Parkinson's disease begins. Lancet 2003; 362:712.

170. During MJ, Kaplitt MG, Stern MB, Eidelberg D. Subthalamic GAD gene transfer in Parkinson disease patients who are candidates for deep brain stimulation. Hum Gene Ther 2001; 12:1589–1591.

171. Smith L, Byers JF. Gene therapy in the post-Gelsinger era. JONAS Healthc Law Ethics Regul 2002; 4:104–110.

172. Somia N, Verma IM. Gene therapy: trials and tribulations. Nat Rev Genet 2000; 1:91–99.

173. Hacein-Bey-Abina S, von Kalle C, Schmidt M, Le Deist F, Wulffraat N, McIntyre E, Radford I, Villeval JL, Fraser CC, Cavazzana-Calvo M, Fischer A. A serious adverse event after successful gene therapy for X-linked severe combined immunodeficiency. N Engl J Med 2003; 348:255–256.

174. Hacein-Bey-Abina S, Von Kalle C, Schmidt M, McCormack MP, Wulffraat N, Leboulch P, Lim A, Osborne CS, Pawliuk R, Morillon E, Sorensen R, Forster A, Fraser P, Cohen JI, de Saint Basile G, Alexander I, Wintergerst U, Frebourg T, Aurias A, Stoppa-Lyonnet D, Romana S, Radford-Weiss I, Gross F, Valensi F, Delabesse E, Macintyre E, Sigaux F, Soulier J, Leiva LE, Wissler M, Prinz C, Rabbitts TH, Le Deist F, Fischer A, Cavazzana-Calvo M. LMO2-associated clonal T cell proliferation in two patients after gene therapy for SCID-X1. Science 2003; 302:415–419.

175. Meyer-Ficca ML, Meyer RG, Kaiser H, Brack AR, Kandolf R, Kupper JH. Comparative analysis of inducible expression systems in transient transfection studies. Anal Biochem 2004; 334:9–19.

176. Harding TC, Geddes BJ, Noel JD, Murphy D, Uney JB. Tetracycline-regulated transgene expression in hippocampal neurones following transfection with adenoviral vectors. J Neurochem 1997; 69:2620–2623.

177. Fitzsimons HL, Bland RJ, During MJ. Promoters and regulatory elements that improve adeno-associated virus transgene expression in the brain. Methods 2002; 28:227–236.

178. Akerud P, Canals JM, Snyder EY, Arenas E. Neuroprotection through delivery of glial cell line-derived neurotrophic factor by neural stem cells in a mouse model of Parkinson's disease. J Neurosci 2001; 21:8108–8118.

179. Kim TE, Lee HS, Lee YB, Hong SH, Lee YS, Ichinose H, Kim SU, Lee MA. Sonic hedgehog and FGF8 collaborate to induce dopaminergic phenotypes in the Nurr1-overexpressing neural stem cell. Biochem Biophys Res Commun 2003; 305:1040–1048.

180. Shim JW, Koh HC, Chang MY, Roh E, Choi CY, Oh YJ, Son H, Lee YS, Studer L, Lee SH. Enhanced in vitro midbrain dopamine neuron differentiation, dopaminergic function, neurite outgrowth, and 1-methyl-4-phenylpyridium resistance in mouse embryonic stem cells overexpressing Bcl-XL. J Neurosci 2004; 24:843–852.

181. Dezawa M, Kanno H, Hoshino M, Cho H, Matsumoto N, Itokazu Y, Tajima N, Yamada H, Sawada H, Ishikawa H, Mimura T, Kitada M, Suzuki Y, Ide C. Specific induction of neuronal cells from bone marrow stromal cells and application for autologous transplantation. J Clin Invest 2004; 113:1701–1710.

182. Burger SR, Kadidlo DM, Basso L, Bostrom N, Orchard PJ. Cellular engineering of HSV-tk transduced, expanded T lymphocytes for graft-versus-host disease management. Acta Haematol 2003; 110:121–131.

183. Schwalb J, Han S, Obrocka M, Tessler A, Murray M, Fischer I. Intraspinal grafting of conditionally immortalized human spinal cord stem cells into adult rats. National Neurotrauma Society, San Diego, CA, November 9–10, 2001.

184. Mohan RR, Possin DE, Sinha S, Wilson SE. Development of genetically engineered tet HPV16-E6/E7 transduced human corneal epithelial clones having tight regulation of proliferation and normal differentiation. Exp Eye Res 2003; 77:395–407.

185. Braak H, Ghebremedhin E, Rub U, Bratzke H, Del Tredici K. Stages in the development of Parkinson's disease-related pathology. Cell Tissue Res 2004; 318:121–134.

186. Lang AE, Obeso JA. Time to move beyond nigrostriatal dopamine deficiency in Parkinson's disease. Ann Neurol 2004; 55:761–765.

187. Beal MF. Experimental models of Parkinson's disease. Nat Rev Neurosci 2001; 2:325–334.

188. Freed CR. Will embryonic stem cells be a useful source of dopamine neurons for transplant into patients with Parkinson's disease? Proc Natl Acad Sci USA 2002; 99:1755–1757.

6

Essential Tremor: Patient Selection, Technique, and Surgical Results

Eun-Kyung Won

Department of Neurosurgery, University of Minnesota, Minneapolis, Minnesota, U.S.A.

Habib E. Ellamushi

The Royal Hospital of St. Bartholomew and The Royal London Hospital, London, U.K.

Uzma Samadani

Department of Neurosurgery, University of Pennsylvania, Philadelphia, Pennsylvania, U.S.A.

Gordon H. Baltuch

Department of Neurosurgery, Penn Neurological Institute, University of Pennsylvania School of Medicine, Philadelphia, Pennsylvania, U.S.A.

1. INTRODUCTION

Essential tremor (ET) is a common movement disorder affecting from 1% to 6% of the population. In this chapter we review its clinical characteristics, epidemiology, genetics, and etiology. We discuss how lesion or stimulation of nuclei within the thalamus may aid with treatment of ET in light of its pathophysiology. Finally, we review both the pharmacologic and surgical treatment options for ET.

2. CLINICAL CHARACTERISTICS AND EPIDEMIOLOGY

ET is more prevalent than Parkinson's or Alzheimer's disease, and is the most common movement disorder of adulthood (1–7). It is characterized by a postural and kinetic tremor typically involving the hands, forearms, and head with an oscillation frequency ranging from 4 to 12 Hz. Though tremor oscillation frequency decreases with age, amplitude increases, resulting in more severe disability (8–10). Thus, persons who are affected by ET for a longer period of time tend to be more severely affected, and the most severe forms are observed in older adults who acquired ET early in life (8). People with ET may experience depression or anxiety due to impaired ability to work, communicate, or perform activities of daily living and recreation requiring manual dexterity (11–13). One-fifth of individuals with ET are forced to leave their jobs or change job responsibilities because of tremor-related disability (13).

Mild to moderate asymmetry of tremor between the upper extremities is characteristic of ET. Community-based studies suggest tremor occurs more often in the nondominant arm, while clinic-based studies have reported greater tremor in the dominant arm, suggesting that patients with dominant arm ET are more likely to seek medical attention (14,15).

Head tremor is one of the major expressions of ET; for unknown reasons it is more frequently observed in women than men with ET, independent of disease duration (16–19). Such gender predilections are speculated to reflect differences in the distribution of disease pathology within the brain (17). Tandem gait dysfunction, or ataxia, is also seen in about half of all ET patients (20).

The differential diagnosis of ET includes medication-induced tremor. Tricyclic antidepressants, valproate, serotonin reuptake inhibitors, steroids, lithium, cyclosporine, beta-adrenergic agonists, ephedrine, theophyline, and antipsychotics can all cause a kinetic tremor. ET is distinguished from Parkinsonian tremor because the latter occurs at rest, has a lower frequency (3–5 Hz) and is often accompanied by rigidity, bradykinesia, or postural instability.

ET affects both young and old; however, there is a substantial rise in prevalence in older age groups. The prevalence estimates in different studies worldwide range from 0.4% to 3.9% for the general population to 1.3% to 5.1% for the age group above 60 years (4,7,21–23). In the United States, the prevalence of ET has been reported to differ considerably in individuals living in various regions ranging from urban New York to rural Mississippi with estimates for ages ≥60 years from 1.3% to 20.5% (23,24). These widely disparate reports could reflect methodological differences between studies such as differences in screening questions and/or differences in study populations in terms of age, environmental exposures, and genetic susceptibilities (4,25). The wide range of reported prevalence may also be due to the fact that some people with ET may be only mildly affected and not seek medical attention, or their disorder may be incorrectly ascribed to other medical conditions, such as Parkinson's disease (PD). Furthermore, mild forms of ET may be dismissed as incidental, particularly in the elderly. For these reasons, surveys that ascertain their study subjects from treatment settings or use medical records of patients evaluated at a clinic or hospital may underestimate the prevalence of ET (4,26).

A trend for higher prevalence was observed in Caucasians than in African Americans (3,23,24). In a recent study, Louis et al. reported a four-fold greater incidence of ET among Caucasians vs. African Americans (1.7% vs. 0.4) (27). In this study, physician-diagnosed ET was associated with Caucasian ethnicity but not with age, gender, education, mental status or depression scores, income, smoking status, or alcohol consumption. These differences in prevalence could reflect ethnically related differences in genetic or environmental risk factors.

3. GENETICS AND ETIOLOGY

Estimates of the proportion of ET patients with an afflicted first degree relative vary from 17% to as high as 96% depending on how the study was conducted (28–30). Family studies frequently show a pattern of aggregation corresponding to an autosomal dominant mode of inheritance of ET (5,6,10). Linkage studies have identified two susceptibility genes for ET. Familial ET gene FET1 or ETM1 maps to chromosome 3q13 (31) and ETM2 maps to chromosome 2p24.1 (32–34). Analyses of large families with autosomal dominant ET suggest that at least one other autosomal dominant susceptibility gene must exist (34,35).

Specific environmental factors predisposing patients to ET have not been identified, although exposure to pesticides, lead, and other toxins has been found in association with action tremor (36,37). Though some agricultural chemicals may play a role in development of ET, statistically significant data have not been reported (38). The serotonin antagonist harmaline is used to mimic ET in animal models (39–42).

Clinically, ET is exacerbated by stress, fatigue, or conditions where vigilance is required (43–46). The development of phobic-like behavior in some persons with ET has been reported (47). In a personality assessment study, patients with ET scored higher on the harm avoidance subscale than control subjects (48). Harm avoidance subscale scores did not correlate with the severity of tremor or with subjective and objective scales of disability, suggesting that the personality profile observed was not entirely related to functional disability caused by the tremor. These observations suggest that ET is under biobehavioral control (47). Patients with ET also have increased hearing disability compared to patients with PD and normal controls, which correlates with tremor severity (49).

4. PATHOPHYSIOLOGY

The etiology and pathogenesis of ET are as yet unknown. One hypothesis proposes a disturbance of olivocerebellar pathways with enhanced olivocerebellar oscillation (39). Abnormal olivary oscillations may be transmitted or amplified through the cerebellum, resulting in an entrainment of the thalamus, motor cortex and the brain stem nuclei (50–52). In support of this hypothesis, neuroimaging studies showed higher resting blood flow values in the cerebellar hemispheres of ET patients compared to normal subjects (53). In ET, there is corticomuscular coherence at the tremor frequencies in simultaneous EEG-EMG recordings, thus demonstrating that the sensorimotor cortex is involved in ET generation (52). Neurophysiological properties of ET are consistent with a central oscillator with only a weak influence from somatosensory pathways. Central oscillators are defined as autonomous neuronal networks with frequencies independent of sensory feedback, limb mechanics, and reflex arc length (54). In ET, the tremor frequency is not a function of the reflex arc length (54). The rhythmic activity of a single group of neurons within the inferior olive or the thalamus may be candidates for the oscillator.

A second possible mechanism proposed for ET is that oscillations might be generated within loops consisting of different nuclei and their connections (55).

Microelectrode recordings during sterotactic surgery have shown that tremor disorders are characterized by the presence of neurons in the ventral thalamus that have a spontaneous rate of discharge known as TRA cells or tremor cells (56). These TRA cells are thalamic neurons firing at frequencies synchronous with tremor, suggesting a role in the generation and maintenance of tremor. Indeed, the aim of surgical interventions for the treatment of tremor disorders is to disrupt the activity of TRA cells in the region of the ventralis intermedius (VIM). Even though the overall distribution of TRA cells was widespread through the ventral lateral thalamus, most of these cells are concentrated in the lower half of the VIM. There were no large differences in the locations of TRA cells among the different diagnostic classes of tremor found in PD, ET, and multiple sclerosis (MS), although there was a difference in the incidence of TRA cells in patients with PD, who had greater than 3.8 times more cells per thalamic trajectory than patients with ET and approximately five times more cells than patients with MS or cerebellar disorders (56).

Lee et al. investigated the characteristics of the neuronal activities of the motor thalamus [VIM and ventralis oralis posterior (Vop)] in ET patients, and compared the results with those of PD patients (57). The kinetic (Ki) neurons were found mainly in the VIM, whereas the voluntary (Vo) neurons were found principally in the Vop of ET patients. The mean firing rates of the ET patients were higher than those of the PD patients. In addition, the mean firing rates of the Ki neurons of the ET patients were higher than those of the PD patients in the VIM nuclei. However, the mean firing rates of the ventralis caudalis (Vc) neurons, which respond to sensory stimulation, were similar in each group. An analysis of the incidence of bursting neurons revealed that the Vop nucleus of the ET patients had less bursting neurons than in the PD patients. However, in the VIM nucleus, both groups possessed bursting neurons even though the incidence was slightly different. Tremor cells were observed less frequently in the VIM nucleus of ET patients than in the PD patients. The full meaning of these characteristic features of the neuronal activities of ET patients compared to those of PD patients is not known. Continued research will give us clues to understanding the impact on society, identifying genetic and environmental contributors to the disease, understanding the significance of a sporadic case, the phenotypic spectrum and timing of presentation, and the relationship with other neurologic disorders. Because the condition is both clinically and genetically heterogeneous and there is overlap with these other disorders, such as dystonia, parkinsonism, peripheral neuropathy, and migraine, the definition of phenotype plagues research in this area (58).

5. PHARMACOLOGICAL TREATMENT FOR ESSENTIAL TREMOR

Alcohol ingestion reduces tremor intensity in 50–70% of patients (59). The beneficial response to ethanol as a secondary criterion for the diagnosis of ET has been suggested (60,61). It has been shown that ethanol specifically reduces ET at low blood levels with a reduction in tremor up to 67%, whereas in Parkinson's tremor and cerebellar tremor there was no significant reduction in amplitude (61). In contrast, diazepam has little, if any, effect on the tremor (62).

Kirsten et al. suggested that the improvement in tremor after ethanol ingestion was due, at least in part, to an effect on the central oscillator (63). Decreased tremor amplitude in the central component after ethanol ingestion suggests that ethanol specifically affects the central oscillator, whose location remains unknown. Physiological and neuroimaging studies were conducted to determine the origin of the central oscillator and the effect of ethanol in patients with ET (51). After ethanol was given, both normal subjects and ET patients showed reduced cerebellar regional cerebral blood flow (rCBF), though the ET patients demonstrated less of a reduction. In addition, only ET patients showed a marked bilateral increase in the medullary rCBF in the region of the inferior olivary nucleus after alcohol (53). The authors concluded that ethanol might cause a decreased inhibitory input from the cerebellar cortex to the deep nuclei, which could in turn lead to increased cerebellar nuclear inhibitory output to the inferior olive via direct pathways. This might be the mechanism for tremor suppression, and would be manifest in the accelerometry as a specific effect on central oscillation.

Pharmacological treatment for ET is initiated when the tremor becomes sufficiently symptomatic that the patient cannot perform activities of daily living or develops anxiety or psychological distress. Two treatment options are the anticonvulsant primidone, which reduces tremor by an unknown mechanism, and β-adrenergic antagonists such as propranolol hydrochloride (64,65). These agents have demonstrated efficacy in many patients, but certain populations such as the elderly, do not benefit from these drugs, because of contraindications, adverse effects, or a failure to achieve adequate tremor control (65–69).Topiramate, another anticonvulsant that functions by blocking sodium channels and potentiating GABA, has also been used in the treatment of ET (70). The short-acting benzodiazepine alprazolam has shown efficacy in treating ET (71), but its long-term efficacy may be limited by its abuse potential. The atypical neuroleptic clozapine (72,73) is efficacious against ET, but its use is balanced by its risk of causing agranulocytosis. Clonidine, barbiturates, methazolamide, 1-octanol, and arotinolol hydrochloride (a nonselective and hydrophilic β-blocker that has difficulty crossing the blood–brain barrier) have shown limited efficacy (74–77).

Some authors propose that the impact of pharmacologic treatment effects on ET is overestimated because the measures used to evaluate tremor have questionable validity and reliability (i.e., clinical ratings, spectral analysis, and accelerometry) (78). Moreover, head tremor and hand tremor do not necessarily respond in the same way to treatments, such as β-blockade (79).

In view of limitations regarding pharmacotherapy and the strong relationship between environmental stressors and tremor severity, biobehavioral (i.e., relaxation training and EMG biofeed-back) intervention has been suggested. Progressive muscle relaxation and behavioral techniques have been helpful in reducing ET (47,80,81).

6. SURGICAL THERAPY FOR ET

In patients with medically refractory tremor, alternative therapies, including surgery may be considered. Thalamotomy using chemical or electric ablation of nuclei within the ventrolateral thalamus has been performed for ET treatment for 30 years (82,83). More recently, deep brain stimulation (DBS) of thalamic nuclei has become the procedure of choice for surgical management of ET based on reversibility of its effects and reduced complication profile (84–86). Most surgeries have targeted the VIM thalamus (ventral intermediate nucleus) which can only be unilaterally lesioned due to the risk of dysphagia from bilateral lesions. Efficacy has also been demonstrated with subthalamic white matter stimulation, which has the advantage of being bilaterally lesionable, and may be more effective for treatment of head tremor (87,88). Numerous outcome measures demonstrate about 80% efficacy for VIM DBS (89–92), with results demonstrable at up to 7 years after lead placement (93). Recently, some have proposed that as many as half of all patients requiring treatment for ET should receive DBS rather than pharmacologic therapy alone (94).

Reported complications of DBS include the risk of hematoma and its sequelae, seizures, and device-related complications (90,95,96).

REFERENCES

1. Deuschl G, Koller WC. Introduction: Essential tremor. Neurology 2000; 54:S1.
2. Koller WC, Huber SJ. Tremor disorders of aging: diagnosis and management. Geriatrics 1989; 44:33–36, 41.
3. Louis ED, Ford B, Lee H, et al. Diagnostic criteria for essential tremor: a population perspective. Arch Neurol 1998; 55:823–828.
4. Louis ED, Ottman R, Hauser WA. How common is the most common adult movement disorder? Estimates of the prevalence of essential tremor throughout the world. Mov Disord 1998; 13:5–10.
5. Rajput AH, Offord KP, Beard CM, et al. Essential tremor in Rochester, Minnesota: a 45-year study. J Neurol Neurosurg Psychiatry 1984; 47:466–470.
6. Rautakorpi I, Takala J, Marttila RJ, et al. Essential tremor in a Finnish population. Acta Neurol Scand 1982; 66:58–67.
7. Salemi G, Savettieri G, Rocca WA, et al. Prevalence of essential tremor: a door-to-door survey in Terrasini, Sicily. Sicilian Neuro-Epidemiologic Study Group. Neurology 1994; 44:61–64.
8. Elble RJ. Essential tremor frequency decreases with time. Neurology 2000; 55:1547–1551.
9. Koller WC, Busenbark K, Gray C, et al. Classification of essential tremor. Clin Neuropharmacol 1992; 15:81–87.
10. Larsson T, Sjogren T. Essential tremor: a clinical and genetic population study. Acta Psychiatr Scand 1960; 36(suppl 144):1–176.
11. Auff E, Doppelbauer A, Fertl E. Essential tremor: functional disability vs. subjective impairment. J Neural Transm Suppl 1991; 33:105–110.
12. Busenbark KL, Nash J, Nash S, et al. Is essential tremor benign? Neurology 1991; 41:1982–1983.
13. Metzer WS. Severe essential tremor compared with Parkinson's disease in male veterans: diagnostic characteristics, treatment, and psychosocial complications. South Med J 1992; 85:825–828.
14. Biary N, Koller W. Handedness and essential tremor. Arch Neurol 1985; 42: 1082–1083.
15. Louis ED, Wendt KJ, Pullman SL, et al. Is essential tremor symmetric? Observational data from a community-based study of essential tremor. Arch Neurol 1998; 55:1553–1559.
16. Ashenhurst EM. The nature of essential tremor. Can Med Assoc J 1973; 109: 876–878.
17. Hardesty DE, Maraganore DM, Matsumoto JY, et al. Increased risk of head tremor in women with essential tremor: longitudinal data from the Rochester Epidemiology Project. Mov Disord 2004; 19:529–533.
18. Hubble JP, Busenbark KL, Pahwa R, et al. Clinical expression of essential tremor: effects of gender and age. Mov Disord 1997; 12:969–972.
19. Lou JS, Jankovic J. Essential tremor: clinical correlates in 350 patients. Neurology 1991; 41:234–238.
20. Singer C, Sanchez-Ramos J, Weiner WJ. Gait abnormality in essential tremor. Mov Disord 1994; 9:193–196.

21. Benito-Leon J, Bermejo-Pareja F, Morales JM, et al. Prevalence of essential tremor in three elderly populations of central Spain. Mov Disord 2003; 18: 389–394.
22. Bharucha NE, Bharucha EP, Bharucha AE, et al. Prevalence of essential tremor in the Parsi community of Bombay, India. Arch Neurol 1988; 45:907–908.
23. Louis ED, Marder K, Cote L, et al. Differences in the prevalence of essential tremor among elderly African Americans, whites, and Hispanics in northern Manhattan, NY. Arch Neurol 1995; 52:1201–1205.
24. Haerer AF, Anderson DW, Schoenberg BS. Prevalence of essential tremor. Results from the Copiah County study. Arch Neurol 1982; 39:750–751.
25. Louis ED, Ford B, Lee H, et al. Does a screening questionnaire for essential tremor agree with the physician's examination? Neurology 1998; 50:1351–1357.
26. Findley LJ. Epidemiology and genetics of essential tremor. Neurology 2000; 54:S8–S13.
27. Louis ED, Fried LP, Fitzpatrick AL, et al. Regional and racial differences in the prevalence of physician-diagnosed essential tremor in the United States. Mov Disord 2003; 18:1035–1040.
28. Busenbark K, Barnes P, Lyons K, et al. Accuracy of reported family histories of essential tremor. Neurology 1996; 47:264–265.
29. Louis ED, Ford B, Wendt KJ, et al. Validity of family history data on essential tremor. Mov Disord 1999; 14:456–461.
30. Louis ED, Ottman R. How familial is familial tremor? The genetic epidemiology of essential tremor. Neurology 1996; 46:1200–1205.
31. Gulcher JR, Jonsson P, Kong A, et al. Mapping of a familial essential tremor gene, FET1, to chromosome 3q13. Nat Genet 1997; 17:84–87.
32. Higgins JJ, Jankovic J, Lombardi RQ, et al. Haplotype analysis of the ETM2 locus in familial essential tremor. Neurogenetics 2003; 4:185–189.
33. Higgins JJ, Pho LT, Nee LE. A gene (ETM) for essential tremor maps to chromosome 2p22–p25. Mov Disord 1997; 12:859–864.
34. Illarioshkin SN, Rakhmonov RA, Ivanova-Smolenskaia IA, et al. [Molecular genetic analysis of essential tremor]. Genetika 2002; 38:1704–1709.
35. Abbruzzese G, Pigullo S, Di Maria E, et al. Clinical and genetic study of essential tremor in the Italian population. Neurol Sci 2001; 22:39–40.
36. Louis ED. Etiology of essential tremor: should we be searching for environmental causes? Mov Disord 2001; 16:822–829.
37. Soderlund DM, Clark JM, Sheets LP, et al. Mechanisms of pyrethroid neurotoxicity: implications for cumulative risk assessment. Toxicology 2002; 171:3–59.
38. Salemi G, Aridon P, Calagna G, et al. Population-based case-control study of essential tremor. Ital J Neurol Sci 1998; 19:301–305.
39. Deuschl G, Elble RJ. The pathophysiology of essential tremor. Neurology 2000; 54:S14–S20.
40. Elble RJ. Animal models of action tremor. Mov Disord 1998; 13(suppl 3): 35–39.
41. Martin FC, Thu Le A, Handforth A. Harmaline-induced tremor as a potential preclinical screening method for essential tremor medications. Mov Disord 2005; 3:298–305.

42. Wilms H, Sievers J, Deuschl G. Animal models of tremor. Mov Disord 1999; 14:557–571.
43. Gengo FM, Kalonaros GC, McHugh WB. Attenuation of response to mental stress in patients with essential tremor treated with metoprolol. Arch Neurol 1986; 43:687–689.
44. Koller WC. Propranolol therapy for essential tremor of the head. Neurology 1984; 34:1077–1079.
45. Koller WC, Biary NM. Volitional control of involuntary movements. Mov Disord 1989; 4:153–156.
46. Pohorecky LA. Stress and alcohol interaction: an update of human research. Alcohol Clin Exp Res 1991; 15:438–459.
47. Lundervold DA, Poppen R. Biobehavioral intervention for older adults coping with essential tremor. Appl Psychophysiol Biofeedback 2004; 29:63–73.
48. Chatterjee A, Jurewicz EC, Applegate LM, et al. Personality in essential tremor: further evidence of non-motor manifestations of the disease. J Neurol Neurosurg Psychiatry 2004; 75:958–961.
49. Ondo WG, Sutton L, Dat Vuong K, et al. Hearing impairment in essential tremor. Neurology 2003; 61:1093–1097.
50. Elble RJ, Higgins C, Hughes L. Essential tremor entrains rapid voluntary movements. Exp Neurol 1994; 126:138–143.
51. Growdon JH, Shahani BT, Young RR. The effect of alcohol on essential tremor. Neurology 1975; 25:259–262.
52. Hellwig B, Haussler S, Schelter B, et al. Tremor-correlated cortical activity in essential tremor. Lancet 2001; 357:519–523.
53. Boecker H, Wills AJ, Ceballos-Baumann A, et al. The effect of ethanol on alcohol-responsive essential tremor: a positron emission tomography study. Ann Neurol 1996; 39:650–658.
54. Elble RJ. Central mechanisms of tremor. J Clin Neurophysiol 1996; 13:133–144.
55. Deuschl G, Raethjen J, Lindemann M, et al. The pathophysiology of tremor. Muscle Nerve 2001; 24:716–735.
56. Brodkey JA, Tasker RR, Hamani C, et al. Tremor cells in the human thalamus: differences among neurological disorders. J Neurosurg 2004; 101:43–47.
57. Lee BH, Lee KH, Chung SS, et al. Neurophysiological identification and characterization of thalamic neurons with single unit recording in essential tremor patients. Acta Neurochir Suppl 2003; 87:133–136.
58. Brin MF, Koller W. Epidemiology and genetics of essential tremor. Mov Disord 1998; 13(suppl 3):55–63.
59. Deuschl G. Differential diagnosis of tremor. J Neural Transm Suppl 1999; 56: 211–220.
60. Bain P, Brin M, Deuschl G, et al. Criteria for the diagnosis of essential tremor. Neurology 2000; 54:S7.
61. Koller WC, Biary N. Effect of alcohol on tremors: comparison with propranolol. Neurology 1984; 34:221–222.
62. Koller WC. A new drug for treatment of essential tremor? Time will tell. Mayo Clin Proc 1991; 66:1085–1087.
63. Zeuner KE, Molloy FM, Shoge RO, et al. Effect of ethanol on the central oscillator in essential tremor. Mov Disord 2003; 18:1280–1285.

64. Hubble JP, Busenbark KL, Koller WC. Essential tremor. Clin Neuropharmacol 1989; 12:453–482.

65. Winkler GF, Young RR. Efficacy of chronic propranolol therapy in action tremors of the familial, senile or essential varieties. N Engl J Med 1974; 290: 984–988.

66. Calzetti S, Findley LJ, Perucca E, et al. The response of essential tremor to propranolol: evaluation of clinical variables governing its efficacy on prolonged administration. J Neurol Neurosurg Psychiatry 1983; 46:393–398.

67. Findley LJ, Cleeves L, Calzetti S. Primidone in essential tremor of the hands and head: a double blind controlled clinical study. J Neurol Neurosurg Psychiatry 1985; 48:911–915.

68. Gorman WP, Cooper R, Pocock P, et al. A comparison of primidone, propranolol, and placebo in essential tremor, using quantitative analysis. J Neurol Neurosurg Psychiatry 1986; 49:64–68.

69. Koller WC, Royse VL. Efficacy of primidone in essential tremor. Neurology 1986; 36:121–124.

70. Connor GS. A double-blind placebo-controlled trial of topiramate treatment for essential tremor. Neurology 2002; 59:132–134.

71. Gunal DI, Afsar N, Bekiroglu N, et al. New alternative agents in essential tremor therapy: double-blind placebo-controlled study of alprazolam and acetazolamide. Neurol Sci 2000; 21:315–317.

72. Ceravolo R, Salvetti S, Piccini P, et al. Acute and chronic effects of clozapine in essential tremor. Mov Disord 1999; 14:468–472.

73. Pakkenberg H, Pakkenberg B. Clozapine in the treatment of tremor. Acta Neurol Scand 1986; 73:295–297.

74. Lee KS, Kim JS, Kim JW, et al. A multicenter randomized crossover multiple-dose comparison study of arotinolol and propranolol in essential tremor. Parkinsonism Relat Disord 2003; 9:341–347.

75. Muenter MD, Daube JR, Caviness JN, et al. Treatment of essential tremor with methazolamide. Mayo Clin Proc 1991; 66:991–997.

76. Sasso E, Perucca E, Fava R, et al. Quantitative comparison of barbiturates in essential hand and head tremor. Mov Disord 1991; 6:65–68.

77. Serrano-Duenas M. [Clonidine versus propranolol in the treatment of essential tremor. A double-blind trial with a one-year follow-up]. Neurologia 2003; 18: 248–254.

78. Bain PG. Tremor assessment and quality of life measurements. Neurology 2000; 54:S26–S29.

79. Calzetti S, Sasso E, Negrotti A, et al. Effect of propranolol in head tremor: quantitative study following single-dose and sustained drug administration. Clin Neuropharmacol 1992; 15:470–476.

80. Lundervold DA, Belwood MF, Craney JL, et al. Reduction of tremor severity and disability following behavioral relaxation training. J Behav Ther Exp Psychiatry 1999; 30:119–135.

81. Wake A, Takahashi Y, Onishi T, et al. [Treatment of essential tremor by behavior therapy. Use of Jacobson's progressive relaxation method (author's transl.)]. Seishin Shinkeigaku Zasshi 1974; 76:509–517.

82. Lakie M, Arblaster LA, Roberts RC, et al. Effect of stereotactic thalamic lesion on essential tremor. Lancet 1992; 340:206–207.
83. Nagaseki Y, Shibazaki T, Hirai T, et al. Long-term follow-up results of selective VIM-thalamotomy. J Neurosurg 1986; 65:296–302.
84. Pahwa R, Lyons KE, Wilkinson SB, et al. Comparison of thalamotomy to deep brain stimulation of the thalamus in essential tremor. Mov Disord 2001; 16:140–143.
85. Schuurman PR, Bosch DA, Bossuyt PM, et al. A comparison of continuous thalamic stimulation and thalamotomy for suppression of severe tremor. N Engl J Med 2000; 342:461–468.
86. Tasker RR. Deep brain stimulation is preferable to thalamotomy for tremor suppression. Surg Neurol 1998; 49:145–153; discussion 153–144.
87. Murata J, Kitagawa M, Uesugi H, et al. Electrical stimulation of the posterior subthalamic area for the treatment of intractable proximal tremor. J Neurosurg 2003; 99:708–715.
88. Plaha P, Patel NK, Gill SS. Stimulation of the subthalamic region for essential tremor. J Neurosurg 2004; 101:48–54.
89. Fields JA, Troster AI, Woods SP, et al. Neuropsychological and quality of life outcomes 12 months after unilateral thalamic stimulation for essential tremor. J Neurol Neurosurg Psychiatry 2003; 74:305–311.
90. Koller WC, Lyons KE, Wilkinson SB, et al. Long-term safety and efficacy of unilateral deep brain stimulation of the thalamus in essential tremor. Mov Disord 2001; 16:464–468.
91. Ondo W, Jankovic J, Schwartz K, et al. Unilateral thalamic deep brain stimulation for refractory essential tremor and Parkinson's disease tremor. Neurology 1998; 51:1063–1069.
92. Troster AI, Fields JA, Pahwa R, et al. Neuropsychological and quality of life outcome after thalamic stimulation for essential tremor. Neurology 1999; 53:1774–1780.
93. Rehncrona S, Johnels B, Widner H, et al. Long-term efficacy of thalamic deep brain stimulation for tremor: double-blind assessments. Mov Disord 2003; 18:163–170.
94. Lyons KE, Pahwa R. Deep brain stimulation and essential tremor. J Clin Neurophysiol 2004; 21:2–5.
95. Beric A, Kelly PJ, Rezai A, et al. Complications of deep brain stimulation surgery. Stereotact Funct Neurosurg 2001; 77:73–78.
96. Duff J, Sime E. Surgical interventions in the treatment of Parkinson's disease (PD) and essential tremor (ET): medial pallidotomy in PD and chronic deep brain stimulation (DBS) in PD and ET. Axone 1997; 18:85–89.

7

Tremor: Patient Selection and Surgical Results

Eun-Kyung Won

Department of Neurosurgery, University of Minnesota, Minneapolis, Minnesota, U.S.A.

Uzma Samadani

Department of Neurosurgery, University of Pennsylvania, Philadelphia, Pennsylvania, U.S.A.

Gordon H. Baltuch

Department of Neurosurgery, Penn Neurological Institute, University of Pennsylvania School of Medicine, Philadelphia, Pennsylvania, U.S.A.

1. INTRODUCTION

Tremor is an involuntary, rhythmic, periodic, mechanical oscillation of a body part. Action, or kinetic, tremor appears during voluntary movements, as opposed to resting tremor, which is present in a body part not voluntarily activated and completely supported against gravity. Surgical management of Parkinson's disease (PD) tremor, which classically is a resting tremor, and of essential tremor (ET), which is kinetic, is addressed elsewhere in this book.

Gordon Morgan Holmes, an Irish neurologist at Queens Square in London, described his eponymous tremor in patients with cerebellar gunshot wounds and tumors in 1922 (1). Since then, this action tremor associated with lesions of the cerebellar outflow system, or midbrain, has been given numerous names including rubral tremor, midbrain tremor, thalamic tremor, myorrhythmia, and Benedikt's syndrome. Criteria for Holmes' tremor include: a rest and intention tremor with irregular presentation; a frequency usually less than 4.5 Hz; and a variable delay, typically ranging from 4 weeks to 2 years, between presentation of the tremor and insult to the brain. In many patients with Holmes' tremor, postural tremor is also present, but may not be as rhythmic as other tremors (2).

Pure cerebellar tremors are similar to Holmes' tremor in frequency and the existence of a possible postural component. A cerebellar tremor, however, does not have a resting tremor component (2). Additionally, some Holmes' tremors have been noted to respond to dopaminergic therapy (3) while pure cerebellar tremors do not.

Among the numerous causes of Holmes' and cerebellar tremors are multiple sclerosis (MS), traumatic brain injury, and infarct. In this chapter we review the incidence, characteristics, and pathophysiology of tremor due to these causes as background to a discussion of treatment with functional neurosurgery.

2. TREMOR IN MULTIPLE SCLEROSIS

2.1. Incidence, Characteristics, and Pathophysiology of Tremor in Multiple Sclerosis

Tremor is estimated to occur in 32–75% of MS patients (4–7). The wide range of observed tremor incidence reflects difficulties in studying tremor in this patient population (4,6,7). Relapse and remission of neurologic symptoms are a hallmark of MS, and along with underreporting (8), can contribute to sampling error. Most studies are conducted at secondary and tertiary MS centers, which have a higher percentage of more disabled patients. Differentiating tremor from other complex movement disorders commonly seen in MS patients, such as dysmetria and ataxia, can also be challenging (9).

The most common tremor found in MS patients is a bilateral upper extremity postural or kinetic tremor. Postural tremor of the legs, head, and trunk, in order of decreasing prevalence, can also occur. Upper extremity tremor in MS patients can be subclassified into 32% distal postural tremor, 36% distal postural and kinetic tremor, 16% proximal postural and kinetic tremor; 4% proximal and distal postural and kinetic tremor, and 12% isolated intention tremor (4). Approximately 16% of MS patients have a distal postural tremor resembling physiologic tremor but with frequencies more typical of ET (10).

Exact classification of the tremor afflicting patients with MS remains controversial. Some neurologists consider the primary tremor a severe Holmes' tremor (11–13), while others state that the MS tremor lacks the resting tremor component of Holmes' tremor and is a pure cerebellar tremor (4). The diverse nature of MS suggests that both Holmes' and cerebellar tremors could occur.

Tremor severity ranges from minimal (27%), to mild (16%), moderate/severe (15%), and disabling (13% of patients) (4,6,7,14). Patients with tremor were more likely than those without tremor to be wheelchair dependent, and had worse Expanded Disability Systems Scores (4). Degree of disability correlated with upper limb tremor severity, but not duration of tremor or disease. Proximal tremor was found to be more disabling than distal postural/kinetic tremor, isolated intention tremor, or distal postural tremor (4). The presence of severe cerebellar signs was associated with a poorer prognosis and a high risk of respiratory impairment (6,7).

The action tremor of MS is thought to result from demyelination in the cerebellum or its connections. Coexistence with cerebellar signs, including dysarthria, dysmetria and dysdiadochokinesia, and intact supratentorial functions including normal cognitive function, Barthel disability profile, grip strength, and walking speed, are consistent with a cerebellar rather than supratentorial tremor etiology (4). Tremor affects thalamic neurons differently in PD, ET, and MS. TRA neurons in the vental lateral thalamus and most particularly lower VIM (nucleus ventralis intermedius) have a discharge rate synchronous with the tremor frequency. Brodkey et al. found an increased incidence of TRA neurons along the thalamic trajectory in patients with PD relative to ET (3.8-fold) and MS (five-fold) or other Holmes' tremors (15).

2.2. Medical Treatment of Tremor in MS Patients

Medical management of MS tremor is an ongoing challenge. Sabra et al. proposed isoniazid in 1982 (16), which was also found efficacious by Hallet et al. (17), Morrow et al. (18), and Francis et al. (19); however, further studies showed improvement was insignificant (20,21). Clifford in 1983 showed improvement in two of eight MS patients ingesting tetrahydrocannabinol (22). Sechi et al. showed tremor improvement in 10 patients taking carbamazepine (23). Glutethimide, which was known to be effective for ET, was used for MS tremor by Aisen et al. (24). Henkin and Herishanu presented two case reports using primidone to treat MS tremor in 1991 (25). More recently, intravenous ondansetron was tried in 20 patients with cerebellar tremor mostly caused by MS (26), and the efficacy of cannabis was disproven (27). Weiss et al. demonstrated improvement of bilateral upper extremity tremor in an MS patient being treated with intrathecal baclofen for spasticity (28). No controlled trial has demonstrated the efficacy of any pharmacological agent for the treatment of MS tremor.

2.3. Surgical Treatment of Tremor in MS Patients

Stereotactic thalamotomy for tremor in MS patients has been performed since 1960 (29,30). Thalamotomy has been found to alleviate contralateral limb tremor in 65–100% of MS patients; however, functional arm improvement is seen in a smaller fraction (14,29–35). Improvement is seen in severe axial and proximal arm tremor as well as truncal ataxia (14,35); however, patients with severe arm clumsiness, marked weakness, and/or significant sensory deficits are unlikely to regain functional capacity after thalamotomy (10,34,35). Although tremor suppression via thalamotomy did not improve some specific arm functions such as writing, it was associated with improvement in tremor-related disability (34–37).

Tremor can recur between 1 and 5 years after thalamotomy (32,37), and the procedural morbidity ranges from 0% to 45%. The most common complications are gait deterioration, hemiparesis, and dysarthria; less frequently, epilepsy, sensory disturbances, dysphagia, transient bladder disturbances, confusion, depression, lethargy, and somnolence have been described (12,29, 30,34–41). Dysarthria occurs at higher frequency in patients undergoing bilateral thalamotomy (33,39,42,43).

Initial concerns that thalamotomy could potentially contribute to MS disease progression (31,34) were subsequently found to be without merit (36).

Thalamotomy has also been performed via gamma-knife irradiation in three patients with MS tremor (44). The risks and complications of radiosurgical thalamotomy are discussed in the section on surgical treatment of posttraumatic tremor.

Since 1980 (45), deep brain stimulation (DBS), which is better tolerated bilaterally than thalamotomy, and has been shown in a prospective randomized trial to be less morbid and equally effective for PD and ET (46), has been performed as an alternative to lesional surgery for MS tremor (45–51). The results of a randomized controlled trial of VIM thalamotomy versus stimulation with 10 MS patients demonstrated that stimulation was no better than thalamotomy at suppressing tremor; stimulation also improved disability less than thalamotomy, although these differences were not significant (46). Larger trials are necessary to compare DBS versus thalamotomy for MS patients.

Determining the optimum lesion or DBS target for MS tremor reduction is an area of ongoing research. Lesion of the nucleus ventralis lateralis of the thalamus, a known target for PD and ET tremor suppression, failed to relieve tremor adequately (35). Hirai and colleagues noted that lesions centered in the lower part of nucleus VIM needed to be large to alleviate kinetic tremor, particularly if the tremor was low frequency and high amplitude, or involved proximal or widely distributed muscle groups, which is characteristic of some types of MS sclerosis tremor (52).

The hypothesis that cerebellar tremors, unlike those of PD and ET, are generated by diminished inhibition of the basal ganglia (53–55) has generated interest in eliminating basal ganglia output to the motor cortex via targeting of the ventralis oralis posterior (Vop) (35,52,56). Vop is the basal ganglia output nucleus, while VIM is the cerebellar input nucleus of the thalamus. Liu and colleagues have shown that Vop thalamotomy in MS patients with distal tremor and minimal ataxia resulted in greater than 50% tremor reduction while patients with complex ataxic movement disorders benefited less than 50% (57).

Stimulation of the zona incerta and subthalamic nuclei resulted in marked improvement in contralateral upper limb tremor and manual function in selected cases (36). Medial globus pallidus and the cerebellar nuclei project not only to the thalamus, but also caudally to the upper brainstem, particularly to the fields of Forel, the zona incerta, the pedunculo-pontine nuclei, and the reticular pontine nuclei. Neuronal discharge in these areas correlates with activity of the proximal spinal and limb girdle muscles during reaching and locomotion, and their axons decussate to project directly or indirectly to their corresponding motor neurons in the ventromedial gray matter of the spinal cord. Proximal tremor is mediated not by distal muscles that are controlled predominantly by thalamocortical circuits, but mainly by paraspinal and limb girdle muscles which, as Lawrence and Kuypers first showed in monkeys, are controlled mainly from areas in the medial part of the upper brainstem (58). Hence zona incerta lesions should alleviate proximal MS tremor by interrupting aberrant oscillatory activity in the cerebellar and basal ganglia outputs.

Patient selection and tailoring of the DBS target based on symptoms poses an ongoing challenge for the treatment of MS tremor. Broager and Fog's 1962 observations that the patients most likely to improve are those with symptoms dominated by tremor and hyperkinetic movements, and that those with terminal disease benefit less than those with a longstanding benign course (31,59), still hold true today.

3. POST-TRAUMATIC TREMOR

3.1. Incidence, Characteristics, and Pathophysiology of Tremor After Traumatic Brain Injury

Cerebellar and Holmes' tremors can occur as a late complication after severe head injury (60–63). A study of 221 brain injury survivors who had presented with an initial Glasgow Coma Score (GCS) of 8 or less, revealed that approximately 23% (54 patients) developed movement disorders at a latency from 2 weeks to 6 months after the trauma (62). Nineteen percent (42 patients) had tremors, half of which were transient. For 5% (12 patients), the post-traumatic movement disorder was disabling and consisted of low-frequency kinetic tremor (2.5–4 Hz,) and/or dystonia. Patients with chronic disabling tremors were more likely than nontremulous survivors to have an initial admission GCS less than 6, or have generalized brain edema on admission computed tomograph.

In addition to diffuse cerebral swelling, other risk factors for post-traumatic kinetic tremor include young age, hemorrhagic lesion in the midbrain or its surroundings, intraventricular hemorrhage, or multiple hemorrhagic lesions consistent with diffuse or shearing injury (64). Moderate and mild head injury result in a lower incidence of movement disorders that frequently resolve and rarely require treatment (65).

Post-traumatic kinetic tremor is believed to result from disruption of the cerebellar outflow tracts. Dentate nucleus lesions were noted on magnetic resonance imaging of 18 patients with severe kinetic post-traumatic tremor (66). Lesions were classified into four types: Type I—ipsilateral to the tremor (4%); Types II and III—involving the ipsilateral predecussational dentatothalamic pathway (56%); and Type IV—involving the contralateral post-decussational course (28%). One patient with a mild head trauma had a lesion of the contralateral thalamus. Two of three patients with a parkinsonian-like rest tremor had Type IV lesions involving the substantia nigra. Midbrain damage is consistent with the hypothesis that damage to the dentatothalamic system accounts for the occurrence of intention tremor. Other studies have implicated damage to the red nucleus of the midbrain in generation of post-traumatic tremor (63).

3.2. Medical Treatment of Post-Traumatic Tremor

Most post-traumatic tremors resolve gradually and spontaneously. Persistent and disabling Holmes' tremors may be responsive to clonazepem (67) or propranolol (60). Intention tremors occurring in patients with midbrain injuries have been successfully treated with nadolol (68) and anticholinergic or dopaminergic therapy (63).

3.3. Surgical Treatment of Post-Traumatic Tremor

Stereotactic thalamotomy has been reported to reduce tremor dramatically, improve limb function, and increase independence in patients after trauma (69–72). Procedural morbidity ranged from 50% to 70%. Alternatively, VIM DBS has been performed in a few patients with post-traumatic tremors (56,72–75). We have successfully treated Holmes' tremor via VIM stimulation in one patient after trauma (75), and in a separate patient after resection of a midbrain cavernous angioma (76). Nguyen and Degos implanted electrodes with four stimulation sites in the length of the VIM to demonstrate that stimulation of the lower VIM suppresses distal tremor, while stimulation of the upper VIM reduces proximal symptoms (56). The advantages of DBS over ablative surgery are its reversibility, adjustability, and reduced side effects allowing bilateral procedures, while disadvantages include device-related complications. Further studies, including a randomized prospective trial, are needed to establish the efficacy of DBS versus thalamotomy in the treatment of trauma-induced tremor.

Gamma-knife VIM thalamotomy has been performed for PD, ET, and for at least five patients with post-traumatic tremor (77,78) with half of patients showing improvement when follow-up was obtained. Complications of gamma-knife thalamotomy for PD and ET include dysphagia and aspiration pneumonia, resulting in death, hemiplegia, homonymous hemianopsia, hand weakness, dysarthria, hypophonia, aphasia, arm and face numbness, pseudobulbar laughter (79), and induction of a more disabling complex movement disorder (80).

4. TREMOR AFTER CEREBRAL INFARCT

4.1. Incidence, Characteristics, and Pathophysiology of Tremor After Stroke

Stroke is the second leading cause of death in the world, and affects 700,000 people in the United States annually (81). Movement disorders are a rare complication of acute stroke affecting only 29 of 2500 patients experiencing a first stroke (82). Only 9 of these 29 patients had tremors, asterixis, or limb-shaking disorders, and all but three of 29 experienced resolution of the dystonic symptoms within 6 months (82).

Thalamic infarction can cause disruption of the dentatorubrothalamic tract, resulting in Holmes' tremor in children (83) and adults (84–87). It is more likely to occur after hemorrhagic strokes resulting in dense hemiplegia and sensory loss, and may be part of a more complex movement disorder or delayed-onset cerebellar syndrome occurring at a latency of 3 weeks to 2 years after ischemic insult (88,89).

Infarct in the anterior cerebral artery distribution can also cause supplementary motor area lesions resulting in a resting tremor similar to that of idiopathic PD. Such tremors are levodopa-unresponsive, and resolve spontaneously (90). There are also case reports of anterior thalamic stroke resulting in hand tremor (91), and focal tremor following striatal infarct (92).

4.2. Nonsurgical Treatment of Post-Stroke Tremor

After thalamic stroke, somatotopic reorganization can occur as evidenced by nuclear mapping during stimulation for lead placement (93). Such reorganization may be part of the mechanism underlying spontaneous tremor resolution. Additionally, physical therapy, in conjunction with electromyographic biofeedback, has been shown to be of benefit for post-thalamic stroke movement disorders and their related pain (94). Haloperidol and dopamine therapy have been used to treat post-stroke tremor in a few patients (95).

4.3. Surgical Treatment of Post-Stroke Tremor

The rarity of stroke-related tremor, and likelihood of symptoms resolving spontaneously, contribute to an overall low number of patients with intractable post-stroke tremor. Gamma-knife thalamotomy has been performed in at least one post-stroke patient for tremor (78). DBS for post-stroke tremor with cathodal Vop and anodal VIM revealed that while tremor improved in all six patients, two required dual-lead stimulation and one required a stimulation intensity high enough to provoke unpleasant parasthesias (96). Other studies suggest that while tremor may be improved by Vop or VIM DBS, movement disorder related pain after stroke may require motor cortex stimulation (97).

REFERENCES

1. Holmes G. On the clinical symptoms of cerebellar disease. Lancet 1922; 1: 1177–1182.
2. Deuschl G, Bain P, Brin M. Consensus statement of the Movement Disorder Society on Tremor. Ad Hoc Scientific Committee. Mov Disord 1998; 13(suppl 3): 2–23.
3. Findley LJ, Gresty MA. Suppression of "rubral" tremor with levodopa. Br Med J 1980; 281:1043.
4. Alusi SH, Worthington J, Glickman S, et al. A study of tremor in multiple sclerosis. Brain 2001; 124:720–730.
5. Weinshenker BG. Epidemiology of multiple sclerosis. Neurol Clin 1996; 14: 291–308.
6. Weinshenker BG, Bass B, Rice GP, et al. The natural history of multiple sclerosis: a geographically based study. 2. Predictive value of the early clinical course. Brain 1989; 112(Pt 6):1419–1428.
7. Weinshenker BG, Bass B, Rice GP, et al. The natural history of multiple sclerosis: a geographically based study. I. Clinical course and disability. Brain 1989; 112(Pt 1): 133–146.
8. Alusi SH, Worthington J, Glickman S, et al. Evaluation of three different ways of assessing tremor in multiple sclerosis. J Neurol Neurosurg Psychiatry 2000; 68:756–760.
9. Sabra AF, Hallett M. Action tremor with alternating activity in antagonist muscles. Neurology 1984; 34:151–156.
10. Alusi SH, Glickman S, Aziz TZ, et al. Tremor in multiple sclerosis. J Neurol Neurosurg Psychiatry 1999; 66:131–134.
11. Bain P. A combined clinical and neurophysiological approach to the study of patients with tremor. J Neurol Neurosurg Psychiatry 1993; 56:839–844.
12. Hooper J, Taylor R, Pentland B, et al. Rater reliability of Fahn's tremor rating scale in patients with multiple sclerosis. Arch Phys Med Rehabil 1998; 79: 1076–1079.
13. Hopfensperger K, Koller WC. Non-Parkinsonian tremor. Curr Opin Neurol Neurosurg 1992; 5:321–323.
14. Kandel EI, Hondcarian OA. Surgical treatment of the hyperkinetic form of multiple sclerosis. Acta Neurol (Napoli) 1985; 7:345–347.
15. Brodkey JA, Tasker RR, Hamani C, et al. Tremor cells in the human thalamus: differences among neurological disorders. J Neurosurg 2004; 101:43–47.
16. Sabra AF, Hallett M, Sudarsky L, et al. Treatment of action tremor in multiple sclerosis with isoniazid. Neurology 1982; 32:912–913.

17. Hallett M, Lindsey JW, Adelstein BD, et al. Controlled trial of isoniazid therapy for severe postural cerebellar tremor in multiple sclerosis. Neurology 1985; 35: 1374–1377.
18. Morrow J, McDowell H, Ritchie C, et al. Isoniazid and action tremor in multiple sclerosis. J Neurol Neurosurg Psychiatry 1985; 48:282–283.
19. Francis DA, Grundy D, Heron JR. The response to isoniazid of action tremor in multiple sclerosis and its assessment using polarised light goniometry. J Neurol Neurosurg Psychiatry 1986; 49:87–89.
20. Bozek CB, Kastrukoff LF, Wright JM, et al. A controlled trial of isoniazid therapy for action tremor in multiple sclerosis. J Neurol 1987; 234:36–39.
21. Koller WC. Pharmacologic trials in the treatment of cerebellar tremor. Arch Neurol 1984; 41:280–281.
22. Clifford DB. Tetrahydrocannabinol for tremor in multiple sclerosis. Ann Neurol 1983; 13:669–671.
23. Sechi GP, Zuddas M, Piredda M, et al. Treatment of cerebellar tremors with carbamazepine: a controlled trial with long-term follow-up. Neurology 1989; 39:1113–1115.
24. Aisen ML, Holzer M, Rosen M, et al. Glutethimide treatment of disabling action tremor in patients with multiple sclerosis and traumatic brain injury. Arch Neurol 1991; 48:513–515.
25. Henkin Y, Herishanu YO. Primidone as a treatment for cerebellar tremor in multiple sclerosis—two case reports. Ir J Med Sci 1989; 25:720–721.
26. Rice GP, Lesaux J, Vandervoort P, et al. Ondansetron, a 5-HT3 antagonist, improves cerebellar tremor. J Neurol Neurosurg Psychiatry 1997; 62:282–284.
27. Fox P, Bain PG, Glickman S, et al. The effect of cannabis on tremor in patients with multiple sclerosis. Neurology 2004; 62:1105–1109.
28. Weiss N, North RB, Ohara S, et al. Attenuation of cerebellar tremor with implantation of an intrathecal baclofen pump: the role of gamma-aminobutyric acidergic pathways. Case report. J Neurosurg 2003; 99:768–771.
29. Cooper IS. Neurosurgical alleviation of intention tremor of multiple sclerosis and cerebellar disease. N Engl J Med 1960; 263:441–444.
30. Cooper IS. Neurosurgical relief of intention tremor due to cerebellar disease and multiple sclerosis. Arch Phys Med Rehabil 1960; 41:1–4.
31. Broager B, Fog T. Thalamotomy for the relief of intention tremor in multiple sclerosis. Acta Neurol Scand 1962; 38(suppl 3):153–156.
32. Critchley GR, Richardson PL. VIM thalamotomy for the relief of the intention tremor of multiple sclerosis. Br J Neurosurg 1998; 12:559–562.
33. Krayenbuehl H, Yasargil MG. Relief of intention tremor due to multiple sclerosis by stereotaxic thalamotomy. Confin Neurol 1962; 22:368–374.
34. Speelman JD, Van Manen J. Stereotactic thalamotomy for the relief of intention tremor of multiple sclerosis. J Neurol Neurosurg Psychiatry 1984; 47:596–599.
35. Whittle IR, Haddow LJ. CT guided thalamotomy for movement disorders in multiple sclerosis: problems and paradoxes. Acta Neurochir Suppl 1995; 64: 13–16.
36. Alusi SH, Aziz TZ, Glickman S, et al. Stereotactic lesional surgery for the treatment of tremor in multiple sclerosis: a prospective case-controlled study. Brain 2001; 124:1576–1589.

37. Shahzadi S, Tasker RR, Lozano A. Thalamotomy for essential and cerebellar tremor. Stereotact Funct Neurosurg 1995; 65:11–17.
38. Hariz GM, Bergenheim AT, Hariz MI, et al. Assessment of ability/disability in patients treated with chronic thalamic stimulation for tremor. Mov Disord 1998; 13:78–83.
39. Samra K, Waltz JM, Riklan M, et al. Relief of intention tremor by thalamic surgery. J Neurol Neurosurg Psychiatry 1970; 33:7–15.
40. Siegfried J. Therapeutic stereotactic procedures on the thalamus for motor movement disorders. Acta Neurochir (Wien) 1993; 124:14–18.
41. van Manen J. Stereotaxic operations in cases of hereditary and intention tremor. Acta Neurochir Suppl 1974; 21:49–55.
42. Andrew J, Fowler CJ, Harrison MJ. Stereotaxic thalamotomy in 55 cases of dystonia. Brain 1983; 106(Pt 4):981–1000.
43. Loher TJ, Pohle T, Krauss JK. Functional stereotactic surgery for treatment of cervical dystonia: review of the experience from the lesional era. Stereotact Funct Neurosurg 2004; 82:1–13.
44. Niranjan A, Kondziolka D, Baser S, et al. Functional outcomes after gamma knife thalamotomy for essential tremor and MS-related tremor. Neurology 2000; 55:443–446.
45. Brice J, McLellan L. Suppression of intention tremor by contingent deep-brain stimulation. Lancet 1980; 1:1221–1222.
46. Schuurman PR, Bosch DA, Bossuyt PM, et al. A comparison of continuous thalamic stimulation and thalamotomy for suppression of severe tremor. N Engl J Med 2000; 342:461–468.
47. Geny C, Nguyen JP, Pollin B, et al. Improvement of severe postural cerebellar tremor in multiple sclerosis by chronic thalamic stimulation. Mov Disord 1996; 11:489–494.
48. Nandi D, Aziz TZ. Deep brain stimulation in the management of neuropathic pain and multiple sclerosis tremor. J Clin Neurophysiol 2004; 21:31–39.
49. Schulder M, Sernas TJ, Karimi R. Thalamic stimulation in patients with multiple sclerosis: long-term follow-up. Stereotact Funct Neurosurg 2003; 80:48–55.
50. Whittle IR, Hooper J, Pentland B. Thalamic deep-brain stimulation for movement disorders due to multiple sclerosis. Lancet 1998; 351:109–110.
51. Wishart HA, Roberts DW, Roth RM, et al. Chronic deep brain stimulation for the treatment of tremor in multiple sclerosis: review and case reports. J Neurol Neurosurg Psychiatry 2003; 74:1392–1397.
52. Hirai T, Miyazaki M, Nakajima H, et al. The correlation between tremor characteristics and the predicted volume of effective lesions in stereotaxic nucleus ventralis intermedius thalamotomy. Brain 1983; 106(Pt 4):1001–1018.
53. Cooper IS. Neurosurgical treatment of the dyskinesias. Clin Neurosurg 1977; 24:367–390.
54. Deuschl G, Raethjen J, Lindemann M, et al. The pathophysiology of tremor. Muscle Nerve 2001; 24:716–735.
55. Stein JF, Aziz TZ. Does imbalance between basal ganglia and cerebellar outputs cause movement disorders? Curr Opin Neurol 1999; 12:667–669.
56. Nguyen JP, Degos JD. Thalamic stimulation and proximal tremor. A specific target in the nucleus ventrointermedius thalami. Arch Neurol 1993; 50:498–500.

57. Liu X, Aziz TZ, Miall RC, et al. Frequency analysis of involuntary movements during wrist tracking: a way to identify ms patients with tremor who benefit from thalamotomy. Stereotact Funct Neurosurg 2000; 74:53–62.
58. Lawrence DG, Kuypers HG. The functional organization of the motor system in the monkey. I. The effects of bilateral pyramidal lesions. Brain 1968; 91:1–14.
59. Hauptvogel H, Poser S, Orthner H, et al. [Indications for stereotaxic neurosurgery of patients with multiple sclerosis (author's transl.)]. J Neurol 1975; 210:239–251.
60. Biary N, Cleeves L, Findley L, et al. Post-traumatic tremor. Neurology 1989; 39:103–106.
61. Koller WC, Wong GF, Lang A. Posttraumatic movement disorders: a review. Mov Disord 1989; 4:20–36.
62. Krauss JK, Trankle R, Kopp KH. Post-traumatic movement disorders in survivors of severe head injury. Neurology 1996; 47:1488–1492.
63. Samie MR, Selhorst JB, Koller WC. Post-traumatic midbrain tremors. Neurology 1990; 40:62–66.
64. Iwadate Y, Saeki N, Namba H, et al. Post-traumatic intention tremor—clinical features and CT findings. Neurosurg Rev 1989; 12(suppl 1):500–507.
65. Krauss JK, Trankle R, Kopp KH. Posttraumatic movement disorders after moderate or mild head injury. Mov Disord 1997; 12:428–431.
66. Krauss JK, Wakhloo AK, Nobbe F, et al. Lesion of dentatothalamic pathways in severe post-traumatic tremor. Neurol Res 1995; 17:409–416.
67. Jacob PC, Pratap Chand R. Posttraumatic rubral tremor responsive to clonazepam. Mov Disord 1998; 13:977–978.
68. Sandyk R. Nadolol in posttraumatic intention tremor. J Neurosurg 1986; 64:162.
69. Andrew J, Fowler CJ, Harrison MJ. Tremor after head injury and its treatment by stereotaxic surgery. J Neurol Neurosurg Psychiatry 1982; 45:815–819.
70. Bullard DE, Nashold BS Jr. Stereotaxic thalamotomy for treatment of post-traumatic movement disorders. J Neurosurg 1984; 61:316–321.
71. Goldman MS, Kelly PJ. Symptomatic and functional outcome of stereotactic ventralis lateralis thalamotomy for intention tremor. J Neurosurg 1992; 77:223–229.
72. Krauss JK, Jankovic J. Head injury and posttraumatic movement disorders. Neurosurgery 2002; 50:927–939; discussion 939–940.
73. Broggi G, Brock S, Franzini A, et al. A case of posttraumatic tremor treated by chronic stimulation of the thalamus. Mov Disord 1993; 8:206–208.
74. Krauss JK, Simpson RK Jr, Ondo WG, et al. Concepts and methods in chronic thalamic stimulation for treatment of tremor: technique and application. Neurosurgery 2001; 48:535–541; discussion 541–543.
75. Umemura A, Samadani U, Jaggi JL, et al. Thalamic deep brain stimulation for posttraumatic action tremor. Clin Neurol Neurosurg 2004; 106:280–283.
76. Samadani U, Umemura A, Jaggi JL, et al. Thalamic deep brain stimulation for disabling tremor after excision of a midbrain cavernous angioma. Case report. J Neurosurg 2003; 98:888–890.
77. Ohye C, Shibazaki T, Zhang J, et al. Thalamic lesions produced by gamma thalamotomy for movement disorders. J Neurosurg 2002; 97:600–606.

78. Young RF, Jacques S, Mark R, et al. Gamma knife thalamotomy for treatment of tremor: long-term results. J Neurosurg 2000; 93(suppl 3):128–135.

79. Okun MS, Stover NP, Subramanian T, et al. Complications of gamma knife surgery for Parkinson disease. Arch Neurol 2001; 58:1995–2002.

80. Siderowf A, Gollump SM, Stern MB, et al. Emergence of complex, involuntary movements after gamma knife radiosurgery for essential tremor. Mov Disord 2001; 16:965–967.

81. Ingall T. Stroke—incidence, mortality, morbidity and risk. J Insur Med 2004; 36:143–152.

82. Ghika-Schmid F, Ghika J, Regli F, et al. Hyperkinetic movement disorders during and after acute stroke: the Lausanne Stroke Registry. J Neurol Sci 1997; 146:109–116.

83. Tan H, Turanli G, Ay H, et al. Rubral tremor after thalamic infarction in childhood. Pediatr Neurol 2001; 25:409–412.

84. Ferbert A, Gerwig M. Tremor due to stroke. Mov Disord 1993; 8:179–182.

85. Kim JS. Delayed onset hand tremor caused by cerebral infarction. Stroke 1992; 23:292–294.

86. Lehericy S, Grand S, Pollak P, et al. Clinical characteristics and topography of lesions in movement disorders due to thalamic lesions. Neurology 2001; 57: 1055–1066.

87. Miwa H, Hatori K, Kondo T, et al. Thalamic tremor: case reports and implications of the tremor-generating mechanism. Neurology 1996; 46:75–79.

88. Kim JS. Delayed onset mixed involuntary movements after thalamic stroke: clinical, radiological and pathophysiological findings. Brain 2001; 124:299–309.

89. Louis ED, Lynch T, Ford B, et al. Delayed-onset cerebellar syndrome. Arch Neurol 1996; 53:450–454.

90. Kim JS. Involuntary movements after anterior cerebral artery territory infarction. Stroke 2001; 32:258–261.

91. Cho C, Samkoff LM. A lesion of the anterior thalamus producing dystonic tremor of the hand. Arch Neurol 2000; 57:1353–1355.

92. Brannan T, Yahr MD. Focal tremor following striatal infarct—a case report. Mov Disord 1999; 14:368–370.

93. Ohara S, Lenz FA. Reorganization of somatic sensory function in the human thalamus after stroke. Ann Neurol 2001; 50:800–803.

94. Edwards CL, Sudhakar S, Scales MT, et al. Electromyographic (EMG) biofeedback in the comprehensive treatment of central pain and ataxic tremor following thalamic stroke. Appl Psychophysiol Biofeedback 2000; 25:229–240.

95. Frates EP, Burke DT, Chae H, et al. Post-stroke violent adventitial movement responsive to levo-dopa/carbi-dopa therapy. Brain Inj 2001; 15:911–916.

96. Yamamoto T, Katayama Y, Kano T, et al. Deep brain stimulation for the treatment of parkinsonian, essential, and poststroke tremor: a suitable stimulation method and changes in effective stimulation intensity. J Neurosurg 2004; 101:201–209.

97. Katayama Y, Yamamoto T, Kobayashi K, et al. Deep brain and motor cortex stimulation for post-stroke movement disorders and post-stroke pain. Acta Neurochir Suppl 2003; 87:121–123.

8

Dystonia: Classification, Etiology, and Therapeutic Options

Galit Kleiner-Fisman

Parkinson's Disease Research Education and Clinical Center (PADRECC), Philadelphia Veterans Administration Hospital, University of Pennsylvania, Philadelphia, Pennsylvania, U.S.A.

Santiago Figuereo

Department of Neurosurgery, Philadelphia Veterans Administration Hospital, University of Pennsylvania, Philadelphia, Pennsylvania, U.S.A.

1. INTRODUCTION

Dystonia is characterized by sustained involuntary postures and excessive movements of muscles. The movements may be fixed or mobile and often are increased with voluntary action. In some cases dystonia, especially if axial, is severely disabling. Severe dystonia may compromise individuals' self-care abilities and may be life-threatening. The term "dystonia" can be used to describe a symptom, a sign, a diagnosis, or a syndrome.

This chapter will provide an approach to the classification of dystonia, discuss pathophysiologic and etiological considerations, and outline the best medical therapy for dystonia and its limitations. We will then review surgical indications, anatomical targets, and surgical techniques, followed by a summary of available results of deep brain stimulation (DBS) and ablative surgeries to date. This chapter will exclude cervical dystonia (CD), which is addressed separately in chapter 9.

2. CLASSIFICATION

Dystonia may be classified according to age at onset, anatomical areas affected, or etiology (Table 1). Age of onset and anatomical distribution are independent classifications but are closely linked to disease severity. The earlier the onset, the more likely the dystonia will generalize and lead to disability (2). Age at onset has been found to have a bimodal distribution in a defined and clinically ascertained population. Peaks occur in childhood (age 9) and adulthood (age 45), with a lower incidence in between (median age 27) (3). As such, dystonia has been divided into early- and late-onset disease (4–6).

Anatomic distribution of muscle involvement is another method of approaching classification of dystonias. Categories include focal, segmental, multifocal, and generalized. In some cases, dystonia may present in one distribution (focal), and progress to other distributions (generalized), as in dystonia caused by DYT1 gene mutation (7). This commonly presents in one leg and then progresses to involve multiple limbs and trunk.

Another approach to dystonia classification is according to etiology. Dystonia may be primary or secondary (Table 2). Primary (idiopathic)

Table 1 Classification of Dystonia According to Age of Onset, Distribution, and Etiology

---

Age at onset
Early (<26): Usually starts in a limb (leg > arm) and frequently progresses to involve other regions
Late (>26): Usually starts in the neck, cranial muscles, or arm and tends to remain localized
Distribution
Focal (single body part): Includes writer's cramp, blepharospasm, torticollis, spasmodic dysphonia, and oromandibular dystonia
Segmental (contiguous body regions): Includes face and jaw or, torticollis and writer's cramp
Multifocal (noncontiguous body regions):
  Hemi: Ipsilateral arm and leg
  Generalized: Leg, trunk, and one other region
Etiology
Primary: Dystonia is the only sign except tremor with no other cause to explain the dystonia
Secondary: Signs other than dystonia and/or neurodegeneration distinguished from primary dystonia
Inherited degenerative
Inherited nondegenerative
Symptomatic

Source: Adapted from Ref. 6.

Table 2 Causes of Dystonia

Primary
Autosomal dominant
  Early onset (DYT1)
  Mixed (DYT6, DYT13)
  Late onset (DYT7)
  Other genes to be determined
  Genetic causes due to other inheritance patterns

Secondary
Inherited
  Nondegenerative
  DRD (DYT5-GHC1, DYT14, tyrosine hydroxylase deficiency, other biopterin
    deficiencies)
  Myoclonus-dystonia (DYT11-epsilon sarcoglycan, DYT15–18p locus)
  Rapid-onset dystonia parkinsonism (DYT12)
  Degenerative
  Autosomal dominant (HD, SCAs)
  Autosomal recessive (Wilson's disease, NB1A1, *Parkin* GM1 and GM2
    gangliosidoses)
  X-linked (X-linked dystonia-parkinsonism/Lubag, deafness-dystonia/DDP)
  Mitochondrial
  Complex (PD, MSA, PSP, CBD)
  Symptomatic
  Tardive, perinatal/hypoxic injury, head trauma, infectious and postinfectious,
    tumor, vascular malformation, stroke, MS, central pontine myelinolysis, others

---

Abbreviations: DRD, dopa-responsive dystonia; GCH1, guanosine triphosphate (GTP) cyclohydrolase 1; HD, Huntington's disease; SCA, spinocerebellar ataxia; NBIA1, neurodegeneration with brain iron accumulation; DDP, deafness dystonia peptide.
Source: Adapted from Ref. 6.

classification is defined as dystonia being the sole clinical manifestation attributable to the condition with no evidence of imaging, laboratory, or pathological abnormalities that would suggest an inherited or other underlying cause. Exceptions to this exist as in the case of tremor-accompanying idiopathic (primary torsion) dystonia (8). Individuals who do not meet these criteria (have symptoms other than dystonia) are classified as having secondary dystonia. Secondary causes of dystonia can also be subdivided into inherited (nondegenerative), inherited (degenerative), and acquired or symptomatic causes (Table 2) (6).

As novel gene mutations are recognized, dystonias of previously unknown causes have been demonstrated to have a genetic basis (Table 3). This suggests that the definition of primary dystonia may require modification and re-classification periodically as genetic factors become better understood.

Table 3 Genetic Loci Associated with Dystonia

Gene	Locus	Inheritance	Phenotype	Gene product
DYT1	9q34	AD	Early limb onset	Torsin A
DYT2	Not mapped	AR	Early onset	Not identified
DYT3	Xq13.1	XR	Filipino dystonia/ parkinsonism	Not identified
DYT4	Not mapped	AD	Whispering dysphonia	Not identified
DYT5	14q22.1	AD	DRD/parkinsonism	GCH1
DYT6	8p	AD	Mixed	Not identified
DYT7	18p	AD	Adult cervical	Not identified
DYT8	2q33–35	AD	PDC/PNKD	Not identified
DYT9	1p21	AD	Episodic choreoathetosis/ ataxia, spasticity	Not identified
DYT10	16	AD	PKC/PKD	Not identified
DYT11	7q21	AD	Myoclonus Dystonia	Epsilon-sarcoglycan
DYT12	19q	AD	Rapid-onset dystonia/ parkinsonism	Not identified
DYT13	1p36.13– p36.32	AD	Cervical/cranial/upper limb	Not identified
DYT14	14q13	AD	DRD	Not identified
DYT15	18p11	AD	Myoclonus dystonia	Not identified

Abbreviations: AD, autosomal dominant; AR, autosomal recessive; XR, x-linked recessive; DRD, dopa-responsive dystonia; GCH1, GTP glycohydrolase 1; PDC, paroxysmal dystonic choreoathetosis; PKC, paroxysmal kinesigenic choreoathetosis or dyskinesia; PNKD, paroxymal nonkinesiogenic dyskinesia.
Source: Adapted from Ref. 6.

The number of loci that are now recognized to cause primary dystonia is rapidly increasing and currently include DYT-1, -6, -7, and -13, of which only DYT-1 has a defined gene mutation (TOR1A) and protein product (Torsin A) (9). Nondegenerative inherited causes of secondary dystonia with a now identified genetic basis include dopa-responsive dystonia (DRD) due to the GTP cyclohydrolase deficiency (DYT5-GCH-1) and mutations in the tyrosine hydroxylase gene (10,30), myoclonus dystonia due to the epsilon sarcoglycan mutation (DYT11) and another locus on chromosome 18 (DYT15), and rapid-onset dystonia-parkinsonism (DYT12).

Inherited degenerative conditions manifesting dystonia include dominantly inherited conditions like Huntington's disease, spinocerebellar ataxias, frontotemporal dementia, and neuroferritinopathy, and also recessively inherited conditions such as Wilson's disease, *parkin* mutation, neurodegeneration with brain iron accumulation (NBIA1 or PKAN), GM1 and 2 gangliosidoses, glutaric acidemia, neuroacanthocytosis, and others.

Atypical parkinsonian syndromes including multiple system atrophy, progressive supranuclear palsy, and corticobasal degeneration are also degenerative conditions that manifest dystonia, but whether a definable pattern of inheritance is involved in its etiology, and what the pattern of the inheritance may be, remain complex and unknown.

There are many causes of symptomatic dystonia, including those that result from birth trauma, kernicterus, hypoxia, head injury, tumor, infectious and postinfectious conditions, multiple sclerosis, structural lesions, drugs, toxins, and stroke, amongst others.

Objective, standardized measures for rating disease symptoms and severity have been developed to assess generalized dystonia (GD), and include the Burke–Fahn–Marsden Dystonia Rating Scale (BFM-DRS), Unified Dystonia Rating Scale (UDRS), and the Global Dystonia Scale (GDS). The Toronto Western Spasmodic Torticollis Scale (TWSTRS) is the most common scale used to evaluate CD.

3. ETIOLOGY AND PATHOPHYSIOLOGY

3.1. Electrophysiology

Clinically, dystonia is characterized by involuntary distorted postures and movements. Electromyographic (EMG) studies confirm prolonged bursts with phasic muscle contractions. Co-contraction of agonist and antagonist muscles occur, with overflow activation of other uninvolved muscles during specific actions (11).

Some evidence suggests that dystonia is generated by a loss of inhibition in basal ganglia circuitry (12–17). One model proposes lower globus pallidus internus (GPi) output (18) (Fig. 1) with decreased pallidal inhibition to the thalamus resulting in excessive release of thalamocortical activity. Evidence of a change in the firing pattern in contrast to the actual firing rate also exists with reported changes in the extent of synchronization and sensory responsiveness of neurons in the pallidum (19). In contrast to the tonic pattern of discharge present under normal circumstances, patients with dystonia have irregularly grouped discharges with intermittent pauses (20). The effectiveness of pallidal ablation in improving dystonia suggests that an abnormal pattern of neuronal firing, rather than the absolute firing rate, may be responsible for the dysfunction that causes dystonia (21–24).

Further data suggest that dystonia may be related to defects in "surround inhibition" (25,26). According to this model, when a specific movement is generated, there is simultaneous suppression of unwanted movements. If surround inhibition is impaired, then dystonia may emerge. This is consistent with evidence of decreased dopamine D2 receptor striatal binding in

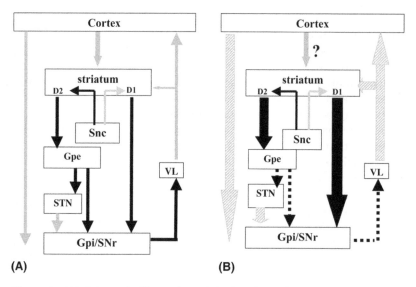

(A)   **(B)**

Figure 1 (A) Schematic illustration of the basal ganglia under normal conditions. (B) A schematic of basal ganglia function in dystonia. Striatal overactivity in both the direct and indirect pathways is postulated to be responsible for the changes in neuronal activity in dystonia. Width of lines represents the relative rate in mean discharge rates compared to normal. Wider lines represent an increase and thinner lines represent a decrease in mean discharge rates. Dotted lines represent the altered patterns and increased synchronization of neuronal activity in the BG thalamocortical circuit, resulting in unregulated cortical output. Black arrows represent inhibitory projections, gray arrows represent excitatory projections. D1, D2, dopamine 1 and 2 receptor subtypes; Snc, substantia nigra compacta; Gpe, globus pallidus externa; Snr, substantia nigra pars reticulata; VL, ventrolateral thalamus. *Source*: Adapted from Vitek JL, Giroux M. Physiology of hypokinetic and hyperkinetic and hypokinetic movement disorders: model for dystonia. Ann Neurol 2000:47:S131–S140.

primates and in people with dystonia (27–29). Dysfunction of the "indirect striato-pallidal pathway" in dystonia, lowering the discharge of subthalamic nucleus (STN)-GPi projections, may explain the findings of reduced Gpi activity and decreased activity in the inhibitory surround (26).

3.2. Pathology and Biochemistry

Aside from electrophysiological considerations, clues from examination of postmortem brains of dystonic patients also suggest an abnormality in the dopaminergic system (30–32). A comprehensive study of markers of dopamine transmission in three specimens of postmortem DYT1 striatum found increased dopamine turnover compared to controls (33). However, no pathological or biochemical abnormalities have consistently been found in DYT1 dystonia (34,35). This is in keeping with a functional, rather than a degenerative or structural, abnormality as the etiology of DYT1 dystonia.

3.3. Imaging

Metabolic studies measuring brain glucose metabolism using fluorodeoxyglucose positron emission tomography (FDG-PET) demonstrate an abnormal metabolic brain network characterized by hypermetabolism of the basal ganglia, supplementary motor area, and the cerebellum in both patients manifesting and those not clinically manifesting DYT1 dystonia. In addition, those that manifest dystonia also show another pattern characterized by increased activity of the midbrain, cerebellum, and pons (36–38). It has been suggested that a clinical correlate of this abnormal metabolic pattern, found even in nonmanifesting DYT1 carriers, is impaired motor sequence learning (39), with an alternate brain network being activated when the task is performed.

3.4. Torsin A

Finally, further insights into the pathophysiology of dystonia may be gained by the examination of the biology of Torsin A, the protein product of the implicated gene (TOR1A) in DYT1 dystonia. A study using in situ hybridization with a Torsin A probe in nondiseased postmortem brain revealed ubiquitous distribution, with greatest protein expression found in the basal ganglia, brain stem, and cerebellum (40,41). The function of this protein, which shows similarity to the AAA+ family of adenosine triphosphatases (ATPases), includes involvement in cellular metabolism, particularly in ATP binding and hydrolysis, but the exact sequence and details of this process are unclear (42–45). The relationship between the ATPase catalytic cycle and the conformational changes leading to biological activity remain to be defined.

In addition to a lack of conclusive knowledge about the function of the normally expressed protein, the consequence of the Δ302/3 mutation (found in DYT1 dystonia), a deleted glutamic acid residue in the C-terminus of Torsin A, is unknown (46–48). Efforts to create a mouse model of dystonia by modifying allelic expression of Torsin A such that there is only 2.5–5% of wild-type protein expression (loss-of-function mutant) have failed to create a dystonic phenotype in the rodent (49), possibly suggesting that this is a necessary but insufficient abnormality to cause dystonia. As such, insights gained from this animal model in its current state are limited.

Recently, preliminary work has been done creating another transgenic mouse model of mutant Torsin A that resulted in a phenotype of abnormal motor function manifesting as fore- and hind-limb clasping, circling, posturing, and head shaking (50). These features were apparent in ≈40% of the transgenic mice, similar to the penetrance in DYT-1 dystonia in humans. Furthermore, in examining the striatum of these transgenic mice, there was evidence of increased dopamine content and turnover, as has been reported in humans with the disease (33). Implications of this work remain to be determined.

3.5. Dopaminergic Transmission

Examination of abnormalities thought to play a role in the pathophysiology of some forms of dystonia, like mutations in the tyrosine hydroxylase gene (30) and the guanosine triphosphate cyclohydrolase gene (31), further support dopamine-mediated dysfunction. Individuals affected with these disorders have limited dopamine synthesis that results in a dystonic phenotype. Despite this, there is currently no evidence pathologically in humans to suggest a relationship between abnormal Torsin A production and dopaminergic function in DYT1 dystonia (49).

4. BEST MEDICAL THERAPY

Treatment options for dystonia are based on etiology and anatomical distribution, each of which influences the effectiveness of therapy. In most cases, dystonia therapy is offered to alleviate symptoms that interfere in activities of daily living and quality of life and is not curative. In rare cases of "dystonic storm," a medical emergency that can manifest in hyperthermia, rhabdomyolysis, and myoglobinuria, medical treatment is crucial and potentially life-saving (51).

The effective treatment of patients with dystonia requires a multidisciplinary and comprehensive approach that includes pharmacologic, nonpharmacologic, and surgical options (for a comprehensive review see Ref. 1). However, there are few randomized, placebo-controlled trials of adequate power to permit definitive recommendations of effective treatment for an individual dystonic patient. An algorithm for the treatment of dystonia is proposed based on the literature available and on clinical experience (Fig. 2).

4.1. Nonpharmacologic Considerations

Emphasis on patient and caregiver education, support, and expectations are important for successful therapy. Physical and occupational therapy may augment the benefit of medical therapy (52,53). In some cases, assistive equipment, such as a mechanical device, have proven useful in alleviating opisthotonus and retrocollis that typically occur in tardive dystonia (54). The introduction of a hand orthosis in writers' cramp has also shown some benefit (55). Recently, there has been some evidence to suggest that immobilization of an affected limb for a brief period of time may result in improvement in dystonia, though whether this effect is sustained is not known (56–58). It is also unknown how immobilization results in symptomatic improvement of dystonia. One possible explanation is that some

TREATMENT OF DYSTONIA

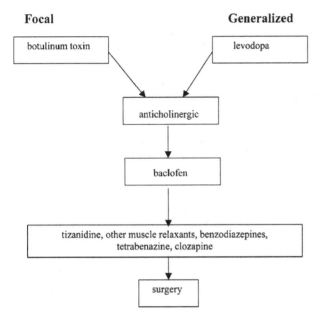

Figure 2 Treatment algorithm for dystonia. *Source*: Adapted from Ref. 1.

patients with dystonia have impaired sensory perception and sensory-motor integration (59,60), and the removal of sensory and motor input to the limb may result in "resetting" and normalizing of the cortical map (61,62). Furthermore, sensory training and mental exercises to restore hand sensory representation have shown benefit in focal limb dystonia (63,64). Finally, in some patients with dystonia, muscle relaxation and sensory feedback therapy can enhance medical or surgical treatments (1,65,66).

4.2. Pharmacologic Interventions

4.2.1. Dopaminergic Therapy

In DRD, supplementation with small doses of levodopa or dopamine agonists provides dramatic improvement in symptoms (53,67). A trial of dopaminergic replacement is appropriate in all childhood-onset dystonia, regardless of whether the clinical presentation is typical of DRD (1,53). A trial of levodopa in adults with non-DRD is also indicated as benefit from dopaminergic therapy exists in 25% of patients with adult-onset primary and secondary dystonias (1).

4.2.2. Antidopaminergic Therapy

While some patients benefit from treatment with dopaminergic therapy, others improve with antidopaminergic treatments (68,69). However, use of these agents that include neuroleptics is often limited by unwanted side effects like parkinsonism, sedation, and tardive dyskinesia or tardive dystonia.

The more recent atypical neuroleptic agents may also prove to be useful in the treatment of dystonia. Clozapine has high D4 receptor affinity with combined serotonergic and dopaminergic effects. It has shown benefit in a small number of patients with segmental and generalized dystonia in an open-label trial (70) using 300–400 mg/day as the optimal dose. However, in some patients treatment was withdrawn due to intolerable side effects such as orthostatic hypotension. Its use is also pragmatically complicated because of a risk of agranulocytosis, requiring weekly blood draws to monitor the white blood cell count.

Risperidone, also considered an atypical neuroleptic despite D2-receptor blocking properties, has also been reported to be efficacious in doses of up to 8 mg/day in the treatment of segmental dystonia in a small number of patients (68,71) and in idiopathic and symptomatic dystonia (69). Tetrabenazine, a presynaptic monoamine-depleting agent and dopamine receptor blocker not available in the United States, is used preferentially in Canada and the United Kingdom for hyperkinetic movement disorders and does not induce tardive dyskinesia (72).

4.2.3. Anticholinergic Therapy

The mainstay of medication treatment for dystonia has been anticholinergic agents, particularly trihexyphenidyl (Artane) (73,74).

Generally, it is necessary to proceed with a slow titration, starting with 1–2 mg at bedtime and usually progressing to 12 mg/day divided over three doses over the course of 4–6 weeks (1). This is to prevent or decrease side effects such as drowsiness, cognitive impairment, and autonomic symptoms such as urinary retention, dry mouth, and blurred vision. In some cases, high doses (60–100 mg) may be needed for the desired effect, though use at the higher doses may not be tolerated due to the aforementioned side effects, especially in the elderly. Pyridostigmine (an anticholinesterase agent), pilocarpine eye-drops, and synthetic saliva may be introduced in order to ameliorate these unwanted anticholinergic effects (1).

4.2.4. Muscle Relaxants

Muscle relaxing agents have proven efficacy in patients with spasticity and may have a role to play in dystonic patients as well. Though there are no trials to attest to their efficacy, drugs such as cyclobenzaprine, metaxalone, carisoprodol, and orphenadrine have been used anecdotally as part of the therapeutic armementarium to treat dystonia. Tizanidine hydrochloride, a centrally acting alpha-adrenergic agonist, is an agent with proven efficacy in spasticity (75) and has sometimes been included as part of a treatment strategy, though its effects in dystonia have not been encouraging. One open-label study of administration of tizanidine did not significantly improve cranial dystonia in 10 patients (76), and another small randomized double-blind cross-over trial of tizanidine treatment in patients with spasmodic torticollis did not show much benefit over a 6-week course with doses up to 12 mg/day (77).

Under certain circumstances, oral baclofen may provide benefit in reducing dystonia by putatively increasing presynaptic inhibition of motor neurons (78,79). An intrathecal baclofen (ITB) pump may also play a limited role in the treatment of medically refractory axial or generalized dystonia (80–84). Evidence from studies conducted in patients with spastic and dystonic cerebral palsy provide support for this practice (85). However, response to an ITB pump is unpredictable. In one series of 14 patients with primary and secondary causes of dystonia, only five patients showed objective benefit as measured by the BFM-DRS. Doses averaged 590 µg/day with a mean length of therapy of 29 months. Tolerance to the drug, device-related complications, and side effects such as constipation, drowsiness, and decreased trunk control (86,87) were identified. The cause of the dystonia did not predict whether or not a patient would respond to an ITB pump.

4.2.5. Other

4.2.5.1. Morphine sulfate: In a series of nine patients (88), slow release morphine sulfate appeared to improve dystonic movements in individuals with tardive and generalized dystonia over and above the improvement due to pain relief. However, the effect seen was transient and is not currently a recommended therapy.

4.2.5.2. Gamma-hydroxy butyric acid (GHB): Subjective improvement of both myoclonus and dystonia in a patient with inherited myoclonic dystonia treated with GHB has been reported (89). Rationale for the use of GHB is based on its therapeutic effects in the treatment of alcohol abuse as it mimics the effects of alcohol. No trials currently support the use of this agent.

4.2.5.3. Mexilitene: In one open-label trial of six patients with spasmodic torticollis, treatment with Mexilitene up to 800 mg/day for a 6-week period resulted in significant improvement in dystonia as measured by the TWSTRS and the BFM-DRS with no significant adverse effects (90). Further experience with this agent in the treatment of dystonia is needed to confirm or refute this finding.

4.2.5.4. Antihistamines: In three of five patients with idiopathic truncal dystonia, treatment with up to 500 mg/kg/day of oral diphenhydramine was found to be beneficial during 20 months of follow-up (91). This result was re-enforced in another small, open-label trial (92). This is in contrast to a double-blind, placebo-controlled study of intravenous chlorpheniramine maleate in 20 patients with adult onset focal dystonia that saw no consistent benefit from this intervention (93). However, given the wide availability of these medications, relative safety, paucity of side effects, and the extent of disability caused by dystonia, a trial of an antihistamine (such as diphenhydramine) is warranted when other treatments have failed (94).

4.2.5.5. Benzodiazepines: Benzodiazepines such as clonazepam, diazepam, and lorazepam may be indicated as alternative or additional agents when other medications such as anticholinergics have failed (95).

4.2.5.6. Summary: Medications in combination are often necessary to achieve satisfactory results. Each patient may require a different combination of medications in varying dosages and the optimal combination for each individual patient is often found by trial and error. The benefits obtained by pharmacologic therapy must always be weighed against the potential for systemic side effects that increase with use of multiple agents. A therapy such as botulinum toxin that acts locally and eliminates the risk of unwanted systemic effects is an attractive alternative under the appropriate circumstances.

4.2.6. Botulinum Toxin

Botulinum toxin has revolutionized the treatment of dystonia and has become the first line agent in some forms of focal dystonias. There are seven isoforms of botulinum neurotoxins identified by the letters A–G that vary with respect to biochemical activity and antigenicity (96,97). Botulinum toxin A (Botox®, Dysport®) received approval from the Food and Drug Administration (FDA) in 1989 for the indications of blepharospasm, hemifacial spasm, and cervical dystonia. Another preparation using a different subunit of the toxin, botulinum toxin B (Myobloc) was FDA approved in the United States in 2000 as treatment for cervical dystonia. Currently, these are the only two isoforms of botulinum toxin that are commercially available and approved by the FDA, though experimental uses of some of the other subunits may show therapeutic promise in the future (98,99).

The therapeutic effect of either botulinum toxin formulation results from denervation in injected muscle. The toxin irreversibly binds to the presynaptic membrane at the neuromuscular junction to prevent acetylcholine release and consequent flaccid weakness (100). Though the binding of the neurotoxin to the terminal is irreversible, the clinical effect of paralysis is not permanent due to synaptic plasticity and nerve sprout regeneration (101,102). Repeated injections are necessary approximately every 3 months to maintain the effect, though a complete return to baseline muscle activity does not usually occur within this time period.

Botulinum toxins A and B are generally believed to be of comparable safety, efficacy, and duration of benefit, though these have not been directly compared in dystonia. A study in healthy volunteers looking at magnitude and duration of paralysis, as measured by M-wave amplitude on EMG at periodic intervals following injection of either botulinum toxin A or B, found that the magnitude and duration of effect was greater in individuals having received botulinum toxin A as compared to botulinum toxin B (103). Whether M-wave amplitude is a valid marker for clinical response to botulinum toxin is unclear (1).

Though initially effective in most patients with focal dystonia, some patients receiving repeated injections of botulinum toxin A develop neutralizing antibodies that confer resistance to the effects of future injections. This phenomenon may be of historical interest, as it appears to be uncommon with the use of the current formulation (104). This more recent formulation contains 5 ng of neurotoxin complex protein/100 units in contrast to the older preparation containing 25 ng/100 units and may therefore be less antigenic.

The risk of development of neutralizing antibodies was found to be increased when larger, more frequent doses were administered and found to occur at a higher incidence in younger individuals (105). Further discussion of botulinum toxins and when to use each is presented in chapter 9 in the context of cervical dystonia.

Safety and therapeutic benefit of botulinum toxin in dystonia has been demonstrated in multiple clinical studies with efficacy and optimal doses varying according to dystonia subtype (106). Experience with botulinum toxin in blepharospasm has been generally excellent with sustained efficacy following repeated use (107) with an average duration of maximum benefit of 16 weeks (1). However, it is not uncommon for patients to experience blurred vision, ptosis, and tearing, especially in the first 2–3 weeks following injections. These usually subside and are dose dependent.

Botulinum toxin can be an effective treatment option in oromandibular dystonia (OMD) with sustained improvement in chewing and speech in ~70% of patients (108) and improved quality of life (109) whether tardive or idiopathic.

OMD manifests as jaw-clenching, bruxism, jaw-opening, or jaw-closing dystonia. In cases of jaw-opening dystonia, EMG-guidance may be required to isolate the lateral pterygoid or the submental muscle complex. Comparison of tardive and idiopathic OMD suggests equivalent benefit from botulinum toxin injections (110). A long-term study (108) of outcomes in OMD with an average follow-up time of 4.4 years used a mean dose of 54.2 ± 15.2 U of botulinum toxin A injected into the masseter muscle and 28.6 ± 16.7 U were administered to the submentalis complex. The average duration of response to injections was 16.4 weeks. Of note, 11% of patients in this study experienced dysphagia and dysarthria following at least one injection during the course of follow-up.

Botulinum toxin has emerged as the treatment of choice in patients with spasmodic dysphonia (laryngeal dystonia). Excellent outcomes with a low risk of adverse events are reported in the majority of patients treated (111), with concomitant improvement in voice-related quality of life (112). These injections need to be performed by experienced practitioners and usually require the use of laryngoscopy.

The first line treatment strategy in action-specific limb dystonia such as writers' cramp is also botulinum toxin (113). In one study, 167 patients presenting with writers' cramp underwent EMG-guided botulinum toxin A injections. The results showed good efficacy and tolerance of this treatment in the long term (up to 10 years) with recovery of normal writing in 46%, partial benefit in 10%, failure in 21%, and loss to follow-up after the first injection in 23% of patients. Amongst those that benefited, EMG-guided injections were repeated approximately every 9 months (114). Though EMG-guidance is often used to isolate the specific muscles involved in the dystonia, evidence suggests that localization with EMG-guidance does not necessarily imply better clinical results than can be achieved using clinical assessment of affected muscle groups (115).

5. SURGICAL THERAPY

Surgical treatment alternatives for patients with dystonia have evolved as a result of mixed or inadequate results of medical therapy. The evolution of surgical approaches has improved along with further understanding of the pathophysiology of the involuntary movements seen in dystonia. Segmental fusions (116) and selective myectomy (117) have been performed or proposed as rare but alternative palliative approaches to refractory dystonia. Most surgical interventions, however, attempt to obtain relief by interrupting the pathways of abnormal motor excitation.

In order to avoid the potential adverse effects of central nervous system interventions, peripheral nerve denervations have been performed for focal dystonia (118,119). Other strategies such as dorsal column stimulation have also given moderate relief to patients with focal (cervical) dystonia (120). Mixed results and frequent complications have discouraged the generalized use of these strategies.

For the past 50 years (121), ablation or DBS of basal ganglia motor nuclei have provided the best outcomes in the surgical treatment of dystonia. Pallidotomy (122–124) and thalamotomy (125,126) have been associated with adequate but inconsistent results as well as complications, particularly dysarthria and dysphagia when performed bilaterally. Better understanding of the functional organization of the basal ganglia, flexibility in adjusting the parameters of stimulation, reversibility of stimulation, and the feasibility of bilateral electrode implantation without unwanted adverse effects make DBS an attractive surgical alternative for the treatment of dystonia.

5.1. Patient Selection

The selection of patients for dystonia surgery is based on identifying those in whom the anticipated benefit of symptomatic improvement outweighs the risks of undergoing brain surgery. Though experience with functional stereotactic brain surgery has increased and the risk of serious surgical morbidity has been reduced to approximately 5% (127), the risk of surgery is only justified in cases of severe dystonia causing intractable pain or disability and when other conservative treatment options have failed.

The main considerations when evaluating a dystonic patient for a neurosurgical intervention are:

1. Determining whether the target symptom is responsible for the disability. For example, if fixed contractures have already occurred, alleviating the dystonia may not provide added benefit.
2. Empirical estimation of the likelihood of improvement of symptoms and quality of life following surgery.
3. Estimation of the surgical risk factors in each individual patient and the likelihood of an adverse event.
4. Assessment of whether the patient's expectations of the surgical outcome are realistic and achievable (128).

6. ANATOMICAL TARGETS IN DBS SURGERY

6.1. GPi

The rationale for the alleviation of dystonia by stimulating the GPi relates to the observed decrease in the firing rate of GPi neurons and abnormal grouping of discharges in a burst–pause pattern in patients with dystonia (18,129). The observation that pallidotomy alleviates levodopa-induced dystonic dyskinesias and OFF period dystonia in Parkinson's disease (PD) patients, combined with reports that pallidotomy may be beneficial in primary generalized dystonia (GD), has lent further support to the role of the GPi as a target in dystonia surgery (22,130–132). Though preliminary studies suggest that the GPi is a promising target especially in GD (Table 4), conclusive data is lacking due to the paucity of large well-designed trials.

6.2. Subthalamic Nucleus

There is minimal experience with STN DBS in dystonia. The theoretical basis for choosing the STN as a target is rooted in the classical model of basal ganglia function (Fig. 1) (159). According to this model, hyperkinetic movement disorders such as dystonia result from overactivity of both the direct and indirect pathways, leading to increased inhibitory activity of the GPi. It is postulated that there is decreased neuronal activity in the globus pallidus

Table 4 Summary of Dystonia DBS Studies

Study number and citation	Study design	Dx	No.	Target	U/L vs. B/L	Follow-up time	% improvement BFM-DRS	Other rating scales
1. (133)		14-GD; 6-CD	20	GPi		GD-8.6 mos (range 3–12); CD-18.9 mos (range 12–24)	GD: 47% (SS); 38% (DS); 46% (TS)	TWSTRS: CD: 64% (SS); 60% (DS); 60% (PS); 60% (TS)
2. (134)		15-DYT1; 17-not known; 21-secondary	53	GPi	B/L	1 yr	71% (CS); 63% (FS); 74% (CS); 49% (FS); 31% (CS); 7% (FS)	
3. (135)	Case series	12-primary GD; 7-CD; 4-MD; 1-TD; 1-posttrauma HD	25		B/L	GD-9.2 mos (range 4–18); CD-19 (range 12–24); Misc 11 (range 4–24)	GD: 47.6% (SS); 37.6% (DS); 45.8% (TS)	TWSTRS: CD: 63.8% (SS); 60% (DA); 60.3% (PS); 59.5% (TS); AIMS misc 37.1%
4. (136)		9-Primary GD (2 DYT1); 10-secondary trauma, stroke, anoxia (NBIA-1)	19	9-Vim; 6-Vim, then GPi; 7-GPi	3 U/L; Vim 6 B/L Vim 6 B/L Gpi 1 B/L GPi	4.5 yrs (4 mos to 11 yrs) 4–36 mos 14 mos 6–24 mos		GF Vim 50% score of 2 or 3 GPi; 70% score of 2 or 3
5. (137)	Case series	5 CD, 3 CD with myelopathy	8	5 GPi; 3 GPi and lamin	B/L	20 mos	63% SS; 69% DS; 50% PS	

	Type	Etiology	N	Target	Laterality	Follow-up	Outcome	Scale
6. (138)	Case series	2 GD; 4 chor due to CP	6	Gpi	B/L	2 yrs	2 GD: 74% SS; 68% DS; 4 chor; 23% DS, 13% DS (2 pts)	
7. (139)	Case series	4 GD (1 DYT-1, 1 IGD, 1 Hunt Dis; 1 TD); 3 CD; 1 HD	8	GPi	7 B/L; 1 U/L	6 mos	GD: 12–35%	TWSTRS; CD: 43–82%
8. (140)	Case series	1 DYT-1 GD; 3 segmental dyst, 2 CD	6	GPi	B/L	1 yr	76%	
9. (141)	Case series	1 DYT-1 GD; 1 IGD	5	GPi	B/L	6 mos	72%	
10. (142)	Case report		2	GPi	B/L	2 yrs	95% DYT-1; 80% IGD	
11. (143)	Case report; double-blind assessment	IGD	1	GPi	B/L	1 yr	67%	
12. (144)	Case report	Posttrauma HD	1	GPi	U/L	4 yrs	Improved–no objective measure	
13. (145)	Case report	Posttrauma CD	1	GPi	U/L	1 yr	Improved–no objective measure	
14. (68)	Case report	Segmental dystonia	1	GPi	B/L	9 mos	86%	
15. (146)	Case report	CD	1	GPi	U/L		Improved–no objective measure	
16. (147)	Case report	Postanoxic GD	1	VOA	B/L	4 mos		UDRS 50%
17. (148)	Case report	ICD, truncal dystonia	1	GPi	B/L	7 wks		TWSTRS 50%
18. (149)	Case report	CD	2	GPi	B/L	24 and 17 mos		64% VAS, 21% Tsui; 55% VAS, 7% Tsui
19. (150)	Case report	IGD	1	GPi	Pall and C/L GPi DBS	1 yr	Worsened–no objective measure	

(Continued)

Table 4 Summary of Dystonia DBS Studies (*Continued*)

Study number and citation	Study design	Dx	No.	Target	U/L vs. B/L	Follow-up time	% improvement BFM-DRS	Other rating scales
20. (151)	Case series	7 DYT-1 GD	7	GPi	B/L	3 mos	90.3%	
21. (152)	Case report	ICD	1	GPi	B/L	1 yr	Improved-no objective measure	
22. (153)	Case series	ICD	3	GPi	B/L	3 mos	Improved-no objective measure	TWSTRS4: 1% (SS); 43% (PS); 52% (DS)
23. (154)	Case report Double-blind	TD	1	Vim and GPi	B/L B/L	6 mos	No change with Vim, 73% GPi	Gpi (AIMS) 54%
24. (155)	Case series	1 IGD, 1 DYT-1 GD, 1 postanoxic at birth	3	GPi	B/L	6–18 mos	DYT-1 34%, IGD 59%; anoxia 14%	
25. (156)	Case series	ICD	3	GPi	B/L	3 mos	Improved-no objective measure	
26. (157)	Case report	FMD	1	GPi	B/L	20 mos	Improved-no objective measure	
27. (158)	Case series	3 NB1A1; 1 IGD	4	STN	B/L	3 mos	No improvement	

Abbreviations: SS, severity score; DS, disability score; PS, pain score; TS, total score; CS, clinical score; FS, functional score; Chor, choreoathetosis; GF, global function outcome; IGD, idiopathic generalized dystonia; ICD, idiopathic cervical dystonia; HD, hemidystonia; TD, tardive dystonia; Hunt Dis, Huntington's disease; NB1A1, neurodegeneration with brain iron deposition; mos, months; yrs, years; wks, weeks; Gpi, globus pallidus internus; VLp, ventral lateral posterior thalamic nucleus; VOA, ventro oralis anterior thalamic nucleus; Vim, ventralis intermedius thalamic nucleus; UDRS, Unified Dystonia Rating Scale; AIMS, Abnormal Involuntary Movement Scale; VAS, visual analogue scale; TWSTRS, Toronto Western Torticollis Rating Scale; BFM-DRS, Burke–Fahn–Marsden Dystonia Rating Scale; FMD, familial myoclonic dystonia; NBIA-1, abnormal brain iron accumulation; pall, pallidotomy; lamin, laminectomy; U/L, unilateral; B/L, bilateral; C/L, contralateral; N/A, not available.

externus (GPe), which increases the excitatory drive to the STN. This in turn further increases GPi inhibitory activity (Fig. 1).

One study in support of this hypothesis shows decreased D2-like binding in the striatum of patients with idiopathic focal dystonia (160). This could result in reduced dopaminergic inhibition and an increase in the activity of striatal neurons in the indirect pathway (19). Other studies, performed using neuronal recording, PET, and TMS, suggest that overactivity of the STN results from both increased cortical activity and increased GPe activity in some forms of dystonia (19,161–166). Again, this would support the use of the STN as a target location for alleviation of dystonic symptoms. Indirect clinical evidence in favor of the STN as a target is provided by the observation that OFF period dystonia resolves in PD patients that have undergone bilateral STN stimulation (158,167–169).

7. SURGICAL TECHNIQUE

The surgical technique for the treatment of dystonia by either ablative or stimulation procedures does not differ significantly from the procedures described elsewhere in the treatment of PD (170–172). Whether the ultimate goal is to create a lesion or to implant a stimulating lead, the adjuvant technology is used with the intention of precisely localizing a target point. Most surgeons will rely on a combination of methods rather than on one particular localization technique. These techniques include imaging, electrophysiological recording, or macrostimulation. Imaging approaches may include fluoroscopy, pneumoencephalography, magnetic resonance imaging (MRI), computed tomography (CT), or a combination of two or more of these. A stereotactic frame is fixed to the patient's head before the imaging study is obtained in order to localize the target's anatomical point in reference to the scaled device. A Leksell Model G stereotactic head frame is most commonly used; however, new navigation technology that integrates imaging studies with computer software may soon popularize frameless localizing devices (173–176). Once a target has been determined, a trajectory devised, and an entry point identified, general surgical technique is used to perform an access Burr hole, traditionally at the level of or just in front of the coronal suture bilaterally. An insertion cannula is placed along the planned trajectory in the brain to guide the microelectrode used for electrophysiologic recordings. Electropysiologic recordings are used to further define the optimal location for placement of the macroelectrode.

Several techniques have been debated in terms of electrophysiological recording. Some proclaim the benefits of accurate delineation of the target organ by multiple electrode recording (either simultaneously or staggered), while others praise the decreased risk of intracerebral hemorrhage with a single electrode pass (177,178). The published data suggest both techniques to be adequately safe and effective. Regardless of the recording technique chosen, the goal is to confirm the coordinates obtained from the imaging studies by identifying the neuronal discharge pattern of the target organ.

Another approach to localization includes stimulation through the implanted macroelectrode to verify an appropriate clinical response in an awake patient. This commonly occurs in PD patients undergoing DBS, but occurs less often in cases of dystonia as the patient is often operated under general anesthesia such that no dystonia is present. Clinical responses used to confirm electrode placement include reduction in muscle tone or a decrease of involuntary repetitive muscle contractions. Conversely, macroelectrode stimulation intraoperatively may be performed in order to detect changes in the neuronal discharge pattern recorded from the electrodes. An example of the latter is the use of flashing lights to elicit a visual evoked response to verify proximity of the optic tract to the final electrode location in the GPi.

Once the target site has been identified by any combination of these methods, the electrodes are used to create the lesion in the case of ablative surgery, or are replaced by permanent electrodes used in DBS. The electrodes are subsequently tunneled under the skin and connected to a generator implanted in the subcutaneous tissue, usually in the chest. The programming of the electrodes occurs days to weeks following electrode implantation and is achieved using a computer-controlled remote device.

8. RESULTS OF SURGERY IN DYSTONIA

8.1. Thalamotomy and Pallidotomy

The thalamus preceded the GPi as a target for dystonia. Thalamotomy outcome studies have shown that dystonia was alleviated in only 1/3 to 1/2 of patients studied and there was an unacceptable rate of intolerable side effects, especially with bilateral procedures (179). Studies comparing the efficacy of surgery on the thalamus versus the GPi have not been performed. Which site is optimal for the indication of dystonia has not been unequivocally determined; however, the current trend, based on previous experience, is toward selecting the GPi as the preferred target.

Since the early 1990s, improvement of dystonia by pallidotomy in the posteroventral medial pallidum has been reported in approximately 75 patients in multiple case reports and case series, with follow-ups ranging from 3 to 42 months (180). Results in these patients have shown that pallidotomy can reduce functional disability that is caused by dystonia with best results demonstrated in patients with primary and tardive causes of dystonia. Both unilateral and bilateral procedures have been performed safely without the cognitive adverse effects experienced by PD patients who underwent bilateral pallidotomy (181). Also, in contrast to the immediate effects of surgery in PD patients, improvement seen following pallidotomy in dystonia was, in some instances, delayed and occurred in a gradual fashion several months after the procedure. However, long-term outcomes have not been reliably documented, and even though there may be benefit that is seen early after the surgical procedure, there are cases of only temporary improvement with recurrent debilitating symptoms (23,182). As such, the results of pallidotomy for dystonia are difficult to predict.

8.2. Deep Brain Stimulation

In dystonia as well as other conditions such as PD, DBS has largely replaced ablative surgery as the surgical treatment of choice because it is both reversible and modifiable.

However, large, blinded, controlled clinical trials are lacking in the field of dystonia DBS surgery. This may be because there are a relatively small number of individuals affected by dystonia severe enough to warrant functional neurosurgery and the fact that DBS is still considered investigational for dystonia. The lack of uniformity among studies in reporting surgical outcomes makes comparison of outcomes between studies difficult. Furthermore, as symptoms of dystonia may be modified by psychological factors, outcomes are likely susceptible to placebo effects (183). In addition to inadequate objective assessment of motor benefit, assessment of quality of life measures following dystonia surgery are also lacking, so the true impact of the procedure is unknown. Notwithstanding these limitations, review of the mostly single case reports or case series published suggests that DBS surgery in carefully selected patients may be a viable treatment option for patients with intractable dystonia.

8.3. Thalamic DBS

In a retrospective study of patients with variable causes of dystonia who had either GPi stimulation or thalamic stimulation, or both (GPi following unsuccessful thalamic stimulation), the patients with pallidal stimulation clearly had a better outcome compared to those implanted in the thalamus (136). Another series of eight patients with heterogeneous causes of dystonia and both ventral intermedius nucleus of the thalamus (Vim) and GPi stimulation reported little benefit in the Vim group, compared to >50% improvement as a result of GPi stimulation (184). In light of the demonstrated better outcomes of GPi DBS compared to Vim DBS, the thalamus as a target site for dystonia has largely been abandoned.

8.3. GPi DBS

Table 4 provides a complete review of the literature with respect to pallidal stimulation.

Unlike PD, where there are clinical tests (levodopa challenge) that may predict response to surgery, no such tests exist for dystonia. In addition, the paucity of conclusive published studies of outcomes in dystonia stereotactic surgery limits the ability to determine which patient is likely to benefit. From the limited reports that do exist, however, there are some clinical factors that suggest a more favorable outcome. As in the pallidotomy experience, review of GPi DBS results suggests that those with primary causes of dystonia tend to have greatest benefit from surgery. Those with DYT-1 genetic mutations have been reported to have up to a 95% reduction in BFM-DRS scores (136,151,155,185).

This is not always the case, however; there have been at least three cases of DYT-1 positive dystonia with poor response to bilateral GPi DBS (186,187). This underscores the point that the mutation itself does not necessarily predict a good outcome from surgery, and that other as yet unidentified factors are likely important as well.

Review of the literature suggests that those with secondary causes of dystonia tend to have a less robust and predictable response to DBS than those with a primary cause (136,155,185,188,189). Nonetheless, even in the secondary dystonia population, which is heterogeneous, there have been reports of dramatic responses to DBS surgery (190–192).

Regardless of the cause, optimal benefit may take several months to achieve. This has been postulated to be due to the gradual resolution of disturbances downstream from the pallidum or due to nervous system plasticity (193). This hypothesis is re-enforced by a study that used PET in a patient with primary dystonia and bilateral GPi DBS placement with significant improvement in the dystonia after the stimulators were turned on. In a blinded fashion the stimulators were turned on and off and PET imaging was performed while performing a motor task. GPi stimulation reversed the abnormal excess activation of multiple brain regions, including primary motor, lateral motor, supplementary motor, anterior cingulate, and prefrontal cortices, leading the authors to propose that GPi stimulation may directly suppress excessive motor area activation (143). Clinically, it has been observed that the mobile component of dystonia tends to resolve earlier than fixed dystonia following DBS (128,136,184). In a study looking at the pattern of recurrence of dystonia following the discontinuation of stimulation, mobile dystonia re-emerged within a few minutes while the tonic component recurred gradually over several hours (194).

8.4. STN DBS

Despite a good theoretical basis for considering STN as a target in dystonia, the only published experience reported disappointing results. PD patients with OFF-period dystonia and four patients with generalized dystonia underwent bilateral STN DBS. Though there was definite relief of OFF-period dystonia in those patients with PD, there was no difference in severity of dystonia in those patients with generalized dystonia that underwent STN DBS. However, three of the four patients suffered from neurodegeneration with brain iron accumulation [also known as pantothenate kinase associated neurodegeneration (PKAN) and formerly as Hallevorden-Spatz disease] (158). It is difficult to deduce from this limited experience and highly select population whether STN DBS is effective in other populations.

9. CONCLUSIONS

Dystonia is a clinically heterogeneous condition with many etiologies. A standard classification and rating system is crucial both for optimal clinical care of patients and for conducting rigorous studies that would further advance therapeutic options. Though medical therapies relieve symptoms to a variable extent, the occurrence of intractable dystonia, causing significant disability and reduction in quality of life, makes development of a safe and effective surgical therapy attractive.

Identification of clinical and pathophysiological factors that predict a good response to surgery is an important research priority. Studies determining the appropriate target site need to be conducted, as the optimal site may vary according to the cause of dystonia, patterns of inheritance, and distribution. Finally, large, prospective, long-term controlled trials using standardized rating and quality of life scales will be an important addition to the current body of knowledge to determine the true efficacy of this procedure.

REFERENCES

1. Jankovic J. Dystonia: medical therapy and botulinum toxin. Adv Neurol 2004; 94:275–285 (Fahn S, Hallett M, DeLong MR Dystonia 4).
2. Greene P, Kang UJ, Fahn S. Spread of symptoms in idiopathic torsion dystonia. Mov Disord 1995; 10(2):143–152.
3. Bressman SB, de Leon D, Brin MF, et al. Idiopathic dystonia among Ashkenazi Jews: evidence for autosomal dominant inheritance. Ann Neurol 1989; 26(5):612–620.
4. Bressman SB. Dystonia. Curr Opin Neurol 1998; 11(4):363–372.
5. Jarman PR, Warner TT. The dystonias. J Med Genet 1998; 35(4):314–318.
6. Bressman SB. Dystonia genotypes, phenotypes, and classification. Adv Neurol 2004; 94:101–107.
7. Bressman SB, Sabatti C, Raymond D, et al. The DYT1 phenotype and guidelines for diagnostic testing. Neurology 2000; 54(9):1746–1752.
8. Dauer WT, Burke RE, Greene P, Fahn S. Current concepts on the clinical features, aetiology and management of idiopathic cervical dystonia. Brain 1998; 121(Pt 4):547–560.
9. Ozelius LJ, Hewett JW, Page CE, et al. The early-onset torsion dystonia gene (DYT1) encodes an ATP-binding protein. Nat Genet 1997; 17(1):40–48.

10. Ludecke B, Dworniczak B, Bartholome K. A point mutation in the tyrosine hydroxylase gene associated with Segawa's syndrome. Hum Genet 1995; 95(1):123–125.

11. Cohen LG, Hallett M. Hand cramps: clinical features and electromyographic patterns in a focal dystonia. Neurology 1988; 38(7):1005–1012.

12. Rothwell JC, Obeso JA, Day BL, Marsden CD. Pathophysiology of dystonias. Adv Neurol 1983; 39:851–863.

13. Nakashima K, Rothwell JC, Day BL, et al. Reciprocal inhibition between forearm muscles in patients with writer's cramp and other occupational cramps, symptomatic hemidystonia and hemiparesis due to stroke. Brain 1989; 112(Pt 3): 681–697.

14. Panizza ME, Hallett M, Nilsson J. Reciprocal inhibition in patients with hand cramps. Neurology 1989; 39(1):85–89.

15. Chen RS, Tsai CH, Lu CS. Reciprocal inhibition in writer's cramp. Mov Disord 1995; 10(5):556–561.

16. Deuschl G, Seifert C, Heinen F, et al. Reciprocal inhibition of forearm flexor muscles in spasmodic torticollis. J Neurol Sci 1992; 113(1):85–90.

17. Valls-Sole J, Hallett M. Modulation of electromyographic activity of wrist flexor and extensor muscles in patients with writer's cramp. Mov Disord 1995; 10(6):741–748.

18. Vitek JL, Chockkan V, Zhang JY, et al. Neuronal activity in the basal ganglia in patients with generalized dystonia and hemiballismus. Ann Neurol 1999; 46(1):22–35.

19. Vitek JL. Pathophysiology of dystonia: a neuronal model. Mov Disord 2002; 17(suppl 3):S49–S62.

20. Vitek JL, Giroux M. Physiology of hypokinetic and hyperkinetic movement disorders: model for dyskinesia. Ann Neurol 2000; 47(4 suppl 1):S131–S140.

21. Gernert M, Bennay M, Fedrowitz M, et al. Altered discharge pattern of basal ganglia output neurons in an animal model of idiopathic dystonia. J Neurosci 2002; 22(16):7244–7253.

22. Lozano AM, Kumar R, Gross RE, et al. Globus pallidus internus pallidotomy for generalized dystonia. Mov Disord 1997; 12(6):865–870.

23. Ondo WG, Desaloms JM, Jankovic J, Grossman RG. Pallidotomy for generalized dystonia. Mov Disord 1998; 13(4):693–698.

24. Vitek JL, Zhang J, Evatt M, et al. GPi pallidotomy for dystonia: clinical outcome and neuronal activity. Adv Neurol 1998; 78:211–219.

25. Hallett M. Dystonia: abnormal movements result from loss of inhibition. Adv Neurol 2004; 94:1–9.

26. Mink JW. The basal banglia and involuntary movements: impaired inhibition of competing motor patterns. Arch Neurol 2003; 60(10):1365–1368.

27. Perlmutter JS, Stambuk MK, Markham J, et al. Decreased [18F]spiperone binding in putamen in idiopathic focal dystonia. J Neurosci 1997; 17(2):843–850.

28. Perlmutter JS, Stambuk MK, Markham J, et al. Decreased [18F]spiperone binding in putamen in dystonia. Adv Neurol 1998; 78:161–168.

29. Naumann M, Pirker W, Reiners K, et al. Imaging the pre- and postsynaptic side of striatal dopaminergic synapses in idiopathic cervical dystonia: a SPECT

study using [123I] epidepride and [123I] beta-CIT. Mov Disord 1998; 13(2): 319–323.

30. Knappskog PM, Flatmark T, Mallet J, et al. Recessively inherited L-DOPA-responsive dystonia caused by a point mutation (Q381K) in the tyrosine hydroxylase gene. Hum Mol Genet 1995; 4(7):1209–1212.

31. Ichinose H, Ohye T, Takahashi E, et al. Hereditary progressive dystonia with marked diurnal fluctuation caused by mutations in the GTP cyclohydrolase I gene. Nat Genet 1994; 8(3):236–242.

32. Burke RE, Fahn S, Jankovic J, et al. Tardive dystonia: late-onset and persistent dystonia caused by antipsychotic drugs. Neurology 1982; 32(12):1335–1346.

33. Augood SJ, Hollingsworth Z, Albers DS, et al. Dopamine transmission in DYT1 dystonia. Adv Neurol 2004; 94:53–60.

34. Walker RH, Brin MF, Sandu D, et al. Torsin A immunoreactivity in brains of patients with DYT1 and non-DYT1 dystonia. Neurology 2002; 58(1):120–124.

35. Rostasy K, Augood SJ, Hewett JW, et al. Torsin A protein and neuropathology in early onset generalized dystonia with GAG deletion. Neurobiol Dis 2003; 12(1):11–24.

36. Eidelberg D, Moeller JR, Ishikawa T, et al. The metabolic topography of idiopathic torsion dystonia. Brain 1995; 118(Pt 6):1473–1484.

37. Eidelberg D, Moeller JR, Antonini A, et al. Functional brain networks in DYT1 dystonia. Ann Neurol 1998; 44(3):303–312.

38. Carbon M, Su S, Dhawan V, et al. Regional metabolism in primary torsion dystonia: effects of penetrance and genotype. Neurology 2004; 62(8): 1384–1390.

39. Ghilardi MF, Carbon M, Silvestri G, et al. Sequence learning is impaired in clinically unaffected carriers of DYT1 mutation. Mov Disord 2002; 17(5):S300.

40. Augood SJ, Penney JB Jr, Friberg IK, et al. Expression of the early-onset torsion dystonia gene (DYT1) in human brain. Ann Neurol 1998; 43(5):669–673.

41. Augood SJ, Martin DM, Ozelius LJ, et al. Distribution of the mRNAs encoding Torsin A and Torsin B in the normal adult human brain. Ann Neurol 1999; 46(5):761–769.

42. Rouiller I, Butel VM, Latterich M, et al. A major conformational change in p97 AAA ATPase upon ATP binding. Mol Cell 2000; 6:1485–1490.

43. Zhang X, Shaw A, Bates PA, et al. Structure of the AAA ATPase p97. Mol Cell 2000; 6:1473–1484.

44. Rouiller I, DeLaBarre B, May AP, et al. Conformational changes of the multifunction p97 AAA ATPase during its ATPase cycle. Nat Struct Biol 2002; 9(12):950–957.

45. Dalal S, Hanson PI. Membrane traffic: what drives the AAA motor? Cell 2001; 104(1):5–8.

46. Kustedjo K, Bracey MH, Cravatt BF. Torsin A and its torsion dystonia-associated mutant forms are lumenal glycoproteins that exhibit distinct subcellular localizations. J Biol Chem 2000; 275(36):27933–27939.

47. Hewett J, Gonzalez-Agosti C, Slater D, et al. Mutant Torsin A, responsible for early-onset torsion dystonia, forms membrane inclusions in cultured neural cells. Hum Mol Genet 2000; 9(9):1403–1413.

48. O'Farrell C, Hernandez DG, Evey C, et al. Normal localization of deltaF323-Y328 mutant Torsin A in transfected human cells. Neurosci Lett 2002; 327(2):75–78.
49. Dauer W, Goodchild R. Mouse models of Torsin A dysfunction. Adv Neurol 2004; 94:67–72.
50. Shashidharan P, Walker RH, McNaught KS, Brin MF, Olanow CW. Transgenic mouse model of childhood-onset dystonia [abstract]. Mov Disord 2004; 19(suppl 9):S86–S87.
51. Opal P, Tintner R, Jankovic J, et al. Intrafamilial phenotypic variability of the DYT1 dystonia: from asymptomatic TOR1A gene carrier status to dystonic storm. Mov Disord 2002; 17(2):339–345.
52. Chen R, Hallett M. Focal dystonia and repetitive motion disorders. Clin Orthop 1998; 351:102–106.
53. Hinson VK, Goetz CG. Torsion Dystonia in Children. Curr Treat Options Neurol 2003; 5(4):291–297.
54. Krack P, Schneider S, Deuschl G. Geste device in tardive dystonia with retrocollis and opisthotonic posturing. Mov Disord 1998; 13(1):155–157.
55. Tas N, Karatas GK, Sepici V. Hand orthosis as a writing aid in writer's cramp. Mov Disord 2001; 16(6):1185–1189.
56. Pesenti A, Barbieri S, Priori A. Limb immobilization for occupational dystonia: a possible alternative treatment for selected patients. Adv Neurol 2004; 94:247–254.
57. Priori A, Pesenti A, Cappellari A, et al. Limb immobilization for the treatment of focal occupational dystonia. Neurology 2001; 57(3):405–409.
58. Candia V, Elbert T, Altenmuller E, et al. Constraint-induced movement therapy for focal hand dystonia in musicians. Lancet 1999; 353(9146):42.
59. Tinazzi M, Rosso T, Fiaschi A. Role of the somatosensory system in primary dystonia. Mov Disord 2003; 18(6):605–622.
60. Abbruzzese G, Berardelli A. Sensorimotor integration in movement disorders. Mov Disord 2003; 18(3):231–240.
61. Levy CE, Nichols DS, Schmalbrock PM, et al. Functional MRI evidence of cortical reorganization in upper-limb stroke hemiplegia treated with constraint-induced movement therapy. Am J Phys Med Rehabil 2001; 80(1): 4–12.
62. Taub E, Uswatte G, Morris DM. Improved motor recovery after stroke and massive cortical reorganization following constraint-induced movement therapy. Phys Med Rehabil Clin N Am 2003; 14(1 suppl):S77–S91.
63. Byl NN, McKenzie A. Treatment effectiveness for patients with a history of repetitive hand use and focal hand dystonia: a planned, prospective follow-up study. J Hand Ther 2000; 13(4):289–301.
64. Byl NN, Nagajaran S, McKenzie AL. Effect of sensory discrimination training on structure and function in patients with focal hand dystonia: a case series. Arch Phys Med Rehabil 2003; 84(10):1505–1514.
65. Jahanshahi M, Sartory G, Marsden CD. EMG biofeedback treatment of torticollis: a controlled outcome study. Biofeedback Self Regul 1991; 16(4): 413–448.

66. Korein J, Brudny J, Grynbaum B, et al. Sensory feedback therapy of spasmodic torticollis and dystonia: results in treatment of 55 patients. Adv Neurol 1976; 14:375–402.
67. Nygaard TG, Marsden CD, Fahn S. Dopa-responsive dystonia: long-term treatment response and prognosis. Neurology 1991; 41(2 Pt 1):174–181.
68. Wohrle JC, Weigel R, Grips E, et al. Risperidone-responsive segmental dystonia and pallidal deep brain stimulation. Neurology 2003; 61(4):546–548.
69. Grassi E, Latorraca S, Piacentini S, et al. Risperidone in idiopathic and symptomatic dystonia: preliminary experience. Neurol Sci 2000; 21(2):121–123.
70. Karp BI, Goldstein SR, Chen R, et al. An open trial of clozapine for dystonia. Mov Disord 1999; 14(4):652–657.
71. Zuddas A, Cianchetti C. Efficacy of risperidone in idiopathic segmental dystonia. Lancet 1996; 347(8994):127–128.
72. Jankovic J, Beach J. Long-term effects of tetrabenazine in hyperkinetic movement disorders. Neurology 1997; 48(2):358–362.
73. Hoon AH Jr, Freese PO, Reinhardt EM, et al. Age-dependent effects of trihexyphenidyl in extrapyramidal cerebral palsy. Pediatr Neurol 2001; 25(1):55–58.
74. Greene P, Shale H, Fahn S. Analysis of open-label trials in torsion dystonia using high dosages of anticholinergics and other drugs. Mov Disord 1988; 3(1):46–60.
75. Nance PW, Bugaresti J, Shellenberger K, et al. Efficacy and safety of tizanidine in the treatment of spasticity in patients with spinal cord injury. North American Tizanidine Study Group. Neurology 1994; 44(11 suppl 9):S44–S51.
76. Lang AE, Riley DE. Tizanidine in cranial dystonia. Clin Neuropharmacol 1992; 15(2):142–147.
77. ten Houten R, Lakke JP, de Jong P, et al. Spasmodic torticollis: treatment with Tizanidine. Acta Neurol Scand 1984; 70(5):373–376.
78. Greene P. Baclofen in the treatment of dystonia. Clin Neuropharmacol 1992; 15(4):276–288.
79. Greene PE, Fahn S. Baclofen in the treatment of idiopathic dystonia in children. Mov Disord 1992; 7(1):48–52.
80. Hou JG, Ondo W, Jankovic J. Intrathecal baclofen for dystonia. Mov Disord 2001; 16(6):1201–1202.
81. van Hilten JJ, Hoff JI, Thang MC, et al. Clinimetric issues of screening for responsiveness to intrathecal baclofen in dystonia. J Neural Transm 1999; 106(9–10):931–941.
82. Ford B, Greene PE, Louis ED, et al. Intrathecal baclofen in the treatment of dystonia. Adv Neurol 1998; 78:199–210.
83. Albright AL, Barry MJ, Fasick P, et al. Continuous intrathecal baclofen infusion for symptomatic generalized dystonia. Neurosurgery 1996; 38(5): 934–938.
84. Narayan RK, Loubser PG, Jankovic J, et al. Intrathecal baclofen for intractable axial dystonia. Neurology 1991; 41(7):1141–1142.
85. Butler C, Campbell S. Evidence of the effects of intrathecal baclofen for spastic and dystonic cerebral palsy. AACPDM Treatment Outcomes Committee Review Panel. Dev Med Child Neurol 2000; 42(9):634–645.

86. Walker RH, Danisi FO, Swope DM, et al. Intrathecal baclofen for dystonia: benefits and complications during six years of experience. Mov Disord 2000; 15(6):1242–1247.

87. Albright AL, Barry MJ, Shafton DH, Ferson SS. Intrathecal baclofen for generalized dystonia. Dev Med Child Neurol 2001; 43(10):652–657.

88. Berg D, Becker G, Naumann M, Reiners K. Morphine in tardive and idiopathic dystonia (short communication). J Neural Transm 2001; 108(8–9): 1035–1041.

89. Priori A, Bertolasi L, Pesenti A, et al. Gamma-hydroxybutyric acid for alcohol-sensitive myoclonus with dystonia. Neurology 2000; 54(8):1706.

90. Lucetti C, Nuti A, Gambaccini G, et al. Mexiletine in the treatment of torticollis and generalized dystonia. Clin Neuropharmacol 2000; 23(4):186–189.

91. Truong DD, Sandroni P, van den NS, Matsumoto RR. Diphenhydramine is effective in the treatment of idiopathic dystonia. Arch Neurol 1995; 52(4): 405–407.

92. Granana N, Ferrea M, Scorticati MC, et al. Beneficial effects of diphenhydramine in dystonia. Medicina (B Aires) 1999; 59(1):38–42.

93. Lang AE, Sheehy MP, Marsden CD. Anticholinergics in adult-onset focal dystonia. Can J Neurol Sci 1982; 9(3):313–319.

94. Lang AE. Antihistaminics in idiopathic dystonia. Arch Neurol 1996; 53(5):405.

95. Boghen DR, Lesser RL. Blepharospasm and hemifacial spasm. Curr Treat Options Neurol 2000; 2(5):393–400.

96. Hatheway CL. Botulism: the present status of the disease. Curr Top Microbiol Immunol 1995; 195:55–75.

97. Smith LD, Sugiyama H. Botulism: the organism, its toxins, the disease. Springfield, IL: C.C. Thomas Publisher, 1988.

98. Eleopra R, Tugnoli V, Quatrale R, et al. Different types of botulinum toxin in humans. Mov Disord 2004; 19(suppl 8):S53–S59.

99. Foran PG, Mohammed N, Lisk GO, et al. Evaluation of the therapeutic usefulness of botulinum neurotoxin B, C1, E, and F compared with the long lasting type A. Basis for distinct durations of inhibition of exocytosis in central neurons. J Biol Chem 2003; 278(2):1363–1371.

100. Rossetto O, Caccin P, Rigoni M, et al. The metalloprotease activity of tetanus and botulinum neurotoxins. In: Brin MF, Jankovic J, Hallett M, eds. Scientific and Therapeutic Aspects of Botulinum Toxin. Philadelphia: Lippincott Williams and Wilkins, 2002:3–10.

101. Angaut-Petit D, Molgo J, Comella JX, et al. Terminal sprouting in mouse neuromuscular junctions poisoned with botulinum type A toxin: morphological and electrophysiological features. Neuroscience 1990; 37(3): 799–808.

102. Meunier FA, Lisk G, Sesardic D, Dolly JO. Dynamics of motor nerve terminal remodeling unveiled using SNARE-cleaving botulinum toxins: the extent and duration are dictated by the sites of SNAP-25 truncation. Mol Cell Neurosci 2003; 22(4):454–466.

103. Sloop RR, Cole BA, Escutin RO. Human response to botulinum toxin injection: type B compared with type A. Neurology 1997; 49(1):189–194.

104. Jankovic J, Vuong KD, Ahsan J. Comparison of efficacy and immunogenicity of original versus current botulinum toxin in cervical dystonia. Neurology 2003; 60(7):1186–1188.
105. Rollnik JD, Wohlfarth K, Dengler R, Bigalke H. Neutralizing botulinum toxin type a antibodies: clinical observations in patients with cervical dystonia. Neurol Clin Neurophysiol 2001; 2001(3):2–4.
106. Hsiung GY, Das SK, Ranawaya R, et al. Long-term efficacy of botulinum toxin A in treatment of various movement disorders over a 10-year period. Mov Disord 2002; 17(6):1288–1293.
107. Calace P, Cortese G, Piscopo R, et al. Treatment of blepharospasm with botulinum neurotoxin type A: long-term results. Eur J Ophthalmol 2003; 13(4): 331–336.
108. Tan EK, Jankovic J. Botulinum toxin A in patients with oromandibular dystonia: long-term follow-up. Neurology 1999; 53(9):2102–2107.
109. Bhattacharyya N, Tarsy D. Impact on quality of life of botulinum toxin treatments for spasmodic dysphonia and oromandibular dystonia. Arch Otolaryngol Head Neck Surg 2001; 127(4):389–392.
110. Tan EK, Jankovic J. Tardive and idiopathic oromandibular dystonia: a clinical comparison. J Neurol Neurosurg Psychiatry 2000; 68(2):186–190.
111. Tisch SH, Brake HM, Law M, et al. Spasmodic dysphonia: clinical features and effects of botulinum toxin therapy in 169 patients—an Australian experience. J Clin Neurosci 2003; 10(4):434–438.
112. Rubin AD, Wodchis WP, Spak C, et al. Longitudinal effects of Botox injections on voice-related quality of life (V-RQOL) for patients with adductory spasmodic dysphonia: part II. Arch Otolaryngol Head Neck Surg 2004; 130(4):415–420.
113. Karp BI. Botulinum toxin treatment of occupational and focal hand dystonia. Mov Disord 2004; 19(suppl 8):S116–S119.
114. Marion MH, Afors K, Sheehy MP. [Problems of treating writer's cramp with botulinum toxin injections: results from 10 years of experience.] Rev Neurol (Paris) 2003; 159(10 Pt 1):923–927.
115. Molloy FM, Shill HA, Kaelin-Lang A, Karp BI. Accuracy of muscle localization without EMG: implications for treatment of limb dystonia. Neurology 2002; 58(5):805–807.
116. Weigel R, Rittmann M, Krauss JK. Spontaneous craniocervical osseous fusion resulting from cervical dystonia. Case report. J Neurosurg 2001; 95 (suppl 1):115–118.
117. Krauss JK, Koller R, Burgunder JM. Partial myotomy/myectomy of the trapezius muscle with an asleep–awake–asleep anesthetic technique for treatment of cervical dystonia. Technical note. J Neurosurg 1999; 91(5):889–891.
118. Freckmann N, Hagenah R, Herrmann HD, Muller D. Bilateral microsurgical lysis of the spinal accessory nerve roots for treatment of spasmodic torticollis. Follow up of 33 cases. Acta Neurochir (Wien) 1986; 83(1–2):47–53.
119. Freckmann N, Hagenah R. Relationship between the spinal accessory nerve and the posterior root of the first cervical nerve in spasmodic torticollis and common autopsy cases. Zentralbl Neurochir 1986; 47(2):134–138.
120. Gildenberg PL. Treatment of spasmodic torticollis by dorsal column stimulation. Appl Neurophysiol 1978; 41(1–4):113–121.

121. Vercueil L. Fifty years of brain surgery for dystonia: revisiting the Irving S. Cooper's legacy, and looking forward. Acta Neurol Belg 2003; 103(3):125–128.
122. Gros C, Frerebeau P, Perez-Dominguez E, et al. Long term results of stereotaxic surgery for infantile dystonia and dyskinesia. Neurochirurgia 1976; 19(4):171–178.
123. Burzaco J. Stereotactic pallidotomy in extrapyramidal disorders. Appl Neurophysiol 1985; 48(1–6):283–287.
124. Ondo WG, Desaloms JM, Jankovic J, Grossman RG. Pallidotomy for generalized dystonia. Mov Disord 1998; 13(4):693–698.
125. Hassler R, Dieckmann G. Stereotactic treatment of different kinds of spasmodic torticollis. Confin Neurol 1970; 32(2):135–143.
126. Andrew J, Fowler CJ, Harrison MJ. Stereotaxic thalamotomy in 55 cases of dystonia. Brain 1983; 106(Pt 4):981–1000.
127. Umemura A, Jaggi JL, Hurtig HI, et al. Deep Brain stimulation for movement disorders: morbidity and mortality in 109 patients. J Neurosurg 2002; 98: 779–784.
128. Volkmann J, Benecke R. Deep brain stimulation for dystonia: patient selection and evaluation. Mov Disord 2002; 17(suppl 3):S112–S115.
129. Lenz FA, Suarez JI, Metman LV, et al. Pallidal activity during dystonia: somatosensory reorganisation and changes with severity. J Neurol Neurosurg Psychiatry 1998; 65(5):767–770.
130. Lozano AM, Lang AE, Galvez-Jimenez N, et al. Effect of GPi pallidotomy on motor function in Parkinson's disease. Lancet 1995; 346(8987): 1383–1387.
131. Iacono RP, Kuniyoshi SM, Lonser RR, et al. Simultaneous bilateral pallidoansotomy for idiopathic dystonia musculorum deformans. Pediatr Neurol 1996; 14(2):145–148.
132. Jankovic J, Lai EC, Krauss J, Grossman R. Surgical treatment of levo-dopa induced dyskinesias Adv Neurol 1999; 80:603–609 (Stern GM. Parkinson's Disease: Advances in Neurology. Stern GM. Philadelphia: Lippincott Raven).
133. Yianni J, Bain PG, Gregory RP, et al. Post-operative progress of dystonia patients following globus pallidus internus deep brain stimulation. Eur J Neurol 2003; 10(3):239–247.
134. Cif L, El Fertit H, Vayssiere N, et al. Treatment of dystonic syndromes by chronic electrical stimulation of the internal globus pallidus. J Neurosurg Sci 2003; 47(1):52–55.
135. Yianni J, Bain P, Giladi N, et al. Globus pallidus internus deep brain stimulation for dystonic conditions: a prospective audit. Mov Disord 2003; 18(4): 436–442.
136. Vercueil L, Pollak P, Fraix V, et al. Deep brain stimulation in the treatment of severe dystonia. J Neurol 2001; 248(8):695–700.
137. Krauss JK, Loher TJ, Pohle T, et al. Pallidal deep brain stimulation in patients with cervical dystonia and severe cervical dyskinesias with cervical myelopathy. J Neurol Neurosurg Psychiatry 2002; 72(2):249–256.
138. Krauss JK, Loher TJ, Weigel R, et al. Chronic stimulation of the globus pallidus internus for treatment of non-DYT1 generalized dystonia and choreoathetosis: 2-year follow up. J Neurosurg 2003; 98(4):785–792.

139. Eltahawy HA, Saint-Cyr J, Giladi N, et al. Primary dystonia is more responsive than secondary dystonia to pallidal interventions: outcome after pallidotomy or pallidal deep brain stimulation. Neurosurgery 2004; 54(3):613–619.
140. Bereznai B, Steude U, Seelos K, Botzel K. Chronic high-frequency globus pallidus internus stimulation in different types of dystonia: a clinical, video, and MRI report of six patients presenting with segmental, cervical, and generalized dystonia. Mov Disord 2002; 17(1):138–144.
141. Katayama Y, Fukaya C, Kobayashi K, et al. Chronic stimulation of the globus pallidus internus for control of primary generalized dystonia. Acta Neurochir Suppl 2003; 87:125–128.
142. Vesper J, Klostermann F, Funk T, et al. Deep brain stimulation of the globus pallidus internus (Gpi) for torsion dystonia—a report of two cases. Acta Neurochir Suppl 2002; 79:83–88.
143. Kumar R, Dagher A, Hutchison WD, et al. Globus pallidus deep brain stimulation for generalized dystonia: clinical and PET investigation. Neurology 1999; 53(4):871–874.
144. Loher TJ, Hasdemir MG, Burgunder JM, Krauss JK. Long-term follow-up study of chronic globus pallidus internus stimulation for post-traumatic hemidystonia. J Neurosurg 2000; 92(3):457–460.
145. Chang JW, Choi JY, Lee BW, et al. Unilateral globus pallidus internus stimulation improves delayed onset post-traumatic cervical dystonia with an ipsilateral focal basal ganglia lesion. J Neurol Neurosurg Psychiatry 2002; 73(5):588–590.
146. Islekel S, Zileli M, Zileli B. Unilateral pallidal stimulation in cervical dystonia. Stereotact Funct Neurosurg 1999; 72(2–4):248–252.
147. Ghika J, Villemure JG, Miklossy J, et al. Postanoxic generalized dystonia improved by bilateral VOA thalamic deep brain stimulation. Neurology 2002; 58(2):311–313.
148. Andaluz N, Taha JM, Dalvi A. Bilateral pallidal deep brain stimulation for cervical and truncal dystonia. Neurology 2001; 57(3):557–558.
149. Kulisevsky J, Lleo A, Gironell A, et al. Bilateral pallidal stimulation for cervical dystonia: dissociated pain and motor improvement. Neurology 2000; 55(11):1754–1755.
150. Cervera A, Vallderiola F, Marti MJ, Molinuevo JL, Pilleri M, Tolosa E. Worsening of dystonia after pallidal surgery [abstr]. Mov Disord 2000; 15(suppl 3):167.
151. Coubes P, Roubertie A, Vayssiere N, et al. Treatment of DYT1-generalised dystonia by stimulation of the internal globus pallidus. Lancet 2000; 355(9222):2220–2221.
152. Islekel S, Cakmur R, Zileli M, Zileli B. Pallidal stimulation: an effective method in the treatment of spasmodic torticollis [abstract]. Mov Disord 2000; 15(suppl 3):162.
153. Krauss JK, Pohle T, Weber S, et al. Bilateral stimulation of globus pallidus internus for treatment of cervical dystonia. Lancet 1999; 354(9181):837–838.
154. Trottenberg T, Paul G, Meissner W, et al. Pallidal and thalamic neurostimulation in severe tardive dystonia. J Neurol Neurosurg Psychiatry 2001; 70(4): 557–559.

155. Tronnier VM, Fogel W. Pallidal stimulation for generalized dystonia. Report of three cases. J Neurosurg 2000; 92(3):453–456.
156. Parkin S, Aziz T, Gregory R, Bain P. Bilateral internal globus pallidus stimulation for the treatment of spasmodic torticollis. Mov Disord 2001; 16(3):489–493.
157. Liu X, Griffin IC, Parkin SG, et al. Involvement of the medial pallidum in focal myoclonic dystonia: a clinical and neurophysiological case study. Mov Disord 2002; 17(2):346–353.
158. Detante O, Vercueil L, Krack P, et al. Off-period dystonia in Parkinson's disease but not generalized dystonia is improved by high-frequency stimulation of the subthalamic nucleus. Adv Neurol 2004; 94:309–314.
159. Albin RL, Young AB, Penney JB. The functional anatomy of basal ganglia disorders. Trends Neurosci 1989; 12(10):366–375.
160. Black KJ, Gado MH, Perlmutter JS. PET measurement of dopamine D2 receptor-mediated changes in striatopallidal function. J Neurosci 1997; 17(9):3168–3177.
161. Hamada I, DeLong MR. Excitotoxic acid lesions of the primate subthalamic nucleus result in reduced pallidal neuronal activity during active holding. J Neurophysiol 1992; 68(5):1859–1866.
162. Hamada I, DeLong MR. Excitotoxic acid lesions of the primate subthalamic nucleus result in transient dyskinesias of the contralateral limbs. J Neurophysiol 1992; 68(5):1850–1858.
163. Eidelberg D, Moeller JR, Ishikawa T, et al. The metabolic topography of idiopathic torsion dystonia. Brain 1995; 118(Pt 6):1473–1484.
164. Ceballos-Baumann A, Brooks D. Activation positron emission tomography scanning in dystonia. Adv Neurol 1998; 78:135–142 (In: Fahn S, Marsden CD, DeLong MR, eds. Philadelphia: Lipincott-Raven, Dystonia 3).
165. Ikoma K, Samii A, Mercuri B, et al. Abnormal cortical motor excitability in dystonia. Neurology 1996; 46(5):1371–1376.
166. Ceballos-Baumann AO, Passingham RE, Warner T, et al. Overactive prefrontal and underactive motor cortical areas in idiopathic dystonia. Ann Neurol 1995; 37(3):363–372.
167. Benabid AL, Koudsie A, Benazzouz A, et al. Deep brain stimulation of the corpus luysi (subthalamic nucleus) and other targets in Parkinson's disease. Extension to new indications such as dystonia and epilepsy. J Neurol 2001; 248(suppl 3):III37–III47.
168. Loher TJ, Burgunder JM, Weber S, et al. Effect of chronic pallidal deep brain stimulation on off period dystonia and sensory symptoms in advanced Parkinson's disease. J Neurol Neurosurg Psychiatry 2002; 73(4):395–399.
169. Krack P, Pollak P, Limousin P, et al. From off-period dystonia to peak-dose chorea. The clinical spectrum of varying subthalamic nucleus activity. Brain 1999; 122(Pt 6):1133–1146.
170. Oh M, Abosch A, Kim S, et al. Long-term hardware-related complications of deep brain stimulation. Neurosurgery 2002; 50(6):1268–1274.
171. Vitek JL, Bakay RA, DeLong MR. Microelectrode-guided pallidotomy for medically intractable Parkinson's disease. Adv Neurol 1997; 74:183–198.
172. Lozano A, Hutchison W, Kiss Z, et al. Methods for microelectrode-guided posteroventral pallidotomy. J Neurosurg 1996; 84(2):194–202.

173. Vinas FC, Zamorano L, Buciuc R, et al. Application accuracy study of a semi-permanent fiducial system for frameless stereotaxis. Comput Aided Surg 1997; 2(5):257–263.
174. Lee MH, Lufkin RB, Borges A, et al. MR-guided procedures using contemporaneous imaging frameless stereotaxis in an open-configuration system. J Comput Assist Tomogr 1998; 22(6):998–1005.
175. Varma TR, Fox SH, Eldridge PR, et al. Deep brain stimulation of the subthalamic nucleus: effectiveness in advanced Parkinson's disease patients previously reliant on apomorphine. J Neurol Neurosurg Psychiatry 2003; 74(2):170–174.
176. Helm PA, Eckel TS. Accuracy of registration methods in frameless stereotaxis. Comput Aided Surg 1998; 3(2):51–56.
177. Hariz MI. Safety and risk of microelectrode recording in surgery for movement disorders. Stereotact Funct Neurosurg 2002; 78(3–4):146–157.
178. Hariz MI, Fodstad H. Do microelectrode techniques increase accuracy or decrease risks in pallidotomy and deep brain stimulation? A critical review of the literature. Stereotact Funct Neurosurg 1999; 72(2–4):157–169.
179. Bejjani BP, Arnulf I, Vidailhet M, et al. Irregular jerky tremor, myoclonus, and thalamus: a study using low-frequency stimulation. Mov Disord 2000; 15(5):919–924.
180. Ford B. Pallidotomy for generalized dystonia. Adv Neurol 2004; 94:287–299.
181. Ghika J, Ghika-Schmid F, Fankhauser H, et al. Bilateral contemporaneous posteroventral pallidotomy for the treatment of Parkinson's disease: neuro-psychological and neurological side effects. Report of four cases and review of the literature. J Neurosurg 1999; 91(2):313–321.
182. Abosch A, Vitek JL, Lozano AM. Pallidotomy and pallidal deep brain stimulation for dystonia. Tarsy D, Vitek JL, Lozano AM, eds. Surgical Treatment of Parkinson's Disease and Other Movement Disorders. Totowa, NJ: Humana Press, 2003:265–274.
183. Krack P, Vercueil L. Review of the functional surgical treatment of dystonia. Eur J Neurol 2001; 8(5):389–399.
184. Kupsch A, Kuehn A, Klaffke S, et al. Deep brain stimulation in dystonia. J Neurol 2003; 250(suppl 1):I47–I52.
185. Tagliati M, Miravite J, Shils SB, Bressman SB, Saunders-Pullman R, Alterman R. Long-term efficacy of pallidal DBS for treatment of medically refractory dystonia [abstract]. Mov Disord 2004; 19(suppl 9):S321–S322.
186. Vercueil L, Krack P, Pollak P. Results of deep brain stimulation for dystonia: a critical reappraisal. Mov Disord 2002; 17(suppl 3):S89–S93.
187. Fogel W, Krause M, Tronnier V. Globus pallidus stimulation in generalized dystonia: clinical data. Mov Disord 2000; 15(suppl 3):S144.
188. Chang JW, Choi JY, Lee BW, et al. Unilateral globus pallidus internus stimulation improves delayed onset post-traumatic cervical dystonia with an ipsilateral focal basal ganglia lesion. J Neurol Neurosurg Psychiatry 2002; 73(5):588–590.
189. Lin JJ, Lin SZ, Chang DC. Pallidotomy and generalized dystonia. Mov Disord 1999; 14(6):1057–1059.

190. Trottenberg T, Paul G, Meissner W, et al. Pallidal and thalamic neurostimulation in severe tardive dystonia. J Neurol Neurosurg Psychiatry 2001; 70(4):557–559.

191. Loher TJ, Hasdemir MG, Burgunder JM, Krauss JK. Long-term follow-up study of chronic globus pallidus internus stimulation for posttraumatic hemidystonia. J Neurosurg 2000; 92(3):457–460.

192. Trottenberg T, Volkmann J, Deuschl G, Schrader B, Schneider GH, Kupsch A. Post-operative progress of severe tardive dystonia and dyskinesia following globus pallidus internus deep brain stimulation [abstract]. Mov Disord 2004; 19(suppl 9):S299.

193. Lozano AM, Abosch A. Pallidal stimulation for dystonia. Adv Neurol 2004; 94:301–308.

194. Grips E, Capelle HH, Blahak C, Hennerici MG, Krauss JK, Wohrle JC. Pattern of recurrence of dystonia after discontinuation of chronic deep brain stimulation [abstract]. Mov Disord 2004; 19(suppl 9):S95.

9

Chemodenervation: Botulinum Toxin

Tanya Simuni

Department of Neurology, Feinberg School of Medicine,
Northwestern University, Chicago, Illinois, U.S.A.

1. INTRODUCTION

Cervical dystonia (CD) is characterized by involuntary spasms of neck muscles that cause abnormal head and neck movements and postures (1). The term spasmodic torticollis is frequently used to describe this condition, but it applies only to one type of CD manifested by jerky (spasmodic) head movement associated with head turning (torticollis). CD is the preferred term to describe focal dystonia that involves neck muscles. CD is the most common type of adult onset focal dystonia (2). CD prevalence is estimated at 9/100,000, but it is likely higher as that number was based on a retrospective chart review (3). The etiology of CD varies. The majority of patients have idiopathic CD, which means that there is no identifiable cause. Some patients with idiopathic CD have a genetic cause; however, genetic contribution to focal dystonia has been much less studied compared to generalized dystonias like DYT1 (4). The most common symptomatic causes of CD are drugs and trauma (5). Drug-induced CD can occur as an acute reaction to neuroleptics or related compounds, which is reversible with discontinuation of the drug, or can be a manifestation of tardive dyskinesia, in which case it is chronic with low chance for remission (6). The relationship between CD and peripheral neck injury remains debated (7,8). A number of patients report "significant" neck injury within a year prior to onset of CD. The causality of such injury has not been established, but the possibility of the

contribution of peripheral mechanisms to development of CD via involvement of the sensory feedback loops cannot be excluded (9,10). A number of
other neurological and non-neurological conditions can present with abnormal head postures and should not be misdiagnosed as CD (11). The most
important conditions for screening include atlanto-axial dislocation, cervical
fracture, or other bone abnormalities of the cervical spine (11). In the majority
of cases, these conditions lead to a fixed and sustained abnormal posture of
the neck, which is atypical for CD. Appropriate imaging of the cervical spine
and brain should be performed when a structural cause of CD is suspected.

  Clinical manifestations of CD are variable. Apart from torticollis (head
turn), the patients can have anterocollis (neck flexion), retrocollis (neck
extension), laterocollis (head tilt), or a combination of above (Fig. 1). CD
is frequently accompanied by dystonic head tremor, which is believed to be
caused by repetitive dystonic contractures of the involved neck muscles (2).
Some patients can have dystonic tremor as the major manifestation of CD.
The diagnosis of CD is based on the clinical examination and observation
of the type of head and neck posturing. Routine imaging is not necessary
unless a symptomatic cause of CD is suspected or the patient has atypical

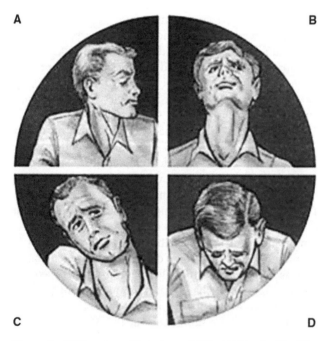

Figure 1 Different manifestations of CD. (A) Torticollis; (B) retrocollis; (C) laterocollis; (D) anterocollis. *Source*: From the National Spasmodic Torticollis Association,
http://torticollis.org/.

findings on the exam. Patients with young onset CD should be screened for Wilson's disease (2).

CD is a chronic condition. Idiopathic CD usually has an insidious onset with gradual progression of symptoms within 3–5 years from onset (12). The majority of patients have stabilization of symptoms at some point. It is not unusual for CD to have segmental spread (involving adjoining muscles of the face or upper limb) but the risk of generalization with an adult onset of CD is low (2). Spontaneous remission of CD is reported in up to 20% of cases, but it is usually short lived and incomplete (13,14).

Treatment choices for CD include oral pharmacotherapy, chemo-denervation by botulinum toxin injections, and surgical intervention. Choices of oral pharmacotherapy include anticholinergics (trihexyphenidyl), anti-spasmodic medications (baclofen or tizanidine), and muscle relaxants (15). Unfortunately, all are only partially effective and are associated with medica-tion-induced side effects, which limit their use (15). Anticholinergics are the most effective drugs for treatment of dystonia. In one study, 39% of patients with CD experienced benefit with trihexyphenidyl, but use of the drug was limited by undesirable side effects of sedation, cognitive changes, urinary retention, and other undesirable anticholinergic side effects (16). Surgical treatment in the form of selective peripheral denervation and pallidal ablative or stimulating procedures is reserved for patients with refractory CD, and will be covered later in this volume. The rest of the chapter will be dedicated to reviewing of the role of chemodenervation in the management of CD.

Chemodenervation with botulinum toxin (BTX Botox®) has become the first-line treatment for management of CD (17–20). It truly has revolutio-nized treatment of CD and other focal dystonias by producing significant and sustained relief of the symptoms. The first monograph on botulinum toxin, then labeled as "sausage poison," was published by Justinus Kerner (21), a German medical officer, in 1820. Even then he envisioned the use of toxin for therapeutic indications (22). However, it was not until the 1980s that use of BTX for chemodenervation was pioneered by Alan Scott, an ophthal-mologist, who demonstrated its efficacy for the treatment of strabismus (23). Originally, BTX-A was approved for management of strabismus and blepha-rospasm, but it is now used for a variety of focal dystonias, including CD.

BTX is a complex protein produced by *Clostridium botulinum*, an anaerobic bacterium. BTX is the most potent known neurotoxic substance, which has a median lethal dose of 40 ng/kg body weight of an adult rat (24). The therapeutic effect of the toxin is via blockade of the presynaptic release of acetylcholine at the neuromuscular junction, which leads to temporary chemodenervation of the injected muscle and results in reduction of muscu-lar contraction (24). There are seven immunologically distinct serotypes of BTX, labeled from A to G (25). BTX A and B are commercially available in the United States and labeled for use in CD.

2. CLINICAL EFFICACY OF BTX-A FOR CD

BTX-A was the only strain of BTX commercially available until approval of BTX-B in 2000. The efficacy and safety of BTX-A for treatment of CD has been demonstrated in a number of controlled and open-label trials (17,19,26–29). Efficacy generally is higher in the open-label trials, which is attributed to potential placebo effect but also to the ability to individualize the dose and injection sites with open-label protocols (18,30). A phase III double-blind randomized placebo-controlled study was conducted by Allergan (31) and enrolled 214 subjects. In order to qualify for the study, the patients had to receive BTX-A for CD before and demonstrated good response and tolerable side effects. The patients were randomized to BTX-A versus placebo and followed for at least 10 weeks postinjection. The primary study outcome was the Cervical Dystonia Severity Scale (CDSS), which is an objective measure of CD severity based on the measurement of angle of head deviation in all three planes as well as change in the Global Assessment Scale (32). The impact of injection on CD pain was also measured. The study demonstrated significant benefit of active treatment versus placebo on all scales but the degree was modest. Most of the patients returned to baseline within 3 months.

In an open-label study of 303 patients with medically refractory CD, Jancovic et al. (33) demonstrated that 92% of the patients had improvement in function and control of head movement, and 93% of patients had marked improvement in pain. The average time to onset of benefit was 1 week, and average duration of sustained benefit 3.5 months. Fourteen percent of patients failed to improve after the first injection, but only 6% had no response with repeated attempts. The same authors have noted that optimal response was more likely if the dose and site for the injection were adjusted at each subsequent visit (29).

The degree of efficacy of BTX-A injections is directly related to the correct selection of the muscles involved and to the appropriate dose of the toxin (33) (Fig. 2). Generally patients with "simple" CD like laterocollis and torticollis as well as those with shorter duration of the symptoms have better response to the injections compared to patients with anterocollis and mixed CD (33). Selection of muscles for the injection usually is made based on the observation of the pattern of CD and palpation of the muscles involved (18). There is a debate regarding utility of electromyography (EMG) guidance for better selection of the muscles (19). Some studies report a better response to the injection when EMG was used for muscles selection (19,34). Comella et al. (19,34) demonstrated that use of EMG-guidance significantly increased the percentage of patients who had marked improvement with injection as determined by the Toronto Western Spasmodic Torticollis Rating Scale (TWSTR) (35). In another study, injection without EMG missed the target muscle in 17% of the 139 injections (36). While EMG is of value in some cases where the muscles involved are difficult to localize, the majority of clinicians

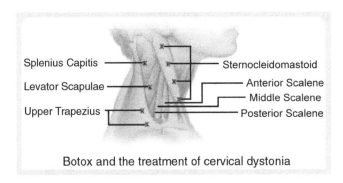

Figure 2 Lateral view of the neck exposing the most commonly injected muscles in CD. *Source*: From Allergan, Inc., Irvine, CA, http://www.botox.com.

perform routine CD injections based on palpation and observation of the involved muscles (18,37).

There are guidelines on the average injected dose of toxin for the most commonly involved muscles in CD (31). The median total dose of BTX-A in a study of 88 patients with good response to the injections was 236 U, with 25th to 75th percentile ranges of 198–300 U (31). The most commonly injected muscles and recommended doses of BTX-A per muscle are listed in Tables 1 and 2. BTX-A is marketed by Allergan, Inc., as Botox in the United States and as Dysport in the United Kingdom. The doses listed in the following text are related to Botox preparation. Most studies support 3:1 dose equivalency ratio for conversion between Dysport and Botox (38,39).

BTX-A is generally very well tolerated when administered in appropriate doses in the correct muscles. The most common injection-related side effects include dysphagia (19%), neck weakness, and local pain (11%), and upper respiratory infection (12%) (31). These are usually transitory and mild.

Table 1 Cervical Muscles Involved in Various Types of CD

Torticollis	Contralateral sternocleidomastoid, ipsilateral splenius, and trapezius
Laterocollis	Ipsilateral sternocleidomastoid, splinius capitis, scalene complex, levator scapulae
Shoulder elevation	Ipsilateral trapezuis and levator scapulae
Retrocollis	Bilateral splenius capitis, trapezuis, deep posterior vertebrals
Anterocollis	Bilateral sternocleidomastoids, scalene complex, submental complex

Source: Adapted from Ref. 5.

Table 2 Cervical Muscles Frequently Injected for CD

Muscle	Number of patients treated in this muscle ($N = 88$)	Mean % dose per muscle	Average dose of Botox per muscle (U)
Splenius capitis	83	38	60–100
Sternocleidomastoid	77	25	40–70
Levator scapulae	52	20	25–60
Trapezius	49	29	25–100
Semispinalis	16	21	30–60
Scalene complex	15	15	15–50
Longissimus	8	29	55–90

Source: Adapted from Botox (botulinum toxin type A), purified neurotoxin complex, product information. http://www.botox.com/prescribing_info.html, accessed 2004.

Jancovic et al. (33) reported their group's long-term experience with BTX-A injections: dysphagia was encountered in 14% of 659 visits but only in five cases was it severe enough to require a change of diet. The mechanism of development of dysphagia is likely related to direct versus hematogenous spread of toxin from the injection site (40). Women with thin necks are more prone to development of that complication. Bilateral injection of sternocleidomastoid muscle also increases the risk of development of swallowing dysfunction (33,41). Other injection-related side effects that have been reported in 2–10% of the patients include flu symptoms, rhinitis, soreness at the injection site, and drowsiness (31). Most side effects resolve spontaneously within 2 weeks (18).

The average duration of benefit of BTX-A injection is 3–4 months (33,42). The beneficial effect of the injections is usually sustained with the repeated injections (43,44). One long-term study showed that 75% of patients had persistent benefit for at least 5 years, and only 7.5% developed secondary unresponsiveness (45). However, one of the major concerns regarding long-term use of BTX-A is the development of secondary resistance to the injections (33,46). That phenomenon is attributed to the development of antibodies that neutralize toxin (47). The rate of development of antibodies has not been well studied. It is believed that antigenicity of BTX is related to the amount of neurotoxin complex protein in the preparation (18). The original Botox® (lot 79–11) contained 25 ng of protein, while the new Botox preparation approved in 1997 contains only 5 ng of protein per 100 units (48). Two preparations have been shown to be equivalent in efficacy and tolerability (49,50). The rate of development of antibodies with the new preparation seems to be lower: in the group of patients who were previously treated for CD with the original strain (lot 79–11), 33 of 192 (17%) were antibody positive while only 2 of 96 patients (2%) who were antibody negative at the baseline developed antibodies after receiving two injections with the new strain (31). Jancovic (18) reported that the new strain decreased the risk of antibody development by a factor of 6. There are several methods to detect antibodies (51). The mouse protection assay (MPA) correlates best with the clinical resistance to BTX (52). However, an immunoprecipitation assay (IPA), which is the quantitative measure of the degree of immunoresistance, has been shown to be more sensitive than MPA and can have a predictive value in determining future or impending unresponsiveness (53). BTX resistance can also be confirmed clinically by performing the unilateral brow injection (UBI) test or frontalis type A toxin (F-TAT) injection (18). Both tests consist of injecting a small dose of BTX-A in the selected forehead muscle on one side. Lack of facial asymmetry at the site of the injected muscle supports BTX-A resistance. The degree of facial asymmetry if the patient is BTX-A responsive is small and usually cosmetically acceptable. Both tests correlate well with MPA results and clinical BTX-A responsiveness (52). These tests can avoid the cost of obtaining the formal immunoassays. Another major determinant of development of BTX-A resistance is the dose and frequency of the injections (33,54). Patients should be injected with the smallest effective dose at an interval of at least 3 months (19). Booster injections are discouraged due to increased risk of development of resistance (19). Some patients who developed antibodies can revert to antibody negative status and again become BTX-A sensitive, but the time to conversion takes on average 30 months (55). Besides, 50% of them lose responsiveness to BTX-A within a relatively short period of time (55). Availability of other strains of BTX offers patients alternative choices. Patients who developed resistance to BTX-A usually respond to injections with the other BTX strains as they are considered immunologically distinct (56–60). However, cross-reactivity between BTX strains cannot be excluded completely (61). Further studies are necessary to determine whether development of antibodies against one strain makes the patients more susceptible to becoming resistant to another strain of BTX (62).

3. BTX-B

BTX-B is an alternative strain of BTX (63). BTX-B is commercially available under the brand name of Myobloc. BTX-B is antigenically different from BTX-A and inhibits acetylcholine release by a different mechanism of action (64). BTX-B was studied for efficacy and safety in CD in three pivotal placebo-controlled randomized studies (57–59). All studies used TWSTRS as the primary outcome measure. Efficacy of BTX-B was evaluated both in BTX-A responsive and resistant patients. BTX-A resistance was determined based on clinical history, presence of antibodies on MPA assay, and positive F-TAT test (58,59). BTX-B was shown to be effective as measured by the change of the TWSTRS score at 4 weeks after the injection, compared to placebo in both groups of patients (57–59). Patients also demonstrated a significant reduction in pain score (57–59). The most effective dose was 10,000 U. The median duration of response was 12–16 weeks.

The most common adverse events included dysphagia and dry mouth (57–59). Dysphagia was reported in up to 28% of patients treated with 10,000 U of BTX-B. The degree of dysphagia was mild to moderate. No cases of severe dysphagia were reported. Dry mouth was reported in 16% of patients in all three studies. The severity was mild to moderate. The other adverse events included pain at the injection site, headache, and flu like symptoms. None of the patients withdrew from the studies due to side effects. The aforementioned studies did not have a direct comparison between BTX-A and -B efficacy in CD. The Dystonia Study Group has recently completed such a study (AB-CD study), but the data have not yet been published. Based on the clinical experience, the efficacy of two preparations is similar when comparable doses are used. The AB-CD study used a conversion ratio of 1 U of BTX-A (Botox) to 50 U of BTX-B (Myobloc). However, a fixed conversion rate should be used with caution as the individual sensitivity of patients to different strains of BTX can vary. Generally, BTX-B is reserved for the patients who developed BTX-A resistance or have insufficient response to it. The injection of BTX-B is more painful due to the higher acidity of the preparation, but has the benefit of the toxin being supplied in the diluted form ready for the injection.

4. OTHER BTX STRAINS

BTX-F is another strain of BTX that is not commercially available but has been studied for efficacy in CD (60,65,66). BTX-F was demonstrated to be effective in a small group of BTX-A-resistant patients (60). However, a subset of patients has subsequently developed resistance to BTX-F as well (60). Besides, BTX-F has a relatively short duration of benefit, averaging 7.9 weeks (65). For those reasons, it is unlikely that BTX-F will become commercially available.

There is very limited experience with use of other strains of BTX in humans (25). BTX-C seems to have a mechanism and duration of action similar to BTX-A (67,68). Injection of two patients with hemifacial spasm and one patient with blepharospasm resulted in sustained benefit and was well tolerated (67). BTX-E is immunologically similar to BTX-A but the duration of effect is much shorter (69,70). Short duration of action makes BTX-E an unlikely alternative to BTX-A in clinical use.

5. CONCLUSIONS

BTX injections are effective and safe for treatment of CD. In order to maximize the benefit and decrease the risk of injections physicians should follow certain guidelines. The Therapeutic and Technology Subcommittee of the American Academy of Neurology (AAN) has proposed specific training guidelines for the use of BTX for treatment of neurological disorders (71). While the AAN does not require special certification for BTX administration, the guidelines highlight the need for prerequisite skills and knowledge of BTX application in clinical practice, familiarity of the physician with clinical presentation of various dystonias, anatomy of the muscles involved, and ability to modify treatment based on the response. Appropriate use of BTX in the smallest effective dose at the longest possible interval in correctly selected muscles increases the benefit of the injections and minimizes the immediate side effects as well as the risk of development of BTX resistance.

REFERENCES

1. Chan J, Brin MF, Fahn S. Idiopathic cervical dystonia: clinical characteristics. Mov Disord 1991; 6(2):119–126.
2. Dauer WT, Burke RE, Greene P, Fahn S. Current concepts on the clinical features, aetiology and management of idiopathic cervical dystonia. Brain 1998; 121(Pt 4):547–560.
3. Nutt JG, Muenter MD, Aronson A, Kurland LT, Melton LJ III. Epidemiology of focal and generalized dystonia in Rochester, Minnesota. Mov Disord 1988; 3(3):188–194.
4. Stacy M. Idiopathic cervical dystonia: an overview. Neurology 2000; 55(12 suppl 5):S2–S8.
5. Jankovic J. Treatment of cervical dystonia. In: Brin MF, Comella CL, Jankovic J, eds. Dystonia: Etiology, Clinical Features, and Treatment. Philadelphia, PA: Lippincott, 2004; 159–166.
6. Adityanjee, Aderibigbe YA, Jampala VC, Mathews T. The current status of tardive dystonia. Biol Psychiatry 1999; 45(6):715–730.
7. Jankovic J. Can peripheral trauma induce dystonia and other movement disorders? Yes! Mov Disord 2001; 16(1):7–12.
8. Weiner WJ. Can peripheral trauma induce dystonia? No! Mov Disord 2001; 16(1):13–22.
9. Tarsy D. Comparison of acute- and delayed-onset posttraumatic cervical dystonia. Mov Disord 1998; 13(3):481–485.
10. Jankovic J. Post-traumatic movement disorders: central and peripheral mechanisms. Neurology 1994; 44(11):2006–2014.
11. Suchowersky O, Calne DB. Non-dystonic causes of torticollis. Adv Neurol 1988; 50:501–508.
12. Lowenstein DH, Aminoff MJ. The clinical course of spasmodic torticollis. Neurology 1988; 38(4):530–532.
13. Jayne D, Lees AJ, Stern GM. Remission in spasmodic torticollis. J Neurol Neurosurg Psychiatry 1984; 47(11):1236–1237.
14. Friedman A, Fahn S. Spontaneous remissions in spasmodic torticollis. Neurology 1986; 36(3):398–400.

15. Jankovic J. Dystonia: medical therapy and botulinum toxin. Adv Neurol 2004; 94:275–286.
16. Greene P, Shale H, Fahn S. Analysis of open-label trials in torsion dystonia using high dosages of anticholinergics and other drugs. Mov Disord 1988; 3:46–60.
17. Poewe W, Schelosky L, Kleedorfer B, Heinen F, Wagner M, Deuschl G. Treatment of spasmodic torticollis with local injections of botulinum toxin. One-year follow-up in 37 patients. J Neurol 1992; 239(1):21–25.
18. Jankovic J. Treatment of cervical dystonia with botulinum toxin. Mov Disord 2004; 19(suppl 8):S109–S115.
19. Comella CL, Jankovic J, Brin MF. Use of botulinum toxin type A in the treatment of cervical dystonia. Neurology 2000; 55(12 suppl 5):S15–S21.
20. Ceballos-Baumann AO. Evidence-based medicine in botulinum toxin therapy for cervical dystonia. J Neurol 2001; 248(suppl 1):14–20.
21. Kerner J. Neue Beobachtungen Uber Die In Wurttemberg so Haufig orfallenden todlichen Vergiftungen durch den Gennus geraucherter Wurste. Tubingen: Osiander, 1820.
22. Erbguth FJ. Botulinum toxin, a historical note. Lancet 1998; 351(9118):1820.
23. Scott AB, Rosenbaum A, Collins CC. Pharmacologic weakening of extraocular muscles. Invest Ophthalmol 1973; 12(12):924–927.
24. Brin MF. Botulinum toxin: chemistry, pharmacology, toxicity, and immunology. Muscle Nerve Suppl 1997; 6:S146–S168.
25. Eleopra R, Tugnoli V, Quatrale R, Rossetto O, Montecucco C. Different types of botulinum toxin in humans. Mov Disord 2004; 19(suppl 8):S53–S59.
26. Blackie JD, Lees AJ. Botulinum toxin treatment in spasmodic torticollis. J Neurol Neurosurg Psychiatry 1990; 53(8):640–643.
27. Greene P, Kang U, Fahn S, Brin M, Moskowitz C, Flaster E. Double-blind, placebo-controlled trial of botulinum toxin injections for the treatment of spasmodic torticollis. Neurology 1990; 40(8):1213–1218.
28. Lorentz IT, Subramaniam SS, Yiannikas C. Treatment of idiopathic spasmodic torticollis with botulinum toxin A: a double-blind study on twenty-three patients. Mov Disord 1991; 6(2):145–150.
29. Jankovic J, Schwartz K. Botulinum toxin injections for cervical dystonia. Neurology 1990; 40(2):277–280.
30. Koller W, Vetere-Overfield B, Gray C, Dubinsky R. Failure of fixed-dose, fixed muscle injection of botulinum toxin in torticollis. Clin Neuropharmacol 1990; 13(4):355–358.
31. Botox (botulinum toxin type A), purified neurotoxin complex, product information. Online at http://www.botox.com.
32. O'Brien C, Brashear A, Cullis P, Truong D, Molho E, Jenkins S, Wojcieszek J, O'Neil T, Factor S, Seeberger L. Cervical dystonia severity scale reliability study. Mov Disord 2001; 16(6):1086–1090.
33. Jankovic J, Schwartz KS. Clinical correlates of response to botulinum toxin injections. Arch Neurol 1991; 48(12):1253–1256.
34. Comella CL, Buchman AS, Tanner CM, Brown-Toms NC, Goetz CG. Botulinum toxin injection for spasmodic torticollis: increased magnitude of benefit with electromyographic assistance. Neurology 1992; 42(4):878–882.

35. Comella CL, Stebbins GT, Goetz CG, Chmura TA, Bressman SB, Lang AE. Teaching tape for the motor section of the Toronto Western Spasmodic Torticollis Scale. Mov Disord 1997; 12(4):570–575.

36. Speelman JD, Brans JW. Cervical dystonia and botulinum treatment: is electromyographic guidance necessary? Mov Disord 1995; 10(6):802.

37. Jankovic J. Needle EMG guidance for injection of botulinum toxin. Needle EMG guidance is rarely required. Muscle Nerve 2001; 24(11):1568–1570.

38. Ranoux D, Gury C, Fondarai J, Mas JL, Zuber M. Respective potencies of Botox and Dysport: a double blind, randomised, crossover study in cervical dystonia. J Neurol Neurosurg Psychiatry 2002; 72(4):459–462.

39. Odergren T, Hjaltason H, Kaakkola S, Solders G, Hanko J, Fehling C, Marttila RJ, Lundh H, Gedin S, Westergren I, Richardson A, Dott C, Cohen H. A double blind, randomised, parallel group study to investigate the dose equivalence of Dysport and Botox in the treatment of cervical dystonia. J Neurol Neurosurg Psychiatry 1998; 64(1):6–12.

40. Borodic GE, Ferrante R, Pearce LB, Smith K. Histologic assessment of dose-related diffusion and muscle fiber response after therapeutic botulinum A toxin injections. Mov Disord 1994; 9(1):31–39.

41. Comella CL, Tanner CM, DeFoor-Hill L, Smith C. Dysphagia after botulinum toxin injections for spasmodic torticollis: clinical and radiologic findings. Neurology 1992; 42(7):1307–1310.

42. Brashear A, Watts MW, Marchetti A, Magar R, Lau H, Wang L. Duration of effect of botulinum toxin type A in adult patients with cervical dystonia: a retrospective chart review. Clin Ther 2000; 22(12):1516–1524.

43. Brashear A, Bergan K, Wojcieszek J, Siemers ER, Ambrosius W. Patients' perception of stopping or continuing treatment of cervical dystonia with botulinum toxin type A. Mov Disord 2000; 15(1):150–153.

44. Jankovic J, Schwartz KS. Longitudinal experience with botulinum toxin injections for treatment of blepharospasm and cervical dystonia. Neurology 1993; 43(4):834–836.

45. Hsiung GY, Das SK, Ranawaya R, Lafontaine AL, Suchowersky O. Long-term efficacy of botulinum toxin A in treatment of various movement disorders over a 10-year period. Mov Disord 2002; 17(6):1288–1293.

46. Borodic G, Johnson E, Goodnough M, Schantz E. Botulinum toxin therapy, immunologic resistance, and problems with available materials. Neurology 1996; 46(1):26–29.

47. Goschel H, Wohlfarth K, Frevert J, Dengler R, Bigalke H. Botulinum A toxin therapy: neutralizing and nonneutralizing antibodies—therapeutic consequences. Exp Neurol 1997; 147(1):96–102.

48. Aoki KR, Guyer B. Botulinum toxin type A and other botulinum toxin serotypes: a comparative review of biochemical and pharmacological actions. Eur J Neurol 2001; 8(suppl 5):21–29.

49. Jankovic J, Vuong KD, Ahsan J. Comparison of efficacy and immunogenicity of original versus current botulinum toxin in cervical dystonia. Neurology 2003; 60(7):1186–1188.

50. Racette BA, McGee-Minnich L, Perlmutter JS. Efficacy and safety of a new bulk toxin of botulinum toxin in cervical dystonia: a blinded evaluation. Clin Neuropharmacol 1999; 22(6):337–339.
51. Sesardic D, Jones RG, Leung T, Alsop T, Tierney R. Detection of antibodies against botulinum toxins. Mov Disord 2004; 19(suppl 8):S85–S91.
52. Hanna PA, Jankovic J. Mouse bioassay versus Western blot assay for botulinum toxin antibodies: correlation with clinical response. Neurology 1998; 50(6):1624–1629.
53. Palace J, Nairne A, Hyman N, Doherty TV, Vincent A. A radioimmuno-precipitation assay for antibodies to botulinum A. Neurology 1998; 50(5): 1463–1466.
54. Zuber M, Sebald M, Bathien N, de Recondo J, Rondot P. Botulinum antibodies in dystonic patients treated with type A botulinum toxin: frequency and significance. Neurology 1993; 43(9):1715–1718.
55. Sankhla C, Jankovic J, Duane D. Variability of the immunologic and clinical response in dystonic patients immunoresistant to botulinum toxin injections. Mov Disord 1998; 13(1):150–154.
56. Truong DD, Cullis PA, O'Brien CF, Koller M, Villegas TP, Wallace JD. BotB (botulinum toxin type B): evaluation of safety and tolerability in botulinum toxin type A-resistant cervical dystonia patients (preliminary study). Mov Disord 1997; 12(5):772–775.
57. Brashear A, Lew MF, Dykstra DD, Comella CL, Factor SA, Rodnitzky RL, Trosch R, Singer C, Brin MF, Murray JJ, Wallace JD, Willmer-Hulme A, Koller M. Safety and efficacy of NeuroBloc (botulinum toxin type B) in type A-responsive cervical dystonia. Neurology 1999; 53(7):1439–1446.
58. Brin MF, Lew MF, Adler CH, Comella CL, Factor SA, Jankovic J, O'Brien C, Murray JJ, Wallace JD, Willmer-Hulme A, Koller M. Safety and efficacy of NeuroBloc (botulinum toxin type B) in type A-resistant cervical dystonia. Neurology 1999; 53(7):1431–1438.
59. Lew MF, Adornato BT, Duane DD, Dykstra DD, Factor SA, Massey JM, Brin MF, Jankovic J, Rodnitzky RL, Singer C, Swenson MR, Tarsy D, Murray JJ, Koller M, Wallace JD. Botulinum toxin type B: a double-blind, placebo-controlled, safety and efficacy study in cervical dystonia. Neurology 1997; 49(3):701–707.
60. Chen R, Karp BI, Hallett M. Botulinum toxin type F for treatment of dystonia: long-term experience. Neurology 1998; 51(5):1494–1496.
61. Atassi MZ, Oshima M. Structure, activity, and immune (T and B cell) recognition of botulinum neurotoxins. Crit Rev Immunol 1999; 19(3):219–260.
62. Dressler D, Bigalke H, Benecke R. Botulinum toxin type B in antibody-induced botulinum toxin type A therapy failure. J Neurol 2003; 250(8):967–969.
63. http://www.myobloc.com/product_information/full_prescribing_info.pdf (accessed June 2004).
64. Schiavo G, Rossetto O, Benfenati F, Poulain B, Montecucco C. Tetanus and botulinum-B neurotoxins block neurotransmitter release by proteolytic cleavage of synaptobrevin. Nature 1992; 359(6398):832–835.
65. Greene PE, Fahn S. Response to botulinum toxin F in seronegative botulinum toxin A-resistant patients. Mov Disord 1996; 11(2):181–184.

66. Houser MK, Sheean GL, Lees AJ. Further studies using higher doses of botulinum toxin type F for torticollis resistant to botulinum toxin type A. J Neurol Neurosurg Psychiatry 1998; 64(5):577–580.
67. Eleopra R, Tugnoli V, Rossetto O, Montecucco C, De Grandis D. Botulinum neurotoxin serotype C: a novel effective botulinum toxin therapy in human. Neurosci Lett 1997; 224(2):91–94.
68. Eleopra R, Tugnoli V, Quatrale R, Gastaldo E, Rossetto O, De Grandis D, Montecucco C. Botulinum neurotoxin serotypes A and C do not affect motor units survival in humans: an electrophysiological study by motor units counting. Clin Neurophysiol 2002; 113(8):1258–1264.
69. Eleopra R, Tugnoli V, Rossetto O, De Grandis D, Montecucco C. Different time courses of recovery after poisoning with botulinum neurotoxin serotypes A and E in humans. Neurosci Lett 1998; 256(3):135–138.
70. Washbourne P, Pellizzari R, Rossetto O, Bortoletto N, Tugnoli V, De Grandis D, Eleopra R, Montecucco C. On the action of botulinum neurotoxins A and E at cholinergic terminals. J Physiol Paris 1998; 92(2):135–139.
71. Report of the Therapeutic and technology Assessment Subcommittee of the American Academy of Neurology. Training guidelines for the use of botulinum toxin for the treatment of neurological disorders. Neurology 1994; 44:2401–2403.

10

Ablative Denervation

Jeff D. Golan and Line Jacques

Division of Neurosurgery, McGill University, Montreal, Quebec, Canada

1. INTRODUCTION

Spasmodic torticollis is the most common form of adult-onset focal dystonia (1). This syndrome is characterized by deviation of the neck due to involuntary contraction of cervical muscles. There may also be spasmodic features such as head jerking or neck spasms. These, however, only manifest in approximately 62% of patients and have led some to use the more accurate term idiopathic cervical dystonia (2). Other forms of torticollis, as well as the possibility of secondary dystonia, must be excluded before arriving at this diagnosis. While its exact etiology is still unclear, there has been much progress in clarifying its clinical features, natural history, genetic predisposition, and association with trauma and vestibular abnormalities. The goals of treatment are to improve the quality of life and prevent secondary complications. Chemodenervation of the involved musculature with botulinum toxin has proven effective in treating this condition. Some patients do not respond well or become resistant to botulinum toxin and require surgical intervention. The most commonly performed surgery is the Bertrand procedure of selective peripheral denervation (3). Refractory cases may be amenable to deep brain stimulation (DBS) or neuroablation. The aim of this chapter is primarily to discuss the surgical indications as well as some of the surgical techniques used in treating this debilitating condition.

2. CLINICAL PRESENTATION

The prevalence of spasmodic torticollis is approximately nine cases per 100,000 population (1). Women are more commonly affected with a male to female ratio of 1:1.5 to 1:1.9 (2,4,5). The disease usually begins between the fourth and sixth decades of life (2,4–6). Symptoms usually begin insidiously with nonspecific neck complaints and progress to a certain degree of head rotation or deviation. Such deviations may occur in a single plane or, more commonly, in a combination of planes. The most common component is rotational torticollis. The left and right sides are equally affected (2,4–6). Other components are laterocollis, retrocollis, and anterocollis. In addition to head jerking or neck spasms, a postural or kinetic hand tremor can be present. The type of tremor that affects the head is either dystonic or essential. The tremor is termed dystonic if there is a directional preponderance and increases in amplitude when the head is deviated away from the direction of involuntary movement. If the tremor is rhythmical, symmetrical, and does not change considerably with head movement, it is essential (7). Dystonic movements can be reduced with sensory tricks or geste antagoniste. These consist of tactile, proprioceptive, or other sensory modulators used by the patient such as touching the involved body part. This sensory stimulation is thought to modulate presynaptic inhibition so as to improve the reciprocal inhibition and the co-contraction of agonist and antagonist muscles (8). Symptoms are commonly exacerbated by activity, fatigue, or stress.

Torticollis tends to worsen for 3–5 years, but the duration of progression is highly variable (9). Partial or even complete spontaneous remissions can occur in 10–20% of patients but are usually not sustained (10). Cervical dystonia can spread segmentally (11) and only rarely becomes generalized. Extracervical manifestations such as oromandibular, blepaharospasm, writers' cramp, and truncal dystonia, are found in approximately 20% of cases (2,4).

Patients with spasmodic torticollis have a wide range of disability. Pain is usually present. As many as 24% of patients develop depression (12). There are also daily functional limitations, such as driving, and avoiding social embarrassment. Complications caused by cervical dystonia include muscular contractures, premature degeneration of the spine, spondylosis, vertebral subluxations and osseous fusions, fractures, radiculopathies, and myelopathies (13).

There are many causes of torticollis that must be excluded. These include lesions of the cerebellum, brainstem, cranial nerves, and cervical spine (14–17), as well as mechanical causes such as C-2,3 dislocations. Psychogenic dystonia can also occur (4) and should be diagnosed with caution (18). In rare cases, a focal dystonia can be drug-induced, as in tardive dystonia, or secondary to a metabolic disturbance, as in Wilson's disease. Differentiating these pathologic entities is crucial. Patients with intra-axial lesions frequently lack pain, the onset is often acute or subacute, and additional findings may be noted on examination (7). Mechanical causes are associated with the persistence of abnormal posture during sleep, continuous pain, the absence of typical provocative or palliative factors, and the lack of appropriate muscle hypertrophy (15). Characteristics suggestive of a psychogenic etiology are abrupt onset, movements that change rapidly or begin as a fixed posture, accompanying bizarre movements, paroxysmal dystonia, and the disappearance of movements with distraction (7).

3. ETIOLOGY

The vast majority of cases of cervical dystonia are idiopathic (19). While the exact pathogenesis of this syndrome remains unknown, there are certain genetic predispositions that have recently been elucidated. As many as 25% of patients with focal dystonia have relatives with dystonia (20). The gene locus on chromosome 9q32–34, has been linked to primary torsional dystonia (21). Several other genes have been associated with dystonia (22). One of these, on chromosome 18p (23), is associated with a dystonia that is usually limited to neck muscles with occasional facial and arm involvement or spasmodic dysphonia.

No consistent morphological abnormalities have been observed in the brains of patients with primary dystonia. Several studies suggest a loss of D2 receptors in the putamen of patients with dystonia (24,25), but the significance of this finding is not yet clear. The mean discharge rate in the globus pallidus internus (GPi) is decreased in dystonia (26–29), which suggests that the inhibitory output from the direct pathway is increased. Dystonia is clearly associated with several changes in neuronal activity in striatal circuits (22).

There are many reports of patients with focal dystonia secondary to trauma (30,31). These injuries are attended by immediate pain followed by the onset of cervical dystonia within several days. Pain may be an important pathogenic factor (32). The fact that peripheral injury can cause dystonia suggests that the sensory system and subsequent alterations in the physiology of the motor system may be important in the pathogenesis of focal dystonia (7). It is possible that genetically predisposed individuals develop dystonia after peripheral injury.

The vestibular system has also been implicated. The vestibulo-ocular reflex is asymmetrical in patients with spasmodic torticollis and fails to correct after treatment with botulinum toxin (33). However, these reflex abnormalities are not found in many patients with cervical dystonia and tend to occur in patients with long disease duration (34). Furthermore, other forms of focal dystonia have not been associated with a vestibular abnormality. These abnormalities are most likely secondary to prolonged abnormal head posture (7).

4. CLINICAL FORMS OF TORTICOLLIS

Spasmodic torticollis is an exaggeration of normal head and neck movements. As such, the pathologic postures encountered are described in relation to the Cartesian axes. Rotatory movements occur along the horizontal axis and give rise to rotational torticollis. Flexion and extension movements occur along the sagittal axis and give rise to retrocollis and anterocollis. Movements of lateral inclination occur along the frontal axis and give rise to laterocollis. Simple movements are those occurring on only one axis. Complex movements may contain a combination of more than one movement, with some being predominant and others relatively secondary. The description of a complex movement must clearly identify which movement is predominant. For example, rotatory retrocollis implies a dominant rotational component with an element of extension. The most common component in complex torticollis is rotational, followed by lateral inclination, retrocollis, and anterocollis. Pure anterocollis is primarily due to bilateral involvement of the sternocleidomastoid muscles, and is an exceptionally rare entity (35).

The main muscle responsible for a specific movement is called an agonist. A muscle that has an action contrary to the agonist is called an antagonist. Their actions are also reinforced by one or more synergistic muscles. At times it can be difficult to establish which muscle is the agonist, the antagonist, or the synergist. A basic understanding of the functional anatomy of the cervical muscles is necessary in defining which muscles are responsible for the various types of movements encountered. A simplified summary of the most commonly involved muscles, their innervation, and their actions is provided in Table 1 (36). The anterior vertebral muscles may act as synergists in anterocollis, but do not contribute significantly to this movement, nor are they easily amenable to surgical or pharmacologic denervation.

5. CLINICAL EVALUATION

Initial evaluation of spasmodic torticollis should focus on a good history, including drug exposure as well as a detailed family history. Some patients may have earlier photographs and videos that will assist in objectively documenting the evolution of their disease. This is also useful for comparison at follow-up. A physical examination may identify neurological signs suggestive of another primary etiology. Cervical radiography is used for excluding spinal abnormalities and documenting the degree of spondylosis. Magnetic resonance of the brain and spine should be considered in all patients (7). Wilson's disease should be excluded in all patients under the age of 50 years by measurement of serum ceruloplasmin and a slit lamp examination (7). Genetic testing and counseling should be done in all those

Table 1 Functional Anatomy of the Cervical Muscles

Muscle	Superior attachment	Inferior attachment	Innervation	Action
Sternocleidomastoid	Mastoid process	Clavicle	CN XI, VR C-2,3	Lateral and anterior flexion
	Mastoid process, occiput	Manubrium streni	CN XI, VR C-2,3	Contralateral rotation, anterior flexion
Trapezius	Medial superior nuchal line, ligamentun nuchae	SP C-7, T-1 to T-12, lateral clavicle, scapular spine	CN XI, VR C-3,4	Posterolateral flexion (when the shoulder is fixed)
Levator scapulae	TP C-1,2, posterior tubercles C-3,4	Medial scapular spine	VR C-3,4,5 via the dorsal scapular nerve	Lateral flexion (when the shoulder is fixed)
Splenius capitis	Mastoid process, lateral superior nuchal line	Ligamentum nuchae, SP C-7 and T-1 to T-6	DR C-2 to C-6	Extension, ipsilateral rotation
Semispinalis capitis	Medial portion between superior and inferior nuchal lines	AP C-4,7, TP T-1 to T-6	DR of lower cervical and upper thoracic spinal nerves	Extension, minimal contralateral rotation
Longissimus capitis	Posterior mastoid process	AP C-4 to C-7, TP T-1 to T-4	DR of lower cervical and upper thoracic spinal nerves	Extension, ipsilateral rotation
Obliquus capitis superior	Between superior and inferior nuchal lines, occipital bone	TP C-1	DR C-1	Posterolateral flexion
Obliquus capitis inferior	TP C-1	SP C-2 and C-2 lamina	DR C-1,2	Ipsilateral rotation
Rectus capitis posterior minor	Medial inferior nuchal line, occipital bone	Posterior C-1 tubercle	DR C-1	Extension
Rectus capitis posterior major	Inferior nuchal line, occipital bone	SP C-2	DR C-1	Extension, ipsilateral rotation

Abbreviations: SP, spinous process; AP, articulating process; TP, transverse process; DR, dorsal rami; VR, ventral rami; CN, cranial nerve.

presenting before the age of 26 years or if the patient has a relative with early-onset symptoms (37).

Several scales have been used to assess the severity of spasmodic torticollis and the response to therapeutic intervention. The Toronto Western Spasmodic Torticollis Rating Scale (38) evaluates severity, disability, and pain in a cumulative score of 0–87. In addition, the Tsui rating scale (39), the visual analog scale, global assessment of change, and pain analog assessments have also been used.

The clinical evaluation is completed by electromyographic analysis of the neck. In order to have an accurate idea of which muscles are responsible for the main abnormal activity, it is mandatory to record simultaneously from at least four muscles. The goals are to determine which are the main agonists and synergists, as well as the condition of the muscles that normally act as antagonists (40,41). Recordings are done with the patient at rest and while the patient attempts voluntary movements. In order to determine the role of the synergists such as the obliqui, recti, and levator scapulae, which are deeply situated, a long bipolar concentric electrode can be inserted to record their activity (42). To verify the contribution of a specific muscle in complex movements, blocks using a local anesthetic agent under electromyographic control may be useful (43).

6. TREATMENT

6.1. Medical Therapy

Pharmacotherapy for spasmodic torticollis is not effective. The administration of anticholinergic medications has been tried with little success (44–48). Dopaminomimetic drugs have an unpredictable response and may cause frequent side effects (49). Dopamine antagonists, such as haloperidol, may be effective but can eventually worsen the dystonia or cause tardive dyskinesia (50). Clozapine has also been shown to be ineffective (51). Most tranquilizers, such as clonazepam, have no specific action in this dystonia (42). Recently, oral mexiletine, an antiarrhythmic drug, has been reported to be safe and effective in treating spasmodic torticollis in a total of 12 patients (52,53). However, experience with this medication is very limited. Physical therapy and various relaxation techniques may be useful in preventing the development of permanent contractures, but these treatment modalities rarely improve function in patients with cervical dystonia (48).

Chemodenervation with botulinum toxin A (BTX-A) has become the first-line treatment for cervical dystonia (48). Injection of this agent into dystonically contracting muscles causes inhibition of acetylcholine release at the neuromuscular junction leading to paralysis. There is satisfactory relief of symptoms in approximately 85% of cases (54,55). The effect of each treatment last 3–4 months (48) and patients require multiple injections per year.

In a recent study (56) of long-term treatment with BTX-A in 100 consecutive patients with cervical dystonia, this modality remained effective and safe for approximately 60% of patients for more than 10 years. Some patients, however, become unresponsive to subsequent treatments. This may be due to the development of neutralizing or blocking antibodies to the medication (57). The use of BTX-A with lower protein loads can reduce this rate of antibody formation (58,59). Other types of BTX have also been tried (54,60). Patients with contractures may not improve with BTX, but may possibly benefit from surgery when denervation is combined with myectomy (61). A substantial number of patients may eventually fail chemodenervation or will choose a surgical intervention to permanently treat their symptoms.

6.2. Surgical Options

The first well-controlled and successful procedure for the treatment of spasmodic torticollis was a unilateral rhizotomy performed by Cushing and McKenzie in 1923 (62). Several surgical techniques have been performed since then with varying degrees of success. Bilateral intradural upper cervical rhizotomy improved symptoms in many patients, but was accompanied by a marked limitation in neck movements, shoulder paresis, cervical subluxations, increased kyphosis, transient myelopathy, and even death (63–65). Epidural cervical stimulation showed some benefit (66), but this was not reproducible in other centers (42,67). Another technique was microvascular lysis of the spinal accessory nerve roots (68). This was done in an attempt to relieve any possible areas of irritation on the nerve. As we now know, there are other muscles responsible for torticollis that must also be addressed. Selective muscle resections have been attempted in various forms, but they do not result in complete denervation and involve extensive resection of the normal muscular structure (42).

The emergence of electromyography has provided a much better appreciation for the muscles involved and permitted the development of selective surgical procedures. Bertrand's technique of selective peripheral denervation (35,69) is the current surgical procedure of choice. It allows for complete denervation of all muscles involved while preserving the innervation to those muscles that do not contribute to the abnormal movements. This is done by the extradural sectioning of the dorsal rami of C-1 to C-6, and peripheral denervation of the accessory nerve via a separate incision. Another technique (70) selectively denervates the anterior nerve roots of C-1 and C-2 intradurally and uses a modified Bertrand approach to denervate C-3 to C-6 as well as the accessory nerve. We do not believe it is justifiable to enter the intradural space and continue to perform extradural sectioning of the C-1 and C-2 dorsal rami.

There has long been an interest in central treatments of cervical dystonia. Initially, thalamic lesions were performed in order to interrupt the cerebello-rubro-thalamo-cortical pathways (71,72). Results were very inconsistent and accompanied by a risk of dysarthria, especially with bilateral lesions. More recently, stereotactic surgery has regained much popularity. Both pallidotomy and DBS of the globus pallidus internus and thalamus are currently being investigated. Current indications for DBS are patients who fail medical therapy and are not candidates for peripheral denervation (73). Patients who do not obtain sufficient relief from selective denervation should also be considered.

7. SELECTIVE PERIPHERAL DENERVATION

7.1. Selection of Patients

This is the most common surgical procedure for spasmodic torticollis. It is offered to the majority of patients who fail conservative therapy and chemodenervation. The dystonic movements must be stable for at least 2 years and should be limited to the cervical region. Patients with generalized dystonia can still be offered selective peripheral denervation if they have a well defined form of torticollis with significant concomitant disability. Such patients should, however, be informed about the possibility of a flare-up of their dystonia after surgery (42). Patients with extracervical involvement may also require special postoperative care to prevent complications associated with exacerbations of their extracervical dystonia (74). Selective denervation will not suppress any head tremor and in fact this may be exacerbated in cases where the abnormal tonic head position served to minimize this tremor (35).

7.2. Surgical Technique

The surgical approach depends on the patient's type of torticollis. Denervation is done for the agonist and synergist muscles. Cases with rotational components require denervation of the contralateral sternocleidomastoid and ipsilateral posterior muscle groups. In complex cases of rotation and retrocollis, the contralateral posterior muscle group may also be denervated, either in the initial surgery or as a second-stage procedure. In some cases of rotational torticollis with a prominent flexion component, the ipsilateral sternocleidomastoid may also need to be denervated in a second-stage procedure. Patients with a component of lateral inclination require denervation of the levator scapulae on the side of the inclination. In pure laterocollis, denervation of the ipsilateral levator scapulae may be sufficient. In laterocollis with a component of anterior flexion, the sternocleidomastoid on the side of the inclination is also denervated. Patients with pure retrocollis require bilateral denervation of the posterior muscle groups. Patients with pure anterocollis require denervation of both sternocleidomastoids.

The procedure is done under light general anesthesia without paralysis. The patient is placed in a sitting position. This allows exposure of the spinal accessory and the posterior nerves in the same surgical field (Fig. 1). The patient's head is fixed in a Gardner headrest with the head in slight forward flexion and rotation to the opposite side of the ramisectomy. This enlarges the space between the posterior arch of C-1 and the occiput. In cases of known patent foramen ovale, a prone or park-bench position is preferred to reduce the risk of venous air embolism (75). In addition to the usual anesthesia monitoring devices, precordial Doppler ultrasonography is used for the possible detection of venous air embolism. In such an event, air can be aspirated by the anesthesiologist from the central venous catheter. Unipolar stimulation is essential in identifying the spinal accessory nerve and its rootlets, as well as in differentiating branches from the ventral and dorsal rami of all cervical roots exposed.

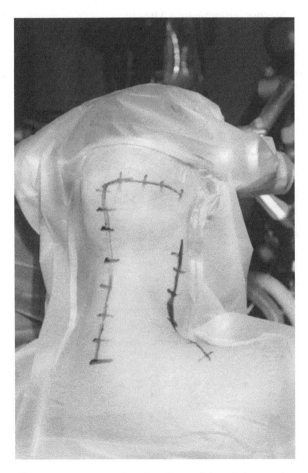

Figure 1 Patient positioning for peripheral denervation.

After the surgery, patients may suffer from severe nausea and usually benefit from antiemetic therapy. Dexamethasone is used in the first 3 days to help control soft tissue edema. Patients get started with active physiotherapy on the third postoperative day and continue for a period of 6–12 weeks. Mirrors are commonly used as visual feedback tools in regaining head and neck proprioception. The goal is to retrain the antagonist and the non-denervated muscles in order to restore normal neck movements.

The procedures described in the following text are nearly identical to those described by Bertrand and Molina Negro (35,42,43,69,76), who have pioneered this technique. Denervation of the trapezius muscle is not described here because it is rarely required for a successful surgical outcome. Furthermore, its denervation can result in the patient's inability to elevate his or her arm above the horizontal plane (74).

7.3. Denervation of the Sternocleidomastoid Muscle

A skin incision is made at the posterior edge of the sternocleidomastoid muscle, starting at the mastoid process and extending down to the junction of the vertical and horizontal portions of the trapezius. Care is taken to avoid injuring the greater auricular nerve. The spinal accessory nerve is identified with the use of stimulation. The branch to the trapezius is stimulated and identified. All the other branches from the spinal accessory nerve are similarly dissected. Any stimulated branches producing isolated contraction of the sternocleidomastoid are sectioned and distally avulsed (Fig. 2). There are

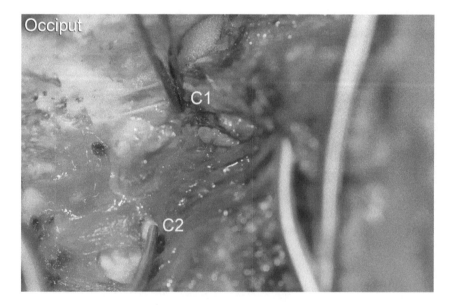

Figure 2 Denervation of the sternocleidomastoid muscle.

usually four to six such branches. The nerve is dissected upward to the level of the styloid process to assure denervation of all possible branches. At the end, only the main trunk remains with one or two branches to the trapezius. Finally, the sternocleidomastoid muscle is completely sectioned. Myectomy is required since this muscle has dual innervation with branches from the cervical descending plexus, which are not easily denervated.

7.4. Posterior Ramisectomy

A midline vertical incision is carried from the external occipital protuber-ance down to the spinous process of C-7. The dissection is continued along the midline to expose the posterior tubercle of C-1 and the spinous processes of C-2 to C-6 (Fig. 3). A 5-cm horizontal incision is made from the external protuberance laterally. This L-shaped incision allows for excellent exposure while minimizing retraction and possible neuropraxic injury. The occipital aponeurosis, trapezius, splenius capitis, and semispinalis capitis muscles are

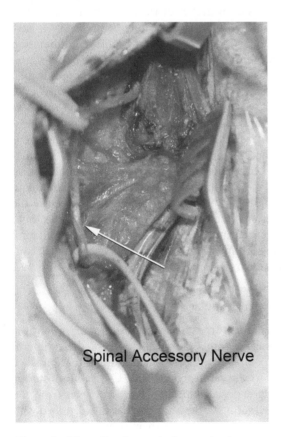

Figure 3 Dissection for posterior ramisectomy.

sectioned 1-cm below their insertions on the occipital bone and are carefully retracted laterally. These large muscles and aponeurosis will be sutured back at the end of the procedure.

There is a natural plane of cleavage along the undersurface of the semispinalis capitis. This plane is followed laterally to expose the articular facets of C-2,3 to C-5,6. The suboccipital triangle, bounded superomedially by the rectus capitis posterior major, superolaterally by the obliquus capitis superior, and inferolaterally by the obliquus capitis inferior, is then identified. The vertebral artery and dorsal ramus of C-1 underneath it are visualized in the middle of the triangle, above the posterior arch of the atlas. Careful stimulation is done to ensure no response from the anterior throat muscles, which are innervated by the anterior ramus and should be spared to prevent swallowing difficulties. Once stimulation of the posterior muscles is confirmed, the C-1 dorsal ramus is sectioned and distally avulsed to minimize the possibility of regeneration.

The C-2 dorsal ramus is more medial and emerges below the obliquus capitus inferior, between the posterior arches of the atlas and the axis. The ventral ramus is deeper, within the two arches. It may be necessary to section obliquus capitus inferior in order to facilitate this exposure. Stimulation is performed to ensure no response from the anterior throat muscles and appropriate response by the posterior muscles. The C-2 dorsal ramus is then sectioned and distally avulsed.

The posterior rami of C-3 to C-6 are found between the articular facets. The longissimus capitis and levator scapulae muscles are cut progressively and retracted laterally in order to expose the facet joints. Each nerve is followed to its point of emergence from the intervertebral foramen. Stimulation is used to confirm the correct ramus as described above. Stimulation of the ventral ramus of C-4 and C-5 can produce elevation of the diaphragm. Early dorsal collateral branches must be identified and sectioned. Once the dorsal rami are taken, stimulation of the periarticular area at each level should not elicit any response in the posterior group of muscles. In cases of bilateral posterior denervation, the ramisectomy is limited to C-5, as C-6 may also contribute to the innervation of the paraspinous muscles.

7.5. Denervation of the Levator Scapulae

The levator scapulae can be accessed from a posterior approach when it is on the same side as the posterior ramisectomy, or from a direct lateral approach. The posterior approach is easily performed in this situation since the four superior attachments (transverse processes of C-1,2 and posterior tubercles of C-3,4) are already exposed and cut. Nerve branches from the ventral rami at C-3 and C-4 innervating the levator scapulae are identified with stimulation. These branches are sectioned once their stimulation produces isolated contractions of the levator scapulae.

The lateral approach is performed through an incision along the posterior border of the sternocleidomastoid muscle. The levator scapulae muscle is located between the posterior portions of the sternocleidomastoid and scalenius medius and the anterior portions of splenius capitis and trapezius. The levator scapulae muscle is found deep to the cervical fascia. Nerve branches from C-3 and C-4 are identified with stimulation. These branches are sectioned if their stimulation produces isolated contractions of the levator scapulae. After denervation, the muscle itself is sectioned.

8. RESULTS

The relief from abnormal movements is apparent immediately after surgery. However, a period of 6–12 weeks of physiotherapy is usually required to restore normal neck movements and at least 6 months for the end result (35). Of 260 patients reviewed by Bertrand (35), 88% had very satisfactory results. Out of the last 50 patients treated in that study, 54% had no detectable abnormal movements and 34% had slight deviation or slight residual abnormal movements. In a study by Cohen-Gadol and colleagues (74), 125 (77%) of 167 patients had moderate to excellent improvement, and pain was markedly improved in 131 (88%). Interestingly, in the latter study, outcome could not be predicted based on preoperative head position, patient sex, severity of abnormal posture of head, symptom duration, presence of tremor or phasic dystonic movements, or failure to respond substantially to botulinum toxin treatment.

In the study by Bertrand, the overall percentage of patients who remained with an appreciable amount of residual movements, whether immediately or delayed, was 12%. This relative failure may be due to residual innervation from early collateral branches at the level of C-3 and C-4. Re-intervention was successful in three of five patients. In three other cases, fibrosis prevented a complete extension of the spine. In two patients, the partial return of rotational torticollis was due to the unopposed action of the contralateral semispinalis muscle. In one of these, a contralateral denervation was required and suppressed the abnormal movements. One patient with severe progressing myoclonic dystonia had a flare up of his symptoms. Two other patients had a poor outcome. One of these patients had severe generalized dystonia and an exacerbation of his symptoms that later also failed thalamotomy. The other patient suffered from retrocollis with marked extension of the entire spine and did not benefit from selective denervation (42). Of the eight other patients with generalized dystonia, three had an excellent result, and five had marked improvement of their posture.

In the study by Cohen-Gadol, 17 (10%) patients underwent a second operation for recurrence of their symptoms. Electromyographic recordings demonstrated reinnervation of previously denervated muscles. Thirteen

(76%) of these 17 patients experienced a marked improvement in their pain and head position after the second surgery, with a mean follow up of 18.3 months. Some muscles may have more than one sources of innervation, and this may only be obvious postoperatively in cases where a complete resection of the dorsal rami does not result in complete denervation of a given muscle. A repeat operation to denervate nerve branches from the anterior rami is often successful in these cases.

Sequelae from a unilateral selective denervation were not significant in Bertrand's study. Some patients developed marked swelling of the neck during the first 24 hour, especially with the posterolateral approach. Most patients did not complain of sensory loss, which, when present, was essentially limited to the distribution of the greater occipital nerve. Cohen-Gadol reported no significant swallowing difficulties and no significant neck muscle weakness that compromised head control. Three of his patients suffered from persistent C-2 distribution dysesthesias. Five patients suffered transient complications that completely resolved. Three patients had nondisabling shoulder weakness that completely resolved in one patient. One patient, with idiopathic myopathy and preexisting chest-wall muscle weakness, suffered a respiratory arrest and eventually died following resuscitation. In a recent study by Girard et al. (75) that was specifically directed at determining the risk of venous air embolism in 342 patients who underwent selective peripheral denervation in the sitting position, the incidence was found to be 2%. None of the patients died.

In assessing long-term outcome, 58 (75%) of 77 patients reviewed by Molina-Negro and Bouvier (77) were satisfied with the surgery after a follow-up period of 3–16 years. In this group, 66 (86%) patients were satisfied immediately after surgery. Persistence of pain was the most common reason for lack of satisfaction, followed by head and neck posture. The reduction in satisfaction over time may be due to the progressive nature of dystonia.

9. SUMMARY

The goals of treatment in spasmodic torticollis are to improve the quality of life and prevent secondary complications. Electromyographic evaluation has greatly improved our ability to recognize and treat all forms of torticollis. Selective peripheral denervation offers long-lasting symptomatic relief with few complications and remains the first-line surgical option if medical treatment fails. In recent years, there have been many advances in our understanding and treatment of this condition. Research in genetics and the pathophysiology of focal dystonia will assist clinicians in the correct diagnosis of this syndrome and in better selecting patients for the most appropriate therapeutic modality.

REFERENCES

1. Nutt JG, Muenter MD, Aronson A, Kurland LT, Melton LJ 3rd. Epidemiology of focal and generalized dystonia in Rochester, Minnesota. Mov Disord 1988; 3(3):188–194.
2. Chan J, Brin MF, Fahn S. Idiopathic cervical dystonia: clinical characteristics. Mov Disord 1991; 6(2):119–126.
3. Bertrand CM, Molina Negro P, Martinez SN. Technical aspects of selective peripheral denervation for spasmodic torticollis. Appl Neurophysiol 1982; 45:326–330.
4. Jankovic J, Leder S, Warner D, Schwartz K. Cervical dystonia: clinical findings and associated movement disorders. Neurology 1991; 41(7):1088–1091.
5. Rondot P, Marchand MP, Dellatolas G. Spasmodic torticollis—review of 220 patients. Can J Neurol Sci 1991; 18(2):143–151.
6. Duane DD. Spasmodic torticollis: clinical and biological features and their implications for focal dystonia. Adv Neurol 1988; 50:473–492.
7. Dauer WT, Burke RE, Greene P, Fahn S. Current concepts on the clinical features, aetiology and management of idiopathic cervical dystonia. Brain 1998; 121:547–560.
8. Madhusudanan M. Dystonia: emerging concepts in pathophysiology. Neurol India 1999; 47(4):263–267.
9. Lowenstein DH, Aminoff MJ. The clinical course of spasmodic torticollis. Neurology 1988; 38(4):530–532.
10. Tranchant C. [Focal dystonia: clinical, etiologic and therapeutic aspects.] Rev Neurol (Paris) 2000; 156(12):1087–1094 (in French).
11. Stacey M. Idiopathic cervical dystonia: an overview. Neurology 2000; 55(suppl 5): S2–S8.
12. Jahanshahi M. Psychosocial factors and depression in torticollis. J Psychosom Res 1991; 35(4–5):493–507.
13. Konrad C, Vollmer-Haase J, Anneken K, Krecht S. Orthopedic and neurological complications of cervical dystonia—review of the literature. Acta Neurol Scand 2004; 109(6):369–373.
14. Kiwak KJ, Deray MJ, Shields WD. Torticollis in three children with syringomyelia and spinal cord tumor. Neurology 1983; 33(7):946–948.
15. Suchowersky O, Calne DB. Non-dystonic causes of torticollis. Adv Neurol 1988; 50:501–508.
16. Isaac K, Cohen JA. Post-traumatic torticollis. Neurology 1989; 39(12):1642–1643.
17. Cammarota A, Gershanik OS, Garcia S, Lera G. Cervical dystonia due to spinal cord ependymoma: involvement of cervical cord segments in the pathogenesis of dystonia. Mov Disord 1995; 10(4):500–503.
18. Lesser RP, Fahn S. Dystonia: a disorder often misdiagnosed as a conversion reaction. Am J Psychiatry 1978; 135(3):349–352.
19. LeDoux MS, Brady KA. Secondary cervical dystonia associated with structural lesions of the central nervous system. Mov Disord 2003; 18(1):60–69.
20. Waddy HM, Fletcher NA, Harding AE, Marsden CD. A genetic study of idiopathic focal dystonias. Ann Neurol 1991; 29(3):320–324.
21. Ozelius LJ, Hewett JW, Page C, Bressman SB, Kramer PL, Shalish C, de Leon D, Brin MF, Raymond D, Corey DP, Fahn S, Risch NJ, Buckler AJ, Gusella JF,

Breakefield XO. The early-onset torsion dystonia gene (DYT1) encodes an ATP-binding protein. Nat Genet 1997; 17(1):40–48.

22. Langlois M, Richer F, Chouinard S. New perspectives on dystonia. Can J Neurol Sci 2003; 30(suppl 1):S34–S44.

23. Leube B, Rudnicki D, Ratzlaff T, Kessler KR, Benecke R, Auburger G. Idiopathic torsion dystonia: assignment of a gene to chromosome 18p in a German family with adult onset, autosomal dominant inheritance and purely focal distribution. Hum Mol Genet 1996; 5:1673–1677.

24. Perlmutter JS, Stambuk MK, Markham J, Black KJ, McGee-Minnick L, Jankovic J, Moerlein SM. Decreased [18F] spiperone binding in putamen in dystonia. Adv Neurol 1998; 78:161–168.

25. Naumann M, Pirker W, Reiners K, Lange KW, Becker G, Brucke T. Imaging the pre- and postsynaptic side of striatal dopaminergic synapses in idiopathic cervical dystonia: a SPECT study using [123I] epidepride and [123I] beta-CIT. Mov Disord 1998; 13(2):319–323.

26. Lozano AM, Kumar R, Gross RE, Giladi N, Hutchison WD, Dostrovsky JO, Lang AE. Globus pallidus internus pallidotomy for generalized dystonia. Mov Disord 1997; 12(6):865–870.

27. Lenz FA, Suarez JI, Metman LV, Reich SG, Karp BI, Hallett M, Rowland LH, Dougherty PM. Pallidal activity during dystonia: somatosensory reorganization and changes with severity. J Neurol Neurosurg Psychiatry 1998; 65(5): 767–770.

28. Vitek JL, Chockkan V, Zhang JY, Kaneoke Y, Evatt M, DeLong MR, Triche S, Mewes K, Hashimoto T, Bakay RA. Neuronal activity in the basal ganglia in patients with generalized dystonia and hemibalismus. Ann Neurol 1999; 46(1): 22–35.

29. Delong MR. Primate models of movement disorders of basal ganglia origin. Trends Neurosci 1990; 13(7):281–285.

30. Schott GD. The relationship of peripheral trauma and pain to dystonia. J Neurol Neurosurg Psychiatry 1985; 48(7):698–701.

31. Jankovic J, Van der Linden C. Dystonia and tremor induced by peripheral trauma: predisposing factors. J Neurol Neurosurg Psychiatry 1988; 51(12):1512–1519.

32. Jankovic J. Post-traumatic movement disorders: central and peripheral mechanisms. Neurology 1994; 44(11):2006–2014.

33. Stell R, Bronstein AM, Marsden CD. Vestibulo-ocular abnormalities in spasmodic torticollis before and after botulinum toxin injections. J Neurol Neurosurg Psychiatry 1989; 52(1):57–62.

34. Colebatch JG, Di Lazzaro V, Quartarone A, Rothwell JC, Gresty M. Click-evoked vestibulocollic reflexes in torticollis. Mov Disord 1995; 10(4):455–459.

35. Bertrand CM. Selective peripheral denervation for spasmodic torticollis: surgical technique, results, and observations in 260 cases. Surg Neurol 1993; 40(2): 96–103.

36. Williams PL, Warwick R, Dyson M, Bannister LH. Gray's Anatomy. 37th edn. New York: Churchill Livingstone, 1989.

37. Bressman SB, Sabatti C, Raymond D, de Leon D, Klein C, Kramer PL, Brin MF, Fahn S, Breakefield X, Ozelius LJ, Risch NJ. The DYT1 phenotype and guidelines for diagnostic testing. Neurology 2000; 54(9):1746–1752.

38. Consky ES, Lang AE. Clinical assessments of patients with cervical dystonia. Jankovic J, Hallett M, eds. Therapy with Botulinum Toxin. New York: Marcel Dekker, 1994:211–237.
39. Tsui JK, Eisen A, Stoessl AJ, Calne S, Calne DB. Double-blind study of botulinum toxin in spasmodic torticollis. Lancet 1986; 2(8501):245–247.
40. Bertrand CM, Molina-Negro P. Selective peripheral denervation in 111 cases of spasmodic torticollis: rationale and results. In: Fahn S, Marsden CD, Calne DB, eds. Advances in Neurology. Vol. 50. Dystonia II. New York: Raven Press, 1988:637–643.
41. Bertrand C, Molina-Negro P, Bouvier G, Gorczyca W. Observations and analysis of results in 131 cases of spasmodic torticollis after selective denervation. Appl Neurophysiol 1987; 50(1–6):319–323.
42. Bertrand C, Molina-Negro P, Bouvier G, Benabou R. Surgical treatment of spasmodic torticollis. Youmans JR, ed. Neurological Surgery. 4th ed. Philadelphia, PA: WB Saunders, 1996:3701–3711.
43. Bouvier G, Molina-Negro P. Selective peripheral denervation for spasmodic torticollis. Winn RH, ed. Youmans Neurological Surgery. 5th ed. Philadelphia, PA: WB Saunders, 2004:2891–2899.
44. Cullis PA, Walker PC. The treatment of spasmodic torticollis. Quinn NP, Jenner PG, eds. Disorders of Movement: Clinical, Pharmacological, and Physiological Aspects. London: Academic Press, 1989:295–301.
45. Fahn S. High dosage anticholinergic therapy in dystonia. Neurology 1983; 33(10):1255–1261.
46. Lee MC. Spasmodic torticollis and other idiopathic torsion dystonias. Medical management. Postgrad Med 1984; 75(7):139–141, 144–146.
47. Marsden CD, Marion MH, Quinn N. The treatment of severe dystonia in children and adults 1984; 47(11):1166–1173.
48. Jankovic J. Treatment of cervical dystonia with botulinum toxin. Mov Disord 2004; 19(suppl 8):S109–S115.
49. Teravainen H, Calne S, Burton K, Beckman J, Calne DB. Efficacy of dopamine agonists in dystonia. Adv Neurol 1988; 50:571–578.
50. Adler CH. Strategies for controlling dystonia. Overview of therapies that may alleviate symptoms. Postgrad Med 2000; 108(5):151–152, 155–156, 159–160.
51. Thiel A, Dressler D, Kistel C, Ruther E. Clozapine treatment of spasmodic torticollis. Neurology 1994; 44(5):957–958.
52. Ohara S, Hayashi R, Momoi H, Miki J, Yanagisawa N. Mexiletine in the treatment of spasmodic torticollis. Mov Disord 1998; 13(6):934–940.
53. Luccetti C, Nuti A, Gambaccini G, Bernadini S, Brotini S, Manca ML, Bonoccelli U. Mexiletine in the treatment of torticollis and generalized dystonia. Clin Neuropharmacol 2000; 23(4):186–189.
54. Comella CL, Jankovic J, Brin MF. Use of botulinum toxin type A in the treatment of cervical dystonia. Neurology 2000; 55(12 suppl 5):S15–S21.
55. Ceballos-Baumann AO. Evidence-based medicine in botulinum toxin therapy for cervical dystonia. J Neurol 2001; 248(suppl 1):14–20.
56. Haussermann P, Marczoch S, Klinger C, Landgrebe M, Conrad B, Ceballos-Baumann A. Long-term follow-up of cervical dystonia patients treated with botulinum toxin A. Mov Disord 2004; 19(3):303–308.

57. Borodic G, Johnson E, Goodnough M, Schantz E. Botulinum toxin therapy, immunologic resistance, and problems with available materials. Neurology 1996; 46(1):26–29.
58. Goeschel H, Wolhfarth K, Frevert J, Dengler R, Bigalke H. Botulinum A toxin therapy: neutralizing and nonneutralizing antibodies—therapeutic consequences. Exp Neurol 1997; 147(1):96–102.
59. Jankovic J, Vuong KD, Ahsan J. Comparison of efficacy and immunogenicity of original versus current botulinum toxin in cervical dystonia. Neurology 2003; 60(7):1186–1188.
60. Priori A, Berardelli A, Mercuri B, Manfredi M. Physiological effects produced by botulinum toxin treatment of upper limb dystonia. Changes in reciprocal inhibition between forearm muscles. Brain 1995; 118(3):801–807.
61. Krauss JK, Toups EG, Jankovic J, Grossman RG. Symptomatic and functional outcome of surgical treatment of cervical dystonia. J Neurol Neurosurg Psychiatry 1997; 63(5):642–648.
62. Rossitch E Jr, Khoshbin S, Black PM, Moore MR, Tyler HR. Kenneth McKenzie, Harvey Cushing, and the early neurosurgical treatment of spasmodic torticollis. Neurosurgery 1991; 28(2):278–282.
63. Hamby WB, Schiffer S. Spasmodic torticollis: results after cervical rhizotomy in 50 cases. J Neurosurg 1969; 31(3):323–326.
64. Perot PL. Upper cervical ventral rhizotomy and selective section of spinal accessory rootlets for spasmodic torticollis. Wilson CB, ed. Neurosurgery Procedures. Baltimore, MD: Williams & Wilkins, 1992:163–168.
65. Friedman AH, Nashold BS Jr, Sharp R, Caputi F, Arruda J. Treatment of spasmodic torticollis with intradural selective rhizotomies. J Neurosurg 1993; 78(1):46–53.
66. Waltz JM, Andreesen WH, Hunt DP. Spinal cord stimulation and motor disorders. Pacing Clin Electrophysiol 1987; 10:180–204.
67. Goetz CG, Penn RD, Tanner CM. Efficacy of cervical cord stimulation in dystonia. Fahn S, Marsden CD, Calne DB, eds. Advances in Neurology. Vol. 50. New York: Raven Press, 1988:645–649.
68. Freckmann N, Hagenah R, Herrmann HD, Muller D. Treatment of neurogenic torticollis by microvascular lysis of the accessory nerve roots—indication, technique, and first results. Acta Neurochir (Wien) 1981; 59:167–175.
69. Bertrand C, Molina Negro P, Martinez SN. Technical aspects of selective peripheral denervation for spasmodic torticollis. Appl Neurophysiol 1982; 45(3): 326–330.
70. Taira T, Kobayashi T, Takahashi K, Hori T. A new denervation procedure for idiopathic cervical dystonia. J Neurosurg 2002; 97(2 suppl):201–206.
71. Cooper PA. Effect of thalamic lesions on torticollis. N Engl J Med 1964; 270:567–572.
72. Hassler R, Hess WR. [Experimental and anatomical findings in rotatory movements and their nervous apparatus.] Arch Psychiatr Nervenkr Z Gesamte Neurol Psychiatr 1954; 192(5):488–526 (in German).
73. Krauss JK, Yianni J, Loher TJ, Aziz TZ. Deep brain stimulation for dystonia. J Clin Neurophysiol 2004; 21(1):18–30.

74. Cohen-Gadol AA, Ahlskog JE, Matsumoto JY, Swenson MA, McClelland RL, Davis DH. Selective peripheral denervation for the treatment of intractable spasmodic torticollis: experience with 168 patients at the Mayo Clinic. J Neurosurg 2003; 98(6):1247–1254.

75. Girard F, Ruel M, McKenty S, Boudreault D, Chouinard P, Todorov A, Molina-Negro P, Bouvier G. Incidences of venous air embolism and patent foramen ovale among patients undergoing selective peripheral denervation in the sitting position. Neurosurgery 2003; 53(2):316–319.

76. Bertrand CM. Operative management of spasmodic torticollis and adult-onset dystonia with emphasis on selective denervation. Schmidek HH, Sweet WH, eds. Operative Neurosurgical Techniques. 2nd edn. Orlando: Grune & Stratton, 1988: 1261–1269.

77. Molina-Negro P, Bouvier G. Surgical treatment of spasmodic torticollis by peripheral denervation. Tarsi D, Vitek JL, Lozano AM, eds. Surgical Treatment of Parkinson's Disease and Other Movement Disorders. Totowa, NJ: Humana Press, 2003:275–286.

11

Deep Brain Stimulation

Atsushi Umemura

Department of Neurosurgery, Nagoya City University Medical School, Mizuho-ku, Nagoya, Japan

1. INTRODUCTION

Spasmodic torticollis (ST) is the most common type of focal dystonia. It involves the muscles of the neck, and is therefore called "cervical dystonia." As a result of abnormal involuntary contractions of the neck muscles, the head may be rotated, tilted, flexed, extended, or any combination of these postures. The movements may be quick, sustained, or patterned, and therefore may be associated with tremor.

ST usually responds poorly to oral medication; therefore, most ST patients are managed by injection of botulinum toxin into the overactive cervical muscles. The availability of botulmum toxin has dramatically improved management for the majority of patients with ST. However, responses are partial and the toxin's effects wear off. Repeat injections at 3–4 monthly intervals are necessary. In addition, botulinum toxin is not effective for 6–14% of ST patients and loses its initial efficacy with continued use in at least 3% due to the development of immunoresistance (1,2).

Surgical treatment has been attempted for medically refractory ST for decades. Surgical alternatives include peripheral denervation and intracranial stereotactic surgery, which includes ablative and deep brain stimulation (DBS) procedures.

Recently, DBS has emerged as an alternative to ablative procedures. DBS seems to reduce the activity of the focal area in a manner similar to ablative surgery by producing a functional lesion in the brain. Compared with ablative surgery, DBS is nondestructive and reversible. Consequently, DBS lessens permanent neurological deficits. In addition, maximal efficacy with minimal adverse events can be obtained by adjusting the stimulation parameters noninvasively. Although this procedure has been widely applied in the treatment of Parkinson's disease and essential tremor, few studies on the efficacy of DBS in ST have been published.

This chapter reviews the results of stereotactic procedure for ST reported in the literature. Some issues concerning methodology and rationale are also discussed.

2. EARLY ATTEMPTS IN ABLATIVE PROCEDURE FOR ST

Stereotactic thermocoagulation procedures have been attempted for treatment of intractable dystonia for the past 50 years (3,4). The two major intracranial targets are the thalamus and globus pallidus. Initially, thalamotomy was the procedure most commonly performed. Cooper performed thermocoagulation of the nucleus ventrointermedius (VIM) thalamus in more than 200 patients with various types of dystonia. He observed sustained improvement in 70% of the patients (5–7). Afterwards, a variety of thalamic targets were attempted (8,9). Pallidotomy was used less frequently than thalamotomy in the early decades (3).

Approximately 300 patients with ST were reported to have undergone functional stereotactic surgery between 1960 and the early 1980s (3). Andrew et al. performed bilateral thalamotomy in 16 patients with ST. They observed improvement in 62% of the patients; however, the incidence of operative complications, in particular dysarthria, was high following bilateral lesions (10). Von Essen et al. reported improvement by unilateral VOI (nucleus ventrooralis internus) thalamotomy in 17 patients with horizontal torticollis (11). Goldhahn and Goldhahn reported benefits for thalamotomy in 58.4% of 24 patients with ST (12). Overall, postoperative improvement was achieved in about 50–70% of the cases in most studies (3).

The fact that "off" dystonia and levodopa-induced dyskinesia in Parkinson's disease were relieved by pallidotomy led to a resurgence of pallidotomy as a treatment for dystonia. Ondo et al. performed bilateral globus pallidus internus (GPi) thermocoagulation in eight patients with generalized dystonia and obtained marked improvements in six patients (13). At present, GPi is much more favored as a target of choice for dystonia (4).

There has been controversy about which side of the brain should be selected for surgery in a particular type of ST. Widespread disturbance of motor control mechanisms may occur in patients with ST. Historically, Cooper recommended lesioning contralateral to the dystonic stemocleidomastoid muscle (SCM) (5). However, Hassler and Dieckmann asserted that the ipsilateral side should be targeted (9). Kavaklis et al. suggested that

VL (nucleus ventralis lateraris) thalamotomy for ST should be performed on the side ipsilateral to the contracting SCM muscle based on results of a study of pallidal and thalamic control of SCM muscles in cats (14). On the basis of a study with transcranial magnetic stimulation in patients with ST, Thickbroom et al. suggested that head turning is chiefly mediated by the hemisphere ipsilateral to the direction of head rotation by means of a corticomotor projection to the contralateral SCM (15).

3. DBS FOR ST

DBS has emerged as a significant therapeutic alternative in intractable ST. In contrast to ablative stereotactic procedures, DBS does not require destructive brain lesions and therefore lessens the risk of permanent postoperative neurological deficits. However, there are some disadvantages of DBS including the risk of infection, the need for frequent visits to adjust stimulation parameters, mechanical problems, and significant equipment costs.

Clinical experience with DBS for ST is very limited. An early DBS target for treatment of ST was the thalamus. Mundinger described the benefits of intermittent unilateral or bilateral DBS in the VOA (nucleus ventro-oralis anterior)/VOI thalamus and the subthaiamic zona incerta in seven patients with ST (16). Andy subsequently reported on chronic unilateral thalamic stimulation in two other patients (17).

Recently, the GPi has been chosen as a more favorable target for ST based on accumulated DBS experience for several types of dystonia (Table 1) (4,7,8,18–25). In most reports, treatment results were assessed with the Toronto Western Spasmodic Torticollis Rating Scale (TWSTRS), which includes a total severity scale (TSS), a disability scale, and a pain scale (26,27).

Krauss et al. first reported on the benefits of bilateral GPi DBS in three patients with severe complex ST (18). Since then, several studies have described favorable results regarding the usefulness of bilateral GPi DBS for treatment of ST. Kulisevsky reported on two patients with idiopathic cervical dystonia treated by bilateral GPi DBS who showed only mild motor improvement but marked amelioration of pain symptoms (20). Parkin et al. reported immediate sense of ease in the neck from activating the stimulator for bilateral GPi DBS, and subsequent improvement in voluntary neck movements and natural head position, which slowly developed over 3 months (22). Goto et al. observed immediate and consistent improvement of ST and associated pain (23). In their patients, the stimulating parameter of pulse width was extremely wide [500 μsec] compared with other studies. Eltahawy et al. found that a structurally normal brain, as seen on preoperative MRI scans, is a predictor of a good response to pallidal interventions (4). It is suggested that the effect of GPi DBS for ST may depend on etiology.

Table 1 Pallidal Deep Brain Stimulation for Spasmodic Torticollis

Series	Patients	Procedure	Stimulation parameters	Follow up	Result (improvement rate)
Krauss et al. (18)	3	Bil GPi DBS	3.1–5.0 V, 130–160 Hz, 210 μsec	6–15 months	41–53% in SS, 49–80% in DS, 25–57% in PS of modified TWSTRS
Islekel et al. (19)	1	Uni GPi DBS	2.5 V, 160 Hz, 90 μsec	3 weeks	Improvement
Kulisevsky et al. (20)	2	Bil GPi DBS	N/A	17–24 months	Mild improvement of torticollis scale, marked improvement of VAS
Andaluz et al. (21)	1	Bil GPi DBS	N/A	8 months	50% improvement in TWSTRS
Parkin et al. (22)	3	Bil GPi DBS	3.0–4.0 V, 130 Hz, 90 μsec, mono- or bipolar	2–6 months	Improvement
Goto et al. (23)	3	Bil GPi DBS	4.5–8.0 V, 50–60 Hz, 500 μsec, bipolar	12 months	73–79% in SS, 63–76 in DS, 100% in PS of TWSTRS
Bereznai et al. (7)	5	Bil GPi DBS	1.8–2.5 V, 130 Hz, 120–180 μsec, monopolar	3–12 months	45–92% improvement in Tsui score
Chang et al. (24)	1	Uni GPi DBS	2.0 V, 160 Hz, 180 μsec	12 months	Improvement
Krauss et al. (8)	5	Bil GPi DBS	3.0–4.5 V, 130–145 Hz, 210 μsec, bipolar	20 months	63% in SS 69%, in DS, 50% in PS of TWSTRS
Yianni et al. (25)	6	Bil GPi DBS	5.8 V, 144 Hz, 169 μsec, bipolar (mean)	18.9 months	64% in SS 60%, in DS, 60% in PS of TWSTRS
Eltahawy et al. (4)	3	Bil GPi DBS	N/A	6 months	58 (43–82)% improvement in TWSTRS

Abbreviations: TWSTRS, Toronto Western Spasmodic Torticollis Rating Scale (SS, severity scale; DS, disability scale; PS, pain scale); VAS, visual analogue scale for pain.

Good results are achieved in patients with primary ST, and poor results are achieved in patients with secondary ST and structural lesions.

Islekel et al. (19) and Chang et al. (24) reported benefits of unilateral GPi DBS in patients with ST. Islekel et al. argued that the target should be the GPi contralateral to the contracted SCM (19). Chang et al. reported on a patient with delayed onset post-traumatic ST (24). The DBS was implanted on the same side as the initial traumatic lesion. However, bilateral DBS seems to be more effective for ST, since transcranial magnetic stimulation studies have confirmed that the corticomotor projection to the SCM follows both contralateral monosynaptic pathways and ipsilateral disynaptic pathways (28). In addition, studies of stemocleidomastoid function during Wada testing have shown that this muscle receives bilateral hemispheric innervation and that maximal input comes from the ipsilateral hemisphere (29).

Considering these small series of studies overall, significant pain reduction and more than 50% improvement in the TWSTRS score can be achieved in patients with ST after pallidal DBS. This procedure seems to be a promising treatment for primary and secondary ST, which are refractory to oral medication or botulinum toxin, but a poor candidate for peripheral denervation. In most series, it takes a few months to obtain the full range of clinical improvement through DBS. This delayed improvement is also seen in patients with other types of dystonia (8).

4. RATIONALE OF DBS FOR ST

The anatomical substrate and pathophysiology of ST remain unknown and the pathophysiological mechanism of GPi DBS is not well understood. It is generally thought that dysfunction of the basal ganglia, which causes the relay of erroneous information from the thalamus to the premotor, supplementary motor, and primary motor cortices, is responsible for the development of dystonia. Patients with primary dystonias have a functional disturbance in basal ganglia outflow that disrupts its targets. Removal of this disturbance, by either pallidotomy or pallidal DBS, allows the motor system to revert to a more normal level of function (3,8).

The primary projection from GPi is inhibitory to the motor thalamus. According to a model of movement disorder, hypokinetic disorders such as Parkinson's disease appear to result from increased mean discharge rates of neurons in the GPi, whereas hyperkinetic disorders such as dystonia are associated with decreased mean discharge rates in the GPi (30). In fact, electrophysiological data has demonstrated that the firing rate of GPi neurons in patients with generalized dystonia was lower than that in patients with Parkinson's disease or in normal primates (31,32). Therefore, it is reasonable to conclude that pallidal DBS, which reduces GPi activity, is effective for Parkinson's disease. However, pallidal DBS is also effective for dystonia.

Regarding this contradiction, Vitek et al. additionally demonstrated changes in the pattern and degree of synchronization of pallidal neurons in dystonia (33). Excessive reductions in mean discharge rates of GPi neurons could lead to changes in the pattern and degree of synchronization of thalamic neuronal activity, which may in turn contribute to the development of dystonia. Therefore, the effectiveness of GPi DBS seems to lie in the fact that it removes the source of inhibitory input to the thalamus and normalizes thalamic neuronal activity (33).

Dysfunction of the basal ganglia is also shown in functional neuroimaging studies. According to a recent PET study, ST patients showed a significantly higher glucose metabolism bilaterally in the lentiform nucleus (34). A recent SPECT study showed that Striatal D2 receptor binding was significantly reduced bilaterally in patients with ST. Altered striatal activity may induce secondary changes in the GPi via direct and indirect striatopallidal pathways (35). It was shown that in patients with idiopathic torsion dystonia, metabolic overactivity of the lentiform nucleus and premotor cortices resulted in dissociation of lentiform and thalamic metabolism (36).

5. TECHNICAL CONSIDERATION OF DBS FOR ST

5.1. Surgical Procedure

The surgical procedure is performed under local or general anesthesia. General anesthesia is chosen when the patient shows continuous hyperkinetic dystonic movement. A DBS electrode is implanted under stereotactic guidance. The target localization is based solely on MR imaging, without physiological refinement by intraoperative microelectrode recording. The coordinates of the GPi (posteroventral pallidum) target, where the lower contact of the electrode is placed, will be 18–22 mm lateral, 2–3 mm anterior to the midcommisural point, and 3–5 mm inferior to AC–PC line. However, there is known to be significant interindividual variability in the position of pallidal structures. Therefore, targeting of the GPi should rely on the direct visualization of the structure by MRI. Visualization of the pallidocapsular border, medial putaminal border, and optic tract are especially important to determine the anatomical target point (37). Surgical planning software is useful in determining the coordinates of the target and the entry point (Fig. 1). Burr holes are made over the coronal suture at the mid-pupillary line in the frontal area, and the DBS leads (Activa 3387; Medtronic, Minneapolis, MN) are implanted at the target point bilaterally. When the patient is under local anesthesia, microelectrode recording is used to refine the target. Microelectrode recording is used to characterize the patterns of activity and receptive field properties of single pallidal neurons and to identify important bordering structures, including the optic tract and internal

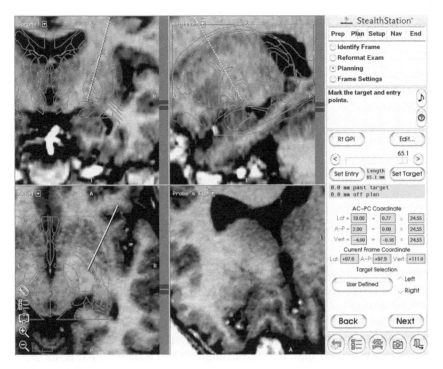

Figure 1 MRI based GPi targeting with surgical planning software (Flame Link; Medtronic, Inc.). This software can easily calculate the coordinates for the target point based on the AC–PC line in 3-D space. The tentative target of GPi is determined as 19 mm lateral, 2 mm anterior to the midcommisural point, and 4 mm inferior to AC–PC line in this case. The anatomical localization of the target point and trajectory are confirmed in the superimposed Schaltenbrand and Wahren Atlas, which is sized to the patient's own MR images.

capsule (38). Generally, the firing rate of pallidal neurons in patients with dystonia (20–50 Hz) is lower than that in patients with Parkinson's disease (80–85 Hz) (32). In the final stage, internal pulse generators (Soletra; Medtronic, Minneapolis, MN) are placed in infraclavicular pockets bilaterally and subcutaneously connected to the DBS leads.

5.2. Postoperative Care

After the operation, MRI is performed to confirm appropriate placement of DBS electrodes in the GPi. Then, the stimulator is activated. The stimulator can deliver pulses with three variable parameters: frequency (0–185 Hz), width (60–420 μsec), and amplitude (0–10.5 V). In most series, stimulation parameters (amplitude, frequency, and pulse width) in patients with ST have been much higher than those in patients with Parkinson's disease (Table 1). This may be due to the severity of the disease or to a different mechanism for the inhibition of GPi activity. Generally, it seems that a much longer pulse width ($>210\,\mu sec$) is required for dystonia (8,23,32). DBS provides the capacity for increasing the intensity of stimulation to yield a better result through the adjustment of parameters.

Regarding the site of stimulation, Goto et al. reported that stimulation of the posteroventral portion of the GPi led to pronounced alleviation of dystonia, while stimulation of the anterodorsal portion or at the dorsal border of the GPi resulted in significant worsening of symptoms (23). They speculated on the existence of at least two different functional zones within the GPi.

In patient with Parkinson's disease, the effect of DBS on tremor, rigidity, or aktnesia is almost immediate. By contrast, some authors have reported that the improvement of dystonia was delayed, taking a few months for the full effect after pallidotomy or DBS to be achieved. Therefore, when a quick response cannot be obtained in patients with ST, it is generally necessary to allow at least 24 hr of continuous stimulation on any one setting before assessing the efficacy of stimulation (39). These differential results suggest that other mechanism of DBS are involved in dystonia. One can speculate that the improvement of dystonia is a phenomenon involving plasticity rather than the simple inhibition of a signal. That is, molecular processes, i.e., protein synthesis, may also play a role in the relief of dystonia during DBS (7,40).

5.3. Surgical Complications

In general, DBS seems to be a relatively safe procedure (41,42). The rate of permanent severe surgical morbidity is less than 2%, and the rate of device-related complications such as infection or skin erosion is less than 5% in centers with extensive experience. Some characteristic symptoms such as cervical movement or head rubbing may expose patients with ST to skin erosions with subsequent infection more frequently than patients with Parkinson's disease (43,44).

REFERENCES

1. Krauss JK, Toups EG, Jankovic J, Grossman RG. Symptomatic and functional outcome of surgical treatment of cervical dystonia. J Neurol Neurosurg Psychiatry 1997; 63:642–648.
2. Jankovic J, Schwartz K. Response and immunoresistance to botulinum toxin injections. Neurology 1995; 45:1743–1746.
3. Krauss JK, Pohle T, Stibal A, Loher T, Burgunder JM. Functional stereotactic surgery for treatment of cervical dystonia. Krauss JK, Jankovic J, Grossman

RG, eds. Surgery for Parkinson's Disease and Movement Disorder. Philadelphia: Lippincott Williams & Wilkins, 2001:343–349.

4. Eltahawy HA, Saint-Cyr J, Giladi N, Lang AE, Lozano AM. Primary dystonia is more responsive than secondary dystonia to pallidal interventions: outcome after pallidotomy or pallidal deep brain stimulation. Neurosurgery 2004; 54: 613–621.

5. Cooper IS. Effect of thalamic lesions upon torticollis. N Engl J Med 1964; 270:567–572.

6. Cooper IS. 20-year follow up study of the neurosurgical treatment of dystonia musculorum deformans. Adv Neurol 1976; 14:423–452.

7. Bereznai B, Steude U, Seelos K, Botzel K. Chronic high-frequency globus pallidus internus stimulation in different types of dystonia: a clinical, video, and MRI report of six patients presenting with segmental, cervical, and generalized dystonia. Mov Disord 2002; 17:138–144.

8. Krauss JK, Loher TJ, Pohle T, Weber S, Taub E, Barlocher CB, Burgunder JM. Pallidal deep brain stimulation in patients with cervical dystonia and severe cervical dyskinesias with cervical myelopathy. J Neurol Neurosurg Psychiatry 2002; 72:249–256.

9. Hassler R, Dieckmann G. Stereotactic treatment of different kinds of spasmodic torticollis. Confin Neurol 1970; 32:135–143.

10. Andrew J, Fowler CJ, Harrison MJG. Stereotactic thalamotomy in 55 cases of dystonia. Brain 1983; 106:981–1000.

11. Von Essen C, Augustinsson LE, Lindqvist G. VOI thalamotomy in spasmodic torticollis. Appl Neurophysiol 1980; 43:159–163.

12. Goldhahn G, Goldhahn WE. Experience with stereotactic brain surgery for spasmodic torticollis. Zentralbl Neurochir 1977; 38:87–96.

13. Ondo WG, Desaloms JM, Jankovic J, Grossman RG. Pallidotomy for generalized dystonia. Mov Disord 1998; 13:693–698.

14. Kavaklis O, Shima F, Kato M, Fukui M. Ipsilateral pallidal control on the sternocleidomastoid muscle in cats: relationship to the side of thalamotomy for torticollis. Neurosurgery 1992; 30:724–731.

15. Thickbroom GW, Byrnes ML, Stell R, Mastaglia FL. Reversible reorganisation of the motor cortical representation of the head in cervical dystonia. Mov Disord 2003; 18:395–402.

16. Mundinger F. New stereotactic treatment of spasmodic torticollis with a brain stimulation system. Med Klin 1977; 72:1982–1986.

17. Andy OJ. Thalamic stimulation for control of movement disorders. Appl Neurophysiol 1983; 46:107–111.

18. Krauss JK, Pohle T, Weber S, Ozdoba C, Burgunder JM. Bilateral stimulation of globus pallidus internus for treatment of cervical dystonia. Lancet 1999; 354:837–838.

19. Islekel S, Zileli M, Zileli B. Unilateral pallidal stimulation in cervical dystonia. Stereotact Funct Neurosurg 1999; 72:248–252.

20. Kulisevsky J, Lleo A, Gironell A, Molet J, Pascual-Sedano B, Pares P. Bilateral pallidal stimulation for cervical dystonia: dissociated pain and motor improvement. Neurology 2000; 55:1754–1755.

21. Andaluz N, Taha JM, Dalvi A. Bilateral pallidal deep brain stimulation for cervical and truncal dystonia. Neurology 2001; 57:557–558.
22. Parkin S, Aziz T, Gregory R, Bain P. Bilateral internal globus pallidus stimulation for the treatment of spasmodic torticollis. Mov Disord 2001; 16:489–493.
23. Goto S, Mita S, Ushio Y. Bilateral pallidal stimulation for cervical dystonia. Stereotact Funct Neurosurg 2002; 79:221–227.
24. Chang JW, Choi JY, Lee BW, Kang UJ, Chung SS. Unilateral globus pallidus internus stimulation improves delayed onset post-traumatic cervical dystonia with an ipsilateral focal basal ganglia lesion. J Neurol Neurosurg Psychiatry 2002; 73:588–590.
25. Yianni J, Bain P, Giladi N, Auca M, Gregory R, Joint C, Nandi D, Stein J, Scott R, Aziz T. Globus pallidus internus deep brain stimulation for dystonic conditions: a prospective audit. Mov Disord 2003; 18:436–442.
26. Consky ES, Lang AE. Clinical assessments of patients with cervical dystonia. Jankovic J, Hallet M, eds. Therapy with Botulinum Toxin. New York: Marcel Dekker, 1994:211–237.
27. Cornelia CL, Stebbins GT, Goetz CG, Chmura TA, Bressman SB, Lang AE. Teaching tape for the motor section of the Tronto Western Spasmodic Torticollis Scale. Mov Disord 1997; 12:570–575.
28. Thompson ML, Thickbroom GW, Mastaglia FL. Corticomotor representation of the sternocleidomastoid muscle. Brain 1997; 120:245–255.
29. DeToledo JC, Dow R. Sternomastoid function during hemispheric suppression by amytal: insights into the inputs to the spinal accessory nerve nucleus. Mov Disord 1998; 13:809–812.
30. Vitek JL. Pathophysiology of dystonia. A neuronal model. Mov Disord 2002; 17(suppl 3):S49–S62.
31. Lozano AM, Kumar R, Gross RE, Giladi N, Hutchinson WD, Dostrovsky JO, Lang AE. Globus pallidus internus pallidotomy for generalized dystonia. Mov Disord 1997; 12:865–870.
32. Lozano AM, Abosch A. Pallidal stimulation for dystonia. Adv Neurol 2004; 94:301–308.
33. Vitek JL, Chockkan V, Zhang JY, Kaneoke Y, Evatt M, DeLong MR, Triche S, Mewes K, Hashimoto T, Bakay RA. Neuronal activity in the basal ganglia in patients with generalized dystonia and hemiballismus. Ann Neurol 1999; 46: 22–35.
34. Magyar-Lehmann S, Antonini A, Roelcke U, Maguire RP, Missimer J, Meyer M, Leenders KL. Cerebral glucose metabolism in patients with spasmodic torticollis. Mov Disord 1997; 12:704–708.
35. Naumann M, Pirker W, Reiners K, Lange KW, Becker G, Brucke T. Imaging the pre- and postsynaptic side of striatal dopaminergic synapses in idiopathic cervical dystonia: a SPECT study using [123I] epidepride and [123I] beta CIT. Mov Disord 1998; 13:319–323.
36. Eidelberg D, Moeller JR, Ishikawa T, Dhawan V, Spetsieris P, Przedborski S, Fahn S. The metabolic topography of idiopathic torsion dystonia. Brain 1995; 118:1473–1484.
37. Hirabayashi H, Tengvar M, Hariz MI. Stereotactic imaging of the pallidal target. Mov Disord 2002; 17(suppl 3):S130–S134.

38. Lozano AM, Hutchinson WD. Microelectrode recordings in the pallidum. Mov Disord 2002; 17(suppl 3):S150–S154.
39. Kumar R. Methods for programming and patient management with deep brain stimulation of the globus pallidus for the treatment of advanced Parkinson's disease and dystonia. Mov Disord 2002; 17(suppl 3):S198–S207.
40. Benabid AL, Koudsie, A, Benazzouz A, Vercueil L, Fraix V, Chabardes S, Lebas JF, Pollak P. Deep brain stimulation of the corpus luysi (subthalamic nucleus) and other targets in Parkinson's disease. Extension to new indications such as dystonia and epilepsy. J Neurol 2001; 248(suppl 3):HI37–H47.
41. Pollak P, Fraix V, Krack P, Moro E, Mendes A, Chabardes S, Koudsie A, Benabid AL. Treatment result: Parkinson's disease. Mov Disord 2002; 17(suppl 3):S75–S83.
42. Umemura A, Jaggi XL, Hurtig H, Siderowf AD, Colcher A, Stern MB, Baltuch GH. Deep brain stimulation for movement disorders: morbidity and mortality in 109 patients. J Neurosurg 2003; 98:779–784.
43. Vercueil L, Krack P, PoUak P. Results of deep brain stimulation for dystonia: a critical reappraisal. Mov Disord 2002; 17(suppl 3):S89–S93.
44. Oh MY, Abosch A, Kim SH, Lang AE, Lozano AM. Long-term hardware-related complications of deep brain stimulation. Neurosurgery 2002; 50: 1268–1276.

12

Tourette's Syndrome Surgical Therapy

Habib E. Ellamushi

The Royal Hospital of St. Bartholomew and The Royal London Hospital, London, U.K.

Gordon H. Baltuch

Department of Neurosurgery, Penn Neurological Institute, University of Pennsylvania School of Medicine, Philadelphia, Pennsylvania, U.S.A.

1. INTRODUCTION

Tourette's syndrome (TS) is a neuropsychiatric disorder with onset in early childhood. TS is named after Georges Albert Edouard Brutus Gilles de la Tourette, a French neuropsychiatrist (1857–1904) (1,2). The syndrome is characterized by motor and vocal tics, which are sudden, brief, intermittent, involuntary or semivoluntary movements (motor tics) or sounds (phonic or vocal tics). Tics usually wax and wane in frequency and intensity during the natural course of the disease. Motor and vocal tics in patients with TS are usually associated with behavioral symptoms such as obsessive–compulsive disorder (OCD) and attention deficit–hyperactivity disorder (AD/HD) (3–5).

It is well known that TS is usually self-limited; however, some patients remain symptomatic and require chronic treatment. The general consensus is that the mean age of onset of tics is 7 years (6). Facial simple motor tics such as eye blinking are thought to be the most common initial symptom. Simple vocal tics occur, on the average, at the age of 11 years. Complex motor tics appear between the ages of 11 and 13 years, and complex vocal tics usually appear a little later, between the ages of 11 and 15 years. The full picture of TS usually develops at about 10 years of age. The severity of tics is thought to peak during the early teens, and thereafter the overall symptoms often go into remission (6,7).

Behavioral disorders such as OCD and AD/HD frequently occur in TS patients. Some studies reported an incidence of more than 50% of AD/HD in TS patients. Other behavioral symptoms such as impulsivity and aggressivity are high in TS patients. Some have reported that 20–30% of TS patients have problems such as physical aggression toward other persons and/or properties (8,9). Anxiety and depression might be more common in TS patients than in healthy controls. Generally, like tics, these associated behavioral symptoms tend to remit with age, possibly by the time the patient reaches 20 years of age or over (8–11).

2. PATHOPHYSIOLOGY OF TOURETTE'S SYNDROME

TS is a heterogeneous disorder with multiple factors possibly involved in its pathogenesis. A number of theories have been proposed concerning the causes of TS including psychogenic, developmental, inflammatory, immune, and genetic factors.

While the pathogenesis at a molecular and cellular level remains largely unknown, several clinical neurophysiological and neuroimaging studies have been performed in an attempt to clarify the pathophysiology of TS (5,12–34). Quantitative analyses of scalp electroencephalography (EEG) (5,12–15), premovement EEG potentials (12), contingent negative variation (16,17), transcranial magnetic stimulation (27–30), and neuroimaging studies (31,32) including echo-planar images and positron emission tomography scans have revealed the likely involvement of the subcortical and the cortical structures, particularly of the basal ganglia and related cortico-striato-thalamo-cortical circuits, in the pathophysiology of TS (35–42). Surface electromyography, evoked potentials, saccadic eye movements (22,23), and polysomnographies (18–20,24,25) have also suggested a dysfunction of the basal ganglia and the brainstem neurons in TS patients. The dysfunction of both motor and nonmotor basal ganglia, thalamus, and cortex circuits were hypothesized to be caused by hypofunction of the dopamine (DA) neurons associated with DA receptor supersensitivity, as well as hypofunction of the serotonergic neurons of the brainstem. It is assumed that the basal ganglia play a major role in the timing and sequencing of motor and behavioral programs by selecting desired and suppressing unwanted programs to be executed (43–46). Uncontrolled movements and vocalizations in TS might be the result of defective inhibitory mechanisms at the level of the basal ganglia, leading to expression of simple or more complex motor or behavioral action. The primary pathology that leads to defective selection mechanisms remains unknown, however intrinsic striatal or extrinsic factors (e.g., excitatory or dopaminergic afferents at the level of the striatum) might play a role (47).

Studies suggested that the activity of DA and 5HT neurons, which have their critical ages of development from late infancy to early childhood, are key elements in pathophysiology of TS. Moreover, TS has a strong genetic component, and considerable progress has been made in understanding the mode of transmission and in identifying potential genomic loci.

3. CONSERVATIVE TREATMENT OF TOURETTE'S SYNDROME

The standard treatment of TS is pharmacologic, using mainly neuroleptics, 2-adrenergic agonists, and sometimes benzodiazepines.

Treatment begins with educational and supportive interventions. However, for severe cases, anti-tic drugs may be necessary. Although there have been only a limited number of double-blind, placebo-controlled trials, neuroleptics are considered to be the most effective remedies. However, limited effectiveness and side effects are major problems of anti-tic treatment (48,49). Two classes of drugs are used most widely to control TS-associated tics: 2-adrenergic agonists such as clonidine and guafacine, and neuroleptics such as tiapride, haloperidol, sulpiride, and pimozide (typical neuroleptic drugs), and olanzapine and risperidone (atypical neuroleptics). 2-adrenergic agonists are generally not as potent as neuroleptics in the suppression of tics; however, their side effects tend to be less severe. The main side effect of 2-adrenergic agonists such as clonidine and guafacine is sedation. The commonly used neuroleptics are tiapride, haloperidol, sulpiride, and pimozide (typical neuroleptics drugs) and olanzapine, risperidone, and ziprasidone (atypical neuroleptics). Long-term treatment with typical neuroleptics is often limited because of the side effects, such as sedation, weight gain, and dysphoria as well as extrapyramidal symptoms. Atypical neuroleptics are less likely to cause extrapyramidal symptoms but they can cause weight gain and sedation (48,49). Ziprasidone is an atypical neuroleptic drug which has been shown to diminish the severity of tics (50), is well tolerated, and does not tend to cause significant weight gain or sedation (51,52).

4. ABLATIVE SURGICAL TREATMENT FOR TOURETTE'S SYNDROME

It is estimated that 1/3 of the patients with TS had persistent disability symptoms in spite of medical therapy. Consequently, there has been an interest in the surgical treatment of intractable symptoms in TS. Many investigators have reported successful suppression of the tics and behavioral symptoms in TS using ablative procedures (53–62), however, the safety and efficacy of such procedures in treating TS are not well documented. Several brain areas have been targeted in lesioning in an attempt to treat intractable TS. These areas include the frontal lobe, the cingulate cortex, and various parts of the thalamic nuclei, particularly the midline intralaminar and ventrolateral nuclei infrathalamic at the level of the H fields of Forel and the zona incerta (ZI), the dentate nucleus, corpus callosum, and caudate–putamen complex. Several ablative procedures have been performed including prefrontal lobotomy and leucotomy, anterior cingulotomy, thalamotomy, and lesioning of the dentate nucleus. Table 1 lists the reports on ablative surgery for TS that have been published in the literature.

In 1962, Baker (63) reported the first leucotomy for intractable TS. The patient was a man with severe vocal and motor tics associated with severe obsessive–compulsive symptoms (OCS). The patient's symptoms improved and after 1 year follow-up the patient had only minimal tics and behavioral symptoms. The patient's surgery was complicated with a brain abscess, which required aspiration.

Cooper (64) reported a case of a 16-year-old girl with intractable tics. The patient underwent right chemothalamectomy followed by a left chemothalamectomy 1 year later. There was significant improvement of the tics following the surgery.

In 1964, Stevens and colleagues (65) reported a case with severe motor and vocal tics and OCS that underwent first prefrontal lobotomy, carried out by James Watts in 1955. The patient had marked improvement of the tics.

In 1969, Cooper et al. reported their experience in the treatment of six patients with severe tics using bilateral thalamic lesioning (66).

Sweet et al. (67) reported the results of treating three patients with intractable TS using bilateral thalamic lesioning of the intralaminar and medial thalamic nuclei, as well as the ventro-oralis internus (VOI). The tics symptoms improved by 100% in Patient 1, 90% in Patient 2, and 70% in Patient 3.

Sawle and colleagues (68) reported a case of intractable TS with severe vocal and motor tics, as well as OCS. The patient had bilateral limbic leucotomy with no effect on the tics initially; however, 19 months after surgery, the tics resolved completely with significant improvement of the OCS.

In 1994, Baer and colleagues (69) reported a patient with TS and OCD who had undergone cingulotomy. The surgery improved the OCS with no effect on the tics. The authors concluded that cingulotomy alone was not an effective treatment for TS.

Babel et al. (70) reported the largest published series of severe intractable TS in 16 patients, with long-term follow-up in 11 patients. Eleven patients underwent lesioning in both the ZI and thalamus, four underwent lesioning of ZI region, and one patient underwent unilateral thalamotomy. There was a significant reduction in vocal and motor tics immediately postoperatively and at long-term follow-up. However, a majority of the patients remained on medical treatment. Several patients developed complications such as hemiparesis and hemiballism.

Temel and Visser-Vandewalle (71) reported a complete review of the literature on the surgical treatment of TS. They found 21 reports and

Table 1 List of the Published Reports on Ablative Surgical Therapy for TS

Author	No. of patients	Surgical procedure	Follow-up (months)	Outcome
Babel et al.	16	Zona incerta and/or thalamotomy	3.5–9.5	45–52% tics reduction
Hassler et al.	15	Intralaminar/ medial/VOI thalamic	Not specified	50–100% tics reduction
Cooper	6	Thalamotomy/ prefrontal lobotomy	22–108	Marked tics reduction
Cappabianca et al.	4	Thalamotomy	Not specified	Temporary improvement
Korzenec et al.	4	Not specified	Not specified	Not specified
Beckers et al.	3	Campotomy/ prefrontal leucotomy	24	Slight improvement
Rauch et al.	3	Anterior cingulotomy	Not specified	90% tics reduction
Asam et al.	2	Zona incerta lesioning	60	Temporary tics relief
Kurlan et al.	2	Cingulotomy	24	No effect on tics
Baker	1	Bilateral frontal leucotomy	12	Marked reduction of tics
Stevens	1	Prefrontal lobotomy	108	Marked tics reduction
Nadvornik et al.	1	Bilateral dentotomy	Not specified	Tics reduction
Moldofsky et al.	1	Leucotomy/ thalamotomy	Not specified	No long-term benefit
Wassman et al.	1	Prefrontal lobotomy	Not specified	Not specified
Robertson et al.	1	Bilateral limbic leucotomy	24	75% tics reduction
Korzen et al.	1	Bilateral thalamotomy	12	Symptoms disappeared
Sawle et al.	1	Bilateral limbic leucotomy	21	Tics disappeared
Leckman et al.	1	Cingulotomy	8	35% tics improvement
Baer et al.	1	Cingulotomy	9	Tics minimally worse

3 descriptions, including about 65 patients in total, who had undergone ablative procedures for intractable TS (71). However, one cannot draw any conclusions on the safety and efficacy of these ablative procedures in these reports for several reasons: (a) lack of information on certainty and confirmation of the target localization in these reports; (b) lack of rationale for choosing specific targets for these ablative procedures; (c) lack of criteria for the diagnosis of TS and lack of evaluation criteria in assessing the tic reduction; (d) lack of blinding and independence of the assessors; (e) many of the patients remained on medical treatment following the surgery, which could influence the outcome of the surgery.

5. DEEP BRAIN STIMULATION FOR TOURETTE'S SYNDROME

Since the introduction of deep brain stimulation (DBS) using permanently implanted brain electrodes by Benabid et al. in 1987 (72), DBS has gained in popularity and has revolutionized the surgical treatment of movement disorders. It is no surprise that DBS is now being used for the treatment of refractory psychiatric disorders. DBS has inherent advantages over the ablative procedures as it is less invasive, reversible, adjustable to the individual, and can be used bilaterally with fewer side effects. Many studies document the safety and efficacy of DBS for treatment of PD, essential tremor, and dystonia. However, reports on using DBS for neuropsychiatric disorders are minimal, comprising several case reports mostly of treating intractable OCD (73–75). To date, there have been only four published cases of bilateral DBS therapy for intractable TS (76–78). The thalamic nuclei were the target in three patients and globus pallidus internus (GPi) in one case.

In 1999, Vandewalle and colleagues (76) reported the first case of intractable TS who underwent DBS therapy. They selected the centromedian nucleus, the intralaminar nucleus, and the ventro-oralis internus (VOI) nucleus as the targets, which are the same group of thalamic nuclei selected by Hassler and Dieckmann for ablative surgery in 1970 (79).

The same authors reported three cases of TS, including the case reported in 1999, all of whom were treated with bilateral thalamic stimulation (77). All three patients were male and suffering from intractable tics. The target selected for stimulation in these cases was at the level of the centromedian nucleus, substantia periventricularis, and the nucleus VOI. At a follow-up of 5 years for Patient 1, 1 year for Patient 2, and 8 months for Patient 3, there was a tic reduction of 90.1% in Patient 1, 72.2% in Patient 2, and 82.6% in Patient 3. Postoperative complications included three revisions of the pulse generator and extension cable. Two patients developed stimulation related side effects which, manifested as increased sexual drive in one patient and reduced sexual potency and ejaculation in another.

In 2002, van der Linden and associates reported a case of TS with motor and vocal tics successfully treated with bilateral internal pallidum (GPi) stimulation (78). The patient underwent bilateral GPi stimulator implantation and, at the same time, bilateral thalamic electrodes were implanted. The patient had test stimulation for 7 days comparing the result of stimulating the thalamus and GPi. The tics improved by 80% with thalamic stimulation and 95% with GPi stimulation. At 6 months follow-up, the GPi stimulation effect remained the same with no postoperative complications or side effects.

6. CONCLUSIONS

For several reasons one cannot draw a conclusion about the safety and efficacy of surgical ablative therapy for intractable TS based on the reports in the literature.

DBS therapy for intractable TS is a new approach with promising initial results in treating tics and associated behavioral symptoms. However, efficacy data are still uncertain, as only a few cases have been reported.

Thus, ablative and DBS surgery for TS continue to be investigational and experimental at this stage. It is clear that more studies with a strict protocol, including well-defined diagnosis criteria, well-defined targets for surgery, and clear specifications of evaluation methods for tics and other symptoms are required.

The increased understanding of the physiology of the basal ganglia and the basal ganglia–thalamocortical circuits, as well as advances in genetics and brain imaging, have provided insight into the possible pathophysiological basis underlying the development of TS. Furthermore, the advances in imaging technology and electrophy-physiological techniques used for localization of brain structures, such as microelectrode mapping, have improved the ability to accurately identify and lesion or stimulate target structures deep in the brain. These developments and data will help increase the degree and consistency of clinical benefit of surgical therapy for TS, as well as contribute to the development of superior methods for treating intractable TS.

REFERENCES

1. Jankovic J. Tourette syndrome. Phenomenology and classification of tics. Neurol Clin 1997; 15:267–275.
2. Lees AJ. Georges Gilles de la Tourette. The man and his times. Rev Neurol (Paris) 1986; 142:808–816.
3. Cummings JL, Frankel M. Gilles de la Tourette syndrome and the neurological basis of obsessions and compulsions. Biol Psychiatry 1985; 20:1117–1126.

4. Jankovic J. Tourette's syndrome. N Engl J Med 2001; 345:1184–1192.
5. Shapiro AK, Shapiro ES, Bruun RD, Sweet RD. Gilles de la Tourette Syndrome. New York, NY: Raven Press, 1978.
6. Bruun RD. The natural history of Tourette's syndrome. Cohen DJ, Bruun RD, Leckman JF, eds. Tourette's Syndrome and Tic Disorders: Clinical Understanding and Treatment. New York, NY: John Wiley & Sons, 1988:22–39.
7. Leckman JF, Zhang H, Vitale A, Lahnin F, Lynch K, Bondi C, Kim YS, Peterson BS. Course of tic severity in Tourette syndrome: the first two decades. Pediatrics 1998; 102:14–19.
8. Comings DE, Comings BG. Tourette syndrome: clinical and psychological aspects. Am J Hum Genet 1985; 37:435–450.
9. Freeman RD, Fast DK, Burd L, Kerbeshian J, Robertson MM, Sandor L. An international perspective on Tourette syndrome: selected findings from 3,500 individuals in 22 countries. Dev Med Child Neurol 2000; 42:436–447.
10. Coffey BJ, Biederman J, Geller DA, Spencer T, Park KS, Shapiro SJ, Garfield SB. The corn-se of Tourette's disorder: a literature review. Harv Rev Psychiatry 2000; 8:192–198.
11. Caine ED, Mcbride MC, Chiverton P, Bamford KA, Redress S, Shiao J. Tourette syndrome in Monroe County school children. Neurology 1988; 38:472–475.
12. Obese JA, Rothwell JC, Marsden CD. The neurophysiology of Tourette syndrome. Adv Neurol 1982; 35:105–114.
13. Stevens A, Gunther W, Lutzenberger W, Bartels M, Muller N. Abnormal topography of EEG microstates in Gilles de la Tourette syndrome. Eur Arch Psychiatry Clin Neurosci 1996; 246:310–316.
14. Gunther W, Muller N, Trapp W, Haag C, Putz A, Straube A. Quantitative EEG analysis during motor function and music perception in Tourette's syndrome. Eur Arch Psychiatry Clin Neurosci 1996; 246:197–202.
15. Hyde TM, Emsellem HA, Randolph C, Rickler KC, Weinberger DR. Electroencephalographic abnormalities in monozygotic twins with Tourette's syndrome. Br J Psychiatry 1994; 164:811–817.
16. Weate SJ, Newell SA, Bongner JE, Andrews JM, Drake ME. Contingent negative variation in Giles de la Tourette syndrome. Clin Electroencephal 1993; 24:188–191.
17. Castellanos FX, Fine EJ, Kaysen D, Marsh WL, Rapoport JL, Hallett M. Sensorimotor gating in boys with Tourette's syndrome and ADHD: preliminary results. Biol Psychiatry 1996; 39:33–41.
18. Straube A, Mennicken JB, Riedel M, Eggert T, Muller N. Saccades in Gilles de la Tourette's syndrome. Mov Disord 1997; 12:536–546.
19. Farber RH, Swerdlow NR, Clementz BA. Saccadic performance characteristics and the behavioural neurology of Tourette's syndrome. J Neurol Neurosurg Psychiatry 1999; 66:305–312.
20. Darsun SM, Burke JG, Reveley MA. Antisaccade eye movement abnormalities in Tourette's syndrome: evidence for cortico-stiriatal network dysfunction. J Psychopharmacol 2000; 14:37–39.
21. Segawa M. Neurophysiology of Tourette's Syndrome: pathophysiological consideration. Brain Dev 2003; 25(suppl I):S62–S69.

22. Hikosaka O, Wurtz RH. The basal ganglia. Wurtz RH, Goldberg ME, eds. The Neurobiology of Saccadic Eye Movements. Amsterdam: Elsevier, 1989:257–281.

23. Hikosaka O, Sakamoto M, Usui S. Functional properties of monkey caudate neurons. Activities related to saccadic eye movements. I Neurophysiol 1989; 61:780–798.

24. Nomura Y. Tics: Gilled de la Tourette syndrome. Sinkeikenkyu No Sinpo 1985; 29:265–275.

25. Fukuda H, Segawa M, Nomura Y, Nishihara K, Ono Y. Phasic activity during REM sleep in movement disorders. Age-Related Dopamine-Dependent Disorders, Monographs in Neural Sciences Vol. 14. Basel: Karger, 1995:69–76.

26. Segawa M. Autism, school refusal and circadian rhythm. Jiritsu shinkei 1998; 35:280–286.

27. Ziemann U, Paulus W, Rothenberger A. Decreased motor inhibition in Tourette's disorder: evidence from transcranial magnetic stimulation. Am J Psychiatry 1997; 154:1277–1284.

28. Ozonoff S, Stayer DL, McMahon WM, Filloux F. Inhibitory deficits in Tourette syndrome: a function of comorbidity and symptom severity. J Child Psychol Psychiatry 1998; 39:1109–1118.

29. Sandyk R. Improvement of right hemispheric functions in a child with Gilles de la Tourette's syndrome by weak electromagnetic fields. Int J Neurosci 1995; 81:199–213.

30. Sandyk R. Reversal of a visuoconstructional disorder by weak electromagnetic fields in a child with Tourette's syndrome. Int J Neurosci 1997; 90:159–167.

31. Braun AR, Randolph C, Stoetter B, Mohr E, Cox C, Vladar K, et al. The functional neuroanatomy of Tourette's syndrome: an FDG-PET study. II: relationships between regional cerebral metabolism and associated behavioral and cognitive features of the illness. Neuropsychopharmacology 1995; 13:151–168.

32. Biswal B, Ulmer JL, Krippendorf RL, Harsch HH, Daniels DL, Hyde JS, et al. Abnormal cerebral activation associated with a motor task in Tourette syndrome. Am J Neuroradiol 1998; 19:1509–1515.

33. Shapiro AK, Shapiro E, Wayne H. Treatment of Tourette's syndrome with haloperidol, review of 34 cases. Arch Gen Psychiatry 1973; 28:92–97.

34. Cohen DJ, Shaywitz BA, Young JG, et al. Central biogenic amine metabolism in children with the syndrome of chronic multiple tics of Gilles de la Tourette: norepinephrine, serotonin, and dopamine. J Am Acad Child Psychiatry 1979; 18:320–341.

35. Braun AR, Stoetter B, Randolph C. The functional neuroanatomy of Tourette's syndrome: an FDG-PET study. Regional changes in cerebral glucose metabolism differentiating patients and controls. Neuropsychopharmacology 1993; 9:277–291.

36. Graybiel AM, Canales JJ. The neurobiology of repetitive behaviors: clues to the neurobiology of Tourette syndrome. Adv Neurol 2001; 85:123–131.

37. Graybiel AM, Rauch SL. Toward a neurobiology of obsessive–compulsive disorder. Neuron 2000; 28:343–347.

38. Leckman JF, Pauls DL, Peterson BS. Pathogenesis of Tourette syndrome: clues from the clinical phenotype and natural history. Adv Neurol 1992; 58:15–24.

39. Peterson B, Riddle MA, Cohen DJ. Reduced basal ganglia volumes in Tourette's syndrome using three-dimensional reconstruction techniques from magnetic resonance images. Neurology 1993; 43:941–949.
40. Rauch SL, Whalen PJ, Curran T. Probing striato-thalamic function in obsessive–compulsive disorder and Tourette syndrome using neuroimaging methods. Adv Neurol 2001; 85:207–224.
41. Singer HS, Butler IJ, Tune LE. Dopaminergic dysfunction in Tourette syndrome. Ann Neurol 1982; 12:361–366.
42. Right CI, Peterson BS, Rauch SL. Neuroimaging studies in Tourette syndrome. CNS Spectr 1999; 4:54–61.
43. Alexander GE, Delong MR, Strick PL. Parallel organization of functionally segregated circuits linking basal ganglia and cortex. Ann Rev Neurosci 1986; 9:357–381.
44. Marsden CD. The mysterious motor function of the basal ganglia: the Robert Wartenberg Lecture. Neurology 1982; 32:514–539.
45. Mink JW. The basal ganglia: focused selection and inhibition of competing motor programs. Prog Neurobiol 1996; 50:381–425.
46. Redgrave P, Prescott TJ, Gurney K. The basal ganglia: a vertebrate solution to the selection problem? Neuroscience 1999; 89:1009–1023.
47. Mink JW. Basal ganglia dysfunction in Tourette's syndrome: a new hypothesis. Pediatr Neurol 2001; 25:190–198.
48. Jankovic J. Tourette's syndrome. N Engl J Med 2001; 345:1184–1192.
49. Leckman JF. Tourette's syndrome. Lancet 2002; 360:1577–1586.
50. Sallee FR, Kurlan R, Goetz CG, Singer H, Scahill L, Law G, Dittman VM, Chappell PB. Ziprasidone treatment of children and adolescents with Tourette's syndrome: a pilot study. J Am Acad Child Adolesc Psychiatry 2000; 39:292–299.
51. Gunasekara NS, Spencer CM, Keating GM. Ziprasidone: a review of its use in schizophrenia and schizoaffective disorder. Drugs 2002; 62:1217–1251.
52. Stimmel GL, Gutierrez MA, Lee V. Ziprasidone: an atypical antipsychotic drug for the treatment of schizophrenia. Clin Ther 2002; 24:21–37.
53. Nadvornik P, Sramka M, Lisy L, Svicka I. Experiences with dentatotomy. Confin Neurol 1972; 34:320–324.
54. Beckers W. [Gilles de la Tourette's disease based on five own observations.] Arch Psychiatr Nervenkr 1973; 217:169–186.
55. Hassler R, Dieckmann G. Relief of obsessive–compulsive disorders, phobias and tics by stereotactic coagulations of the rostral intralaminar and medial-thalamic nuclei. Laitinen LV, Livingston K, eds. Surgical Approaches in Psychiatry. Proceedings of the Third International Congress of Psychosurgery. Cambridge, UK: Garden City Press, 1973:206–212.
56. Hassler R. Stereotaxic surgery for psychiatric disturbances. Schaltenbrand G, Walker AE, eds. Stereotaxy of the Human Brain. New York: Thieme-Stratton Inc., 1982:570–590.
57. Cappabianca P, Spaziante R, Carrabs G, de Divitiis E. Surgical stereotactic treatment for Gilles de la Tourette's syndrome. Acta Neurol (Napoli) 1987; 9:273–280.
58. de Divitiis E, D'Errico A, Cerillo A. Stereotactic surgery in Gilles de la Tourette syndrome. Acta Neurochir (Wien) 1977; 24(suppl.):73.

59. Robertson M, Doran M, Trimble M, Lees AJ. The treatment of Gilles de la Tourette syndrome by limbic leucotomy. J Neurol Neurosurg Psychiatry 1990; 53:691–694.
60. Kurlan R, Kersun J, Ballantine HT Jr, Caine ED. Neurosurgical treatment of severe obsessive–compulsive disorder associated with Tourette's syndrome. Mov Disord 1990; 5:152–155.
61. Kurlan R, Caine ED, Lichter D, Ballantine HT Jr. Surgical treatment of severe obsessive–compulsive disorder associated with Tourette syndrome. Neurology 1988; 38(Suppl):203.
62. Asam U, Karrass W. [Gilles de la Tourette syndrome psychosurgery.] Acta Paedopsychiatr 1981; 47:39–48.
63. Baker EFW. Tourette syndrome treated by biomedical leucotomy. Can Med Assoc J 1962; 86:746–747.
64. Cooper IS. Dystonia reversal by operation in the basal ganglia. Arch Neurol 1962; 7:64–74.
65. Stevens H. The syndrome of Gilles de la Tourette and its treatment. Med Ann District Columbia 1964; 36:277–279.
66. Cooper IS, ed. Involuntary Movement Disorders. New York, NY: Harper and Row, 1969:274–279.
67. Sweet RD, Solomon GE, Wayne H, Shapiro E, Shapiro AK. Neurological features of Gilles de la Tourette's syndrome. J Neurol Neurosurg Psychiatry 1973; 36:1–9.
68. Sawle GV, Lees AJ, Hymas NF, Brooks DJ, Frackowiak RS. The metabolic effects of limbic leucotomy in Gilles de la Tourette syndrome. J Neurol Neurosurg Psychiatry 1993; 56:1016–1019.
69. Baer L, Rauch SL, Ballantine HT Jr, et al. Cingulotomy for intractable obsessive–compulsive disorder. Prospective long-term follow-up of 18 patients. Arch Gen Psychiatry 1995; 52:384–392.
70. Babel TB, Warnke PC, Ostertag CB. Immediate and long term outcome after infrathalamic and thalamic lesioning for intractable Tourette's syndrome. J Neurol Neurosurg Psychiatry 2001; 70:666–671.
71. Temel Y, Visser-Vandwalle V. Surgery in Tourette syndrome. Mov Disord 2004; 19(1):3–14.
72. Benabid AL, Pollak P, Louveau A, Henry S, de Rougemont J. Combined (thalamotomy and stimulation) stereotactic surgery of the VIM thalamic nucleus for bilateral Parkinson disease. Appl Neurophysiol 1987; 50(1–6):344–346.
73. Aouizerate B, Cuny E, Martin-Guehl C, Guehl D, Amieva H, Benazzouz A, Fabrigoule C, Allard M, Rougier A, Bioulac B, Tignol J, Burbaud P. Deep brain stimulation of the ventral caudate nucleus in the treatment of obsessive–compulsive disorder and major depression. Case report. J Neurosurg 2004; 101(4):682–686.
74. Sturm V, Koulousakis A, Trener H, Klien JC, Klosterkotte J. The nucleus accumbens: a target for deep brain stimulation in obsessive–compulsive and anxiety-disorders. J Chem Neuroanat 2003; 26(4):293–299.
75. Gabriels L, Cosyns P, Nuttin B, Demeulemeester H, Gybels J. Deep brain stimulation for treatment-refractory obsessive–compulsive disorder: psychopathological and neuropsychological outcome in three cases. Acta Psychiatr Scand 2003; 107(4):275–282.

76. Vandewalle V, van der Linden C, Groenewegen HJ, Caemaert J. Stereotactic treatment of Gilles de la Tourette syndrome by high frequency stimulation of thalamus. Lancet 1999; 353:724.

77. Visser-Vandewalle V, Temel Y, Boon P, et al. Chronic bilateral thalamic stimulation: a new therapeutic approach in intractable Tourette syndrome. A report of three cases. J Neurosurg 2003; 99:1094–1100.

78. van der Linden C, Colle H, Vandewalle V, Alessi G, Rijckaert D. Successful treatment of tics with bilateral internal pallidum (GPi) stimulation in a 27-year-old male patient with Gilles de la Tourette's syndrome (GTS).

79. Hassler R, Dieckmann G. [Stereotaxic treatment of tics inarticulate cries or coprolalia considered as motor obsessional phenomena in Gilles de la Tourette's disease.] Rev Neurol (Paris) 1970; 123:89–100.

80. Robertson MM, Trimble MR, Lees AJ. The psychopathology of the Gilles de la Tourette syndrome: a phenomenological analysis. Br J Psychiatry 1988; 152:383–390.

13

Botulinum Toxin/Microvascular Decompression—Indication, Technique, and Surgical Results

Frédéric Schils and Nicolas de Tribolet
Department of Neurosurgery, University of Geneva, Geneva, Switzerland

Michel R. Magistris
Department of Neurology, University of Geneva, Geneva, Switzerland

1. INTRODUCTION

Hemifacial spasm is a rare condition of intermittent, painless, involuntary, spasmodic contractions of muscles innervated by the facial nerve on one side of the face only. As other movement disorders, it is responsible for neurological disability with potentially severe social and aesthetic impact on patients' daily quality of life. Hemifacial spasm was categorized by Janetta (1) among hyperactive cranial nerve dysfunction syndromes caused by vascular compression at the root exit or entry zone of the cranial nerve with trigeminal and glossopharyngeal neuralgia. This benign condition was first described more than a century ago by Schultze (2) in 1875 who described a typical case of left hemifacial spasm without other cranial nerve symptoms or signs in a patient who died from a tuberculous pneumonia. Autopsy revealed a compression of the seventh cranial nerve by a small aneurysm of the left vertebral artery. Gowers (3) also described in 1884 a case of hemifacial spasm due to mechanical pressure on the facial nerve by a vertebral artery aneurysm. At that time, the cause of hemifacial spasm was presumed to be idiopathic in most cases or, rarely, to be secondary to gross organic lesions, such as cerebellopontine angle (CPA), neurinomas, cholesteatomas, or meningiomas. At the beginning of the 20th century, Cushing (4) was the first to suggest that palsies of the cranial nerves could be caused by vascular compression. At the same time, many neurosurgeons were working on trigeminal neuralgia, and Dandy in 1929 (5) observed that in trigeminal neuralgia, the fifth nerve was compressed and distorted by a vascular arterial contact of the superior cerebellar artery with the dorsal root of the nerve.

In 1947, Campbell and Keedy (6) reported two patients with tic douloureux and hemifacial spasm and demonstrated vascular arterial compression of the seventh nerve. A year later, Laine and Nayrac (7) also discovered a vascular abnormality (aneurysm of the basilar artery) in a patient with isolated hemifacial spasm. In 1962, Gardner and Sava (8) proposed vascular decompression for the treatment of hemifacial spasm inspired by the treatment of the tic douloureux and the similarities between these two pathologies. By this way, they achieved excellent results with 17 of 19 patients relieved of their symptoms. Fifteen years later (9), a great contribution to our understanding of the pathophysiological mechanism of this rhizopathy was provided by the work of Jannetta et al.

As the vascular compression of the facial nerve at its root exit zone from the brainstem is the etiology, the most logical and curative treatment is microsurgical vascular decompression, which is a widely accepted concept now.

2. EPIDEMIOLOGY

Hemifacial spasm is an uncommon condition. The reported incidence is 0.8 per 100,000 per year, and the prevalences are 7.4 per 100,000 for men and 14.5 per 100,000 for women (10). Other series (11) confirmed these numbers with a male female ratio of 35:65. Hemifacial spasm is not considered a hereditary disease, even though a few familial cases have been reported (12,13). It occurs almost exclusively in adults but may also occur in children aged 18 or younger. In Barker and Jannetta's series, the mean patient age at onset was 44 years (11). In the series of Mooij, the mean patient age at onset was 56 years (14), and in the latest series of Samii, the mean patient age at onset was 54 (15) with an age range between 19 and 80 years. The pathology especially affects the middle-age population. For unknown reasons, all the authors report that the left side is affected more frequently than the right side with a ratio approximately 55:45 (1,16). The symptoms are usually unilateral, even if in some cases both sides were affected (17). The mean duration of symptoms was 6 years prior to surgical procedure. In one study, arterial hypertension was found to be an associated condition among 66.7% of patients (18).

3. SYMPTOMS AND CLINICAL SIGNS

Hemifacial spasm is an induced movement disorder characterized by intermittent, involuntary, irregular, unilateral, tonic, or clonic contractions of muscles innervated by the ipsilateral facial nerve. Although a benign condition, it represents a distressing experience and constitutes a severe handicap for the patient with aesthetic and social impacts on daily life. The condition includes synkinesis (simultaneous contraction of different muscles of the face) and spasms (involuntary sustained contractions) that vary in severity over time. The symptoms experienced by the patient are classically categorized into typical and atypical. The typical spasm, which is observed in the great majority of the patients, with a frequency of 95% in Samii's series (15), starts with involuntary twitching of the orbicularis oculi muscle and gradually progresses downward to involve the orbicularis oris, buccinator, and/or the platysma. The condition usually begins with rare contractions of the orbicularis oculi muscle, and slowly progresses to involve the entire half of the face and increases in frequency. These contractions are synchronous in the involved muscles. After an initial period of clonic movements, a tonic phase usually supervenes, producing a grinning expression called risus sardonicus, better known in generalized tetanus. This phase produces a forced ipsilateral eye closure interfering with binocular vision. During these episodes, pain is not a significant symptom, although some patients may describe an aching discomfort during an attack. In atypical forms, which are quite rare, the spasm starts from the buccinator and orbicularis oris muscles and spreads upward to the orbicularis oculi muscle. Hemifacial spasm and palatal myoclonus are the only involuntary movement disorders that persist during sleep (19). Some trigger factors have been described among which we can mention emotional stress, fatigue, or voluntary contraction of any facial muscle. Over the years, the severity of the affliction, although fluctuating, tends to increase, and a mild facial weakness can develop on the affected side, but this finding requires a careful neurological examination because often only a deficit ability to hide eyelashes on forced eye closure can be discovered. A clinical manifestation reported by Babinski as a specific and early sign of the condition is the closure of the eye on the side of the spasm while the patient is asked to raise the ipsilateral eyebrow (20). The patients have no other symptoms of cranial nerve dysfunction. Hemifacial spasm may be associated with trigeminal neuralgia, geniculate neuralgia, or vestibular and/or cochlear nerve dysfunction.

4. DIAGNOSIS, STAGING, CLASSIFICATION

Although a differential diagnosis must be made, in most cases there is no ambiguity regarding the diagnosis, and hemifacial spasm is easily recognized by those familiar with this disorder. It must be distinguished from facial myokymia (continuous facial spasm), which may be a manifestation of an intrinsic brainstem glioma or of multiple sclerosis. It must also be distinguished from blepharospasm (bilateral spasmodic closure of the orbicularis oculi muscles), which is more common in the elderly, and may be associated with organic brain syndrome. Blepharospasm is notorious for disappearing when the patient presents for medical examination (an "alerting effect"), but may be elicited by asking the patient to gently close the eyes and then rapidly open them, following which a blepharospasm may occur. The differential diagnosis also includes "habit" spasm (volitional), focal motor seizures, synkinesia after nerve injury, tardive dyskinesia, and Meige's syndrome (oromandibular dystonia and blepharospasm) (21,22). There is no evidence that these disorders will respond to microvascular decompression. Before the introduction of magnetic resonance (MR) imaging, computed tomography with bone windows was the only radiological method used; since that time, both methods have been used to evaluate mass lesions. Angiography is not indicated. Magnetic resonance imaging and magnetic resonance angiography may demonstrate the vascular features around the root exit zone and exclude other conditions. It is important to note that the absence of visible vascular compression of the nerve on MR scans does not mean that it does not exist. Clinical classification have been developed by Palfi and Jedynak (23), and the spasms were classified as mild, moderate, or severe: mild, with almost exclusive involvement of the orbicularis oculi muscle; moderate, between mild and severe, including mouth deviation; and severe, complete eye closure, deviation of mouth, and involvement of the platysma.

5. PHYSIOPATHOLOGY

It is now thought that the pathophysiological mechanism of hemifacial spasm is the result of vascular compression of the facial nerve at its root exit zone from the brainstem. Two pathophysiologic mechanisms have been suggested to explain hemifacial spasm: (a) ephaptic transmission between adjacent axons within the facial nerve (24–26) and (b) abnormal hyperexcitability of the facial nucleus (27–32). The ephaptic hypothesis proposed that cross-talk occurs among axons of the facial nerve. This hypothesis has received strong support from several electrophysiologic studies that showed that electrical stimulation of a branch of the facial nerve was able to evoke responses in the territory of other branches (delayed responses or lateral spread responses) (33–39) or within the territory of the same branch (28,35,36,38,40,41). This neurophysiologic investigation may confirm the diagnosis by demonstrating both the typical spontaneous electromyographic pattern and the presence of the so-called abnormal response. The complete resolution of hemifacial spasm that may be obtained by surgical microvascular decompression also speaks in favor of the ephaptic mechanism rather than of a sole nucleus hyperexcitability. The matter nevertheless remains the subject of disputes

(26,29–32,38). Some authors suggested that the combination of a central facial hyperexcitability with impaired afferent conduction in the facial nerve could be the cause of hemifacial spasm (35,36,42,43). By studying responses of single axons of the facial nerve in patients with hemifacial spasm, Roth et al. (44) concluded that ephaptic connections, which may be bidirectional and connect more than two axons, and hyperexcitability of the facial nucleus both play a role in hemifacial spasm. These authors proposed that one mechanism could explain the synkinesis and the spasm observed in hemifacial spasm. Although the ephapse would be responsible for the synkinesis, the variation of excitability of the facial nucleus would modulate the importance of the spasm. In Roth et al.'s theory, F waves play a pivotal role (an F wave is an action potential generated sporadically by the motor neuron in response to an antidromic action potential). F waves are not observed physiologically; they supervene when a motor axon is excited artificially somewhere along its length or when, in many pathologic conditions, including hemifacial spasm, ectopic depolarizations occur on any site along the axon. "F" relates to foot because F responses were first recorded from foot muscles. In hemifacial spasm, when an action potential travels on an axon of the facial nerve (whether it is a potential normally generated by a motor neuron or, in case of an ectopic depolarization, occurring anywhere along the axon), it may be transmitted to an axon (or possibly to several), through the ephaptic connection. The postephaptic pathway conducts the potential orthodromically toward the facial musculature, where it results in a synkinesis if the potentials of the pre- and postephatic axons conduct to different muscles. The postephatic pathway also conducts antidromically toward the facial motor neuron. If the potential that reaches the motor neuron produces an F wave, this wave is transmitted to the whole population of motor axons interconnected through the ephapse.

All these axons are invaded by orthodromic and antidromic waves. It is sufficient that one motor neuron gives rise to another F wave and a self-sustained involuntary activity reaches the muscle, where it results in a short spasm. A more prolonged rhythmic excitation and re-excitation of a population of neurons may result from the higher occurrence of F responses caused by a temporarily increased excitability of the facial nucleus. This increased excitability may be triggered by the antidromic activity itself or may relate to other influences. In hemifacial spasm patients, the occurrence of F waves evoked by electrical stimuli of the facial nerve was observed to be high compared with normal controls (in whom F waves of the facial nerve are uncommon). F waves are more frequent in alert states and during the Jendrassik maneuver. In hemifacial spasm, it is commonly observed that spasms are made worse by increased alertness and emotional tension. Under these influences, the motor neurons probably become more excitable, facilitating the invasion of their soma by the antidromic wave (45) and the subsequent generation of F waves. Spreading of the spasm may result from the excitation of adjacent quiescent axons (46), the rhythmic activity (47), and the ephaptic synchronization of several populations of axons. An amplification of the ephaptic response (34,48), or a mass effect, may result in spatial summation. This spatial summation may cause all axons of the facial nerve to fire together, leading to the disfiguring spasms that are occasionally observed in severe hemifacial spasm. Several subsequent works by Ishikawa et al. (49–53) confirm the finding of Roth et al. (44).

6. SURGICAL ANATOMY

The origin of the acousticofacial complex is located far laterally in the pontomedullar sulcus, anteriorly and slightly superiorly to the end of the lateral recess of the rhomboid fossa of the fourth ventricule, inferolaterally to the peduncle of the cerebellar flocculus, and above the rootlets of the glossopharyngeal nerve (54). This complex is composed of three nerves: the facial nerve anteriorly, the vestibulocochlear posteriorly, and the nervus intermedius in the middle and posterosuperiorly to the facial nerve. Just after leaving the pontomedullary sulcus, the facial nerve remains in close contact with the pons over a few millimeters in length at the subpial course of the facial nerve that can be visualized during microvascular decompression when the compressing artery is lifted from the nerve; the distal portion of the facial nerve is attached to the artery, while the subpial part remains closely attached to the pons. The end of this subpial part corresponds to the point of contact between the nerve and the pons that usually is hidden by the cerebellar flocculus and choroid plexus.

From the brainstem, the seventh cranial nerve enters the pontocerebellar cistern and courses anterosuperiorly into the posterior fossa. It crosses the vestibulocochlear nerve anterosuperiorly before reaching the internal auditory meatus. The compression of the facial nerve at its root exit zone is often due to the anterior inferior cerebellar artery (AICA) (55–58). The AICA arises at the lowest third of the basilar artery mostly as a single vessel but can be duplicated or triplicated and rarely is absent (59). The proximal part of the AICA courses backward and slightly caudally around the pons, crossing the abducens nerve either ventrally or dorsally. It then proceeds to the CPA, where it divides into two major trunks, rostral and caudal, before or after reaching the acoustical complex. One or more of these trunks course in close relationship with the seventh and eighth cranial nerves and are said to be nerve related. Distally, these two trunks anastomose with the superior cerebellar artery and the posterior inferior cerebellar artery (PICA). The nerve related trunks of the AICA are divided in different segments composed of one or two arterial trunks. The premeatal segment starts at the basilar artery to finish in the vicinity of the internal acoustic meatus, where the meatal segment begins. This segment forms a convex loop directed toward or through the porus acousticus. This loop is under the acousticofacial bundle in 46% of cases, between in

36%, and above in 6% (60). The postmeatal segment returns medially toward the pons to supply the cerebellum and the brainstem. The distal premeatal, meatal, and proximal postmeatal segments are of clinical relevance because they are the portions of the AICA that potentially can compress the facial nerve in the CPA, causing hemifacial spasm.

The internal auditory artery, or the labyrinthine artery, derives from the nerve-related segments of the AICA, mostly from the proximal limb or the apex of the meatal loop medially to the canal. This artery commonly courses inferiorly or anteroinferiorly to the acoustical bundle as far as the meatus, where it terminates by giving off branches to supply the inner ear. Several other small important arteries come off these nerve-related segments, such as subarcuate or the recurrent perforating arteries. The PICA represents a frequent source of hemifacial spasm, being a compressing vessel at least as frequently (61,62) as, or even more frequently than, the AICA (11,63). Its origin from the vertebral artery is mostly above the level of the foramen magnum at the level of the olive, anteroinferiorly to the pyramid within the premedulary cistern (64). Rarely, the PICA can originate from below the foramen magnum. The artery courses in various ways with the hypoglossal nerve and reaches the fila of cranial nerves 9, 10, and 11 at the posterolateral margins of the medulla. This lateral medullary segment interacts in different ways with these nerves within the pontomedullary cistern, passing mostly between the rootlets of the accessory nerve. This segment is usually the source of glossopharyngeal neuralgia but can be involved in the genesis of hemifacial spasm in compressing the root exit zone of the facial nerve as described by Janetta et al. (9). The artery continues its courses around the cerebellar tonsil. Veins and the vertebral artery are also found among compressive vascular structures, and there are multiple cases where the compression is attributable to more than one vessel (AICA and vertebral artery; PICA and vertebral artery; AICA and PICA; AICA, PICA and vertebral artery; and AICA with veins).

Observation of the histology of the facial nerve shows that two different types of myelin are present during its course from the brainstem to the porous acousticus. The proximal portion of the nerve root is covered by the central myelin synthesized by the oligodendrocytes, whereas the Schwann cells produce a thinner myelin sheet that covers the peripheral segment. The zone of transition between the central segment and the peripheral segment corresponds to the root exit zone of the facial nerve or the Redlich–Obersteiner zone. These two types of myelin are differentiated easily with myelin-specific staining. At the root entry zone, the central myelin forms a dome-shaped projection into the peripheral myelin. The measurement of this projection shows a great variability among authors, ranging from 0.8 to 2.5 mm (65,66). This zone forms a kind of funnel or ring (the so-called pial ring of Tarlov) that is reinforced by a plexus of neuroglial and connective tissue fibers (65). It has been proposed that the passage of this pial ring produces a constriction of numerous axons that could explain the diminution of myelin observed in this zone.

Similar to the other cranial nerves, the facial nerve has no perineurium or epineurium, in contrast to the peripheral nerves, but still possesses an endoneurium, which contributes to its sensitivity toward traction or compression. Ruby and Janetta (67) examined the ultrastructural changes of the facial nerve induced by a vascular compression and commented:

> The most apparent changes were observed in the medium to large sized fibers. The most obvious pathology was a "proliferation" or hypermyelination of many of the myelin sheaths with a concomitant disorganization of the myelin lamellar structure . . . the axis cylinders were usually eccentrically placed and the denuded side was in direct contact with the extracellular collagen. Totally denuded, tortuous, hypertrophic axis cylinders exhibiting an appearance suggestive of early microneuroma formation were also encountered.

7. TREATMENT

7.1. Medical

The main objective in the treatment of hemifacial spasm is to decrease or end the annoying twitches of one side of the face. The nonsurgical treatments of hemifacial spasm vary from simple massage and the application of heating pads to different types of medications, including carbamazepine, baclofen, clonazepam, felbamate, gabapentin, and botulin toxin injections. Before considering surgical approaches for patients with hemifacial spasm, a trial of medical therapy should be undertaken. Many neurologists use the botulinum toxin, which exerts its effects by a paralytic action. There are isolated reports of spasm relief by drugs such as carbamazepine, but oral medication is unlikely to be helpful. Botulinum toxin type A (BTX-A) is the preferred medical treatment in hemifacial spasm patients. After endocytosis, the toxin undergoes disulfide cleavage. The remaining light chain enters the cytosol and blocks normal binding of vesicles to the axon's presynaptic terminal membrane. By strongly binding to presynaptic neuromuscular cholinergic receptors, the toxin decreases the frequency of acetylcholine release. Although much work is yet to be done in this area, some general conclusions can be derived. Assuming proper technique is used, local side effects from botulinum toxin are rare. The two most common local side effects from orofacial injection of botulinum toxin are alteration in salivary consistency and inadvertent weakness of the swallowing, speech and facial muscles. These complications are injection-site specific (e.g., more common with lateral pterygoid injections and palatal and tongue muscle injections) and dose dependent problems. Dysphagia is the most common worrisome side effect, and it is caused primarily by spread of toxin to pharyngeal muscles. Nausea, general malaise, and weakness, as well as allergic reactions and the development of antibodies to BTX-A, have also been reported. Report of successful therapy is mostly case series based, but randomized, blinded, controlled studies are needed to establish the true efficacy of this method. For BTX-A, the duration of the effect is 2 or 3 months, and patients typically require injections every 3–6 months. It is recommended that injection be done no more than once every 12 weeks to avoid the development of antibodies against the toxin. Clinical trials report that facial hemispasm may be treated with repeated injections of botulinum toxin with a high success rate and relatively low complications (68). In some patients, relief from spasm can only be obtained at the cost of an ipsilateral upper lip droop of varying severity (69). Some clinical series have been published in the literature evaluating the efficacy of botulinum toxin A for the treatment of hemifacial spasm. Defazio et al. (70) presented a retrospective review with a 95% response rate and an overall mean duration of improvement of 12.6 weeks with limited local adverse effects (upper lid ptosis, facial weakness, diplopia). Other series (71–73) advanced similar results with a relief response between 88% and 98% and a benefit duration superior to 2 months with a range between 2 and 13 months. They conclude that botulinum toxin injection is an effective and safe treatment for patients with hemifacial spasm and provides effective, safe, and long-lasting relief of spasms.

In a minority of patients, botulinum toxin is either ineffective or poorly tolerated. In this group of patients, a trial with oral medication is warranted. A partial alcoholization sometimes helps to achieve an improvement, as does carbamazepine.

Recently, some authors described the use of doxorubicin in hemifacial spasm (74). They proposed chemical rhizotomy of facial nerve under local anesthesia in a subgroup of patients with hemifacial spasm, especially elderly patients and those in the high-risk group for general anesthesia and intracranial neurosurgery. They reported no major complications and no recurrence of spasm 3 years after the procedure in a patient with unsuccessful treatment with antiepileptic medicine. They did not observe regrowth of nerve fibers after this chemical rhizotomy. But again this successful therapy is case series based, and randomized, blinded, controlled studies are needed to establish the true efficacy of this method.

7.2. Surgical

The patient is placed in the lateral position with the upper shoulder pulled down and anteriorly. The head is flexed slightly and tilted toward the floor and fixed in a three point head holder. The longitudinal skin incision is 6 cm long, 1 cm medial to the mastoid tip. The incision continues through the muscle to the bone. The occipital artery is coagulated and cut as it courses below the mastoid tip. The muscle is separated from the bone, and the orifice of the emissary vein medial to the mastoid is obliterated with bone wax. While drilling the bone, this emissary vein leads to the sigmoid sinus. A craniotomy or craniectomy, 3 cm in diameter, is performed medially and slightly inferiorly to the mastoid. The lateral edge of the craniotomy must expose the posteromedial border of the sigmoid sinus. The transverse sinus need not be exposed. The opened air cells are packed carefully with bone wax. Cerebrospinal fluid can be drained through a lumbar catheter placed at the beginning of the surgical procedure to obtain a slack dura. At this point, the microscope is installed. A curvilinear incision of the dura that remains attached to the sigmoid sinus is performed, and the dural flap is tacked up laterally. The cerebellum is carefully lifted rostromedially to expose the arachnoid of the cerebellomedullary cistern. Opening the arachnoid allows the escape of cerebrospinal fluid and obtains a relaxed cerebellum. No retractors are used during the procedure because they are more in the way than helpful. Cranial nerve 11 is identified and followed until cranial nerves 10 and 9 are visualized. At this point, the vertebral artery is also in the view. The arachnoid covering these nerves and the flocculus behind them must be dissected carefully. Deep (anterior) to the flocculus, the choroids plexus of the foramen of Luschka is seen. Approximately 5 mm rostral to the origin of cranial nerve 9, the origin of cranial nerve 8, and deeper to it, cranial nerve 7, can be identified.

The facial nerve is recognizable because of its slightly grayish color. In typical cases, its origin is hidden by the offending artery.

If a large loop of the vertebral artery seemingly is compressing the origin of the nerve, it is important to check that the PICA is not causing additional compression. Using a microdissector or the bipolar forceps, the offending artery is lifted carefully away from the brainstem (Fig. 1). The subpial course of cranial nerve 7 now can be seen. To keep the artery away, we use a fluffy Polytef (Teflon) pledget (Fig. 2). The artery also can be fixed to the dura with a sling and fibrin glue. Care must be taken to push it against the artery and not the nerve. In a compression caused by a large artery such as the vertebral, it is helpful to use two or three pledgets pushed caudally as suggested by McLaughlin et al. (75). During this delicate part of the procedure, the surgeon must absolutely avoid tearing small vessels vascularizing the pons or the nerves, particularly the internal auditory artery. Bipolar coagulation should not be used.

As mentioned previously, retractors are not used because they are in the way. The suction, set at low power, is used as an intermittent retractor. During this phase of the procedure, monitoring auditory evoked potentials can be helpful. When the surgeon is satisfied with separation of the artery from the nerve, the Teflon pleget is fixed in place with fibrin glue. There must be no compression of the nerve by the pledget. If a clear arterial compression has been identified proximally, which should be the case, the nerve does not need to be explored distally. At the beginning of his experience, the senior author had to reoperate on two patients who failed to respond and found that he had not explored proximally enough the first time. Closure is performed with

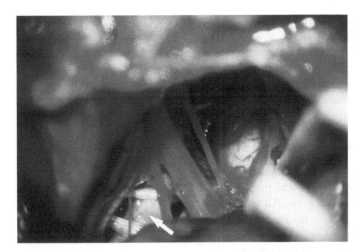

Figure 1 Left cerebellopontine angle under surgical microscope. The bipolar forceps points to the origin of the facial nerve. The vertebral artery (*arrow*) is seen between cranial nerves 11 and 10. The offending artery (posterior inferior cerebellar artery) is lifted carefully.

a running suture on the dura, the bone flap is fixed with miniplates, and the skin sutured in two layers without subcutaneous drainage. In some cases the exact site of vascular compression may be unclear. For this reason, some authors proposed the use of intraoperative monitoring to improve the results of vascular decompression in hemifacial spasm. Mooij et al. presented a

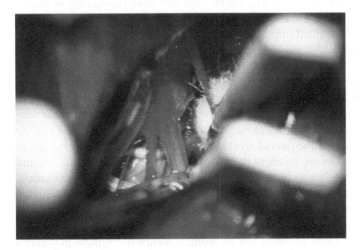

Figure 2 Same case as Figure 1, the fluffy Teflon has been inserted between the origin of cranial nerve 7 and the posterior inferior cerebellar artery.

74-patient series (14) and demonstrated the applicability and usefulness of intraoperative facial nerve monitoring in microvascular decompression operations for hemifacial spasm. A guiding role of intraoperative monitoring was apparent in 33.8% of patients, and a confirming role was demonstrated in 52.7% of patients, which resulted in a positive contribution of approximately 87% for intraoperative facial monitoring in microvascular decompression for hemifacial spasm.

8. CONTRAINDICATIONS TO SURGERY

Relative contraindications to intracranial procedures include coagulopathy, use of antiplatelet agents, and poorly controlled hypertension. These must be considered before surgery. All aspirin-type products are discontinued ten days before surgery. Intraoperatively, it is essential to monitor the patient's systolic blood pressure, because hypertension will significantly increase the risk of an intracerebral hemorrhage.

9. RESULTS

For several reasons, caution must be applied during the analysis of the clinical results of microvascular decompression. First, only a few important prospective studies have been conducted. Second, the end points, which are most of the time quoted as excellent, partial relief, and failure of surgery, are difficult to compare because their definitions differ from study to study, or simply do not exist. Third, the time elapsed between the evaluations of these different end points varies. Nevertheless, these different studies designed to evaluate the yields of surgery not only show the superiority of microvascular decompression over other forms of surgical treatment, but also show the efficacy of microvascular decompression in curing hemifacial spasm. Barker et al. (11) in 1995 published one of the most important studies, comprising 612 patients followed for 1 year or more (average 8 years) after microvascular decompression. The initial results at 1 month were gratifying.

Of the patients, 86% had excellent results, 5% were partial successes, and in 9% the operation failed. Barker et al. (11) first evaluated the long-term results (at 10 years) of the initial procedure only: 79% of patients reported excellent results, 5% were partial successes, and in 16% the operation failed. Then the investigators reported the overall treatment results, including all operations in all patients. Results were excellent in 84% of cases, partial successes in 7%, and failures in 9%. Nearly all failures occurred within 24 months of the operation, and the percentage of reoperation was 9%. A statistically significant higher probability of excellent results was shown in patients with typical hemifacial spasm vs. patients with atypical hemifacial spasm (88% versus 59% of excellent results at 5 years) and for men versus women within the typical hemifacial spasm group (93% versus 83% at 10 years). Chun et al. (16) reported in 1992 the results of microvascular decompression in 310 Chinese patients. Follow-up varied from 6 months to 8 years (average 4.3 years). The immediate results at 3 days postoperatively were excellent for 273 patients (88%). They found no improvement in 37 patients (12%). Of these 37 cases of failure, 16 (5.2%) presented with spontaneous relief 4–22 months (average 21 days) after the surgery and 5 (1.6%) improved to partial relief. All of the 16 patients (5.2%) with no improvement after surgery were reoperated. Thirteen had complete immediate relief. Shin et al. (76) conducted a prospective study enrolling 261 patients. Of these, 226 patients were followed for 6 months to 2 years. One week after microvascular decompression, excellent outcomes were reported in 61.1% of patients. Shin et al. found that the percentage of excellent results increased to 82.7% when the patients were followed for more than 6 months. The authors concluded that time significantly ($P < 0.5$) improves the clinical pictures of hemifacial spasm after microvascular decompression. Illingworth et al. (77) published one of the longest prospective studies to evaluate the long-term benefit of microvascular decompression in a population of 83 patients. Of operated patients, 78 were followed for an average of 8 years. The authors noted the absence of any spasm in 72 (92%) and reported minor intermittent muscles twitches in 2 (3%); 3 (4%) had recurrent of hemifacial spasm. One patient's operation was not completed.

In their study, Payner and Tew (57), in addition to reporting their own results of microvascular decompression, reviewed the literature concerning the recurrence of hemifacial spasm in more than 600 operated patients. In their own retrospective study, they enrolled 34 patients followed for 1–14 years (average 6.2 years). Complete resolution was noted in 29 patients (85%), partial relief in 3 (9%), and failure in 2 (6%). Excellent results were obtained for 25 patients immediately after operation, and for three patients, excellent results were obtained within 3 months to 3 years. For the patients relieved initially, some degree of spasm recurred in 10.3%, but no patient developed a recurrence after 24 months. The literature review by Payner and Tew (57) suggested that the recurrence rate is 7.0% of 751 patients. These authors also concluded that patients without signs of spasm after 2 years have a 0.1% risk of developing a spasm again.

Samii et al. (15) reported their long-term results for 145 cases treated with microvascular decompression. At discharge, 59% were spasm-free, 41% experienced further spasm. At 6 months, the number of spasm-free patients had increased to 92.3% whereas 7.7% complained of hemifacial spasm. The level of recurrence was 7.7%.

10. COMPLICATIONS

The complications reported in the literature are those that can be expected from an operation aiming to reach the cerebellopontine angle. Barker et al. (11) reported 21 cases (3%) of hearing deficit out of the 648 first operations. Seventeen patients (2.6%) were deaf, and mild to moderate hearing loss was present in

4 (0.7%). The introduction of intraoperative monitoring of brainstem evoked responses showed a trend in diminishing this complication, but it did not reach statistical significance ($P = 0.05$). The atypical spasms were associated significantly ($P = 0.04$) with an increased risk of hearing loss. On reoperation, a lesion of the acoustic nerve seems more frequent, reaching 3% of all reoperated patients (differences not statistically significant). Twenty-five patients (3.9%) suffered a transitory facial weakness, and 25 (3.4%) suffered a permanent facial weakness. Intraoperative measurement (monitoring of facial nerve function and brainstem evoked responses) lowered the rate of facial injury significantly. If the compressing vessel was a labyrinthine artery, a facial weakness was more frequent ($P = 0.002$). Reoperation was associated with a fivefold increased risk of severe facial weakness. Other complications were cerebrospinal fluid leaks in 21 patients (2.7%) and aseptic meningitides affecting 16% of patients. Wound infection, transient dysphagia, and hoarseness were infrequent. One patient (0.1%) died during the operation.

In another large study (16), deafness was present in five (1.6%) patients and transient hearing loss in two (0.6%). Facial weakness was the most frequently encountered complication, being mild in 10 patients (3.2%) and moderate in 5 (1.6%). Eight (2.6%) patients suffered from cerebrospinal fluid rhinorrhea. This last complication was no longer a problem because the exposed mastoid air cells were routinely and immediately sealed with bone wax and muscle pledgets. No surgical deaths were reported. In 1983, Loeser and Chen (42) reviewed 16 series encompassing 450 microvascular decompression procedures done on 433 patients. They found a total of 109 (24%) complications: 38 (8%) were temporary and 71 were permanent. Auditory nerve dysfunction in 58 (13%) patients was two times more frequent than the 26 (6%) facial nerve dysfunctions reported. Loser and Chen (42) reported one death (0.2%).

In Samii's series (15), complications included deafness (8.3%), reduction in auditory acuity (7.6), vertigo (9.6%), facial nerve weakness (2.7%), and cerebrospinal fluid leaks (4.8%).

11. CONCLUSIONS

The treatment of hemifacial spasm is a challenging but rewarding area for neurosurgeons. The proper selection of surgical candidates is critical to achieving positive outcomes. Both the selection of patients and the follow-up evaluation can be facilitated with the use of standardized evaluation scales. Through multidisciplinary collaboration, neurosurgeons are able to improve the quality of life of patients who have a variety of movement disorders.

Analysis of the series in the literature demonstrates that microvascular decompression to treat hemifacial spasm involves very low risk, is well tolerated, is associated with a very low recurrence rate, and represents the definitive treatment for more than 90% of cases.

REFERENCES

1. Jannetta PJ. Cranial rhizopathies. Youmans JR, ed. Neurological Surgery. 3rd ed. Philadelphia, PA: W.B. Saunders, 1990:4169–4182.
2. Schultze F. Linksseitiger fatialiskrampf in folge eines aneurisma der arteria vertebralis sinistra. Virchows Arch 1875; 65:385–391.
3. Gowers R, ed. Manual of Diseases of the Nervous System. London: J&A Churchill, 1888.
4. Cushing H. Strangulation of the nervi abducentes by lateral branches of the basilar artery in case of brain tumor. Brain 1911; 33:204–235.
5. Dandy WE. An operation for the cure of tic douloureux: partial section of the sensory root at the pons. Arch Surg 1929; 18:687–734.
6. Campbell E, Keedy C. Hemifacial spasm: a note on the aetiology in two cases. J Neurosurg 1947; 4:342–347.
7. Laine E, Nayrac P. Hémispasme facial guéri par intervention sur la fosse postérieure. Rev Neurol 1948; 80:38–40.
8. Gardner WJ, Sava GA. Hemifacial spasm: a reversible pathophysiological state. J Neurosurg 1962; 19:240–247.
9. Jannetta PJ, Abbasy M, Maroon JC, Ramos FM, Albin MS. Etiology and definitive microsurgical treatment of hemifacial spasm. Operative techniques and results in 47 patients. J Neurosurg 1977; 47(3):321–328.
10. Auger RG, Whisnant JP. Hemifacial spasm in Rochester and Olmsted County, Minnesota, 1960 to 1984. Arch Neurol 1990; 47:1233–1234.
11. Barker FG II, Jannetta PJ, Bissonette DJ, Shields PT, Larkins MV, Jho HD. Microvascular decompression for hemifacial spasm. J Neurosurg 1995; 82: 201–210.
12. Carter JB, Patrinely JR, Jankovic J, McCrary JA III, Boniuk M. Familial hemifacial spasm. Arch Ophthalmol 1990; 108:249–250.
13. Friedman A, Jamrozik Z, Bojakowski J. Familial hemifacial spasm. Mov disord 1989; 4:213–218.
14. Mooij JJ, Mustafa MK, van Weerden TW. Hemifacial spasm: intraoperative electromyographic monitoring as a guide for microvascular decompression. Neurosurgery 2001; 49:1365–1371.
15. Samii M, Gunther T, Iaconetta G, Muehling M, Vorkapic P, Samii A. Microvascular decompression to treat hemifacial spasm: long term results for a consecutive series of 143 patients. Neurosurgery 2002; 50:712–718.
16. Chun IH, Ih-Hsin C, Liang-Shong L. Microvascular decompression for hemifacial spasm: analyses of operative findings and results in 310 patients. Neurosurgery 1992; 30:53–57.
17. Ehni G, Woltman HW. Hemifacial spasm: a review of hundred and six cases. Arch Neurol Psychiatry 1945; 53:205–211.
18. Oliveira LD, Cardoso F, Vargas AP. Hemifacial spasm and arterial hypertension. Mov Disord 1999; 14:832–835.
19. Tew JM, Yeh HS. Hemifacial spasm [abstr]. Neurosurgery 1983; 2:267–278.
20. Dwoize JL. "The other" Babinski's sign: paradoxal raising of the eyebrow in hemifacial spasm. J Neurol Neurosurg Psychiatry 2001; 70:516.
21. Blair RL, Berry H. Spontaneous facial movement. J Otolaryngol 1981; 10:459–462.
22. Wilkins RH. Hemifacial spasm: a review. Surg Neurol 1991; 36:251–277.

23. Palfi S, Jedynak CP. Hemifacial spasm and other hemifacial abnormal movements: Clinical aspects. Sindou M, Keravel Y, Moller AR, eds. Hemifacial Spasm: A Multidisciplinary Approach. Vienna: Springer-Verlag, 1997:45–49.

24. Woltman HW, Williams HL, Lambert EH. An attempt to relieve hemifacial spasm by neurolysis of the facial nerves; a report of two cases of hemifacial spasm with reflections on the nature of the spasm, the contracture and mass movement. Mayo Clin Proc 1951; 26(13):236–240.

25. Williams HL, Lambert EH, Woltman HW. The problem of synkinesis and contracture in case of hemifacial spasm and Bell's palsy. Ann Otol Rhinol Laryngol 1952; 61(3):850–872.

26. Ravits J, Hallett M. Pathophysiology of hemifacial spasm. Neurology 1986; 36(4):591–593.

27. Wartenberg R. Hemifacial Spasm: A Clinical and Pathological Study. New York: Oxford University Press, 1952:86.

28. Ferguson JH. Hemifacial spasm and facial nuceus. Ann Neurol 1978; 4:97–103.

29. Moller AR, Jannetta PJ. On the origin of synkinesis in hemifacial spasm: results of intracranial recordings. J Neurosurg 1984; 61(3):569–576.

30. Moller AR, Jannetta PJ. Synkinesis in hemifacial spasm: results of recording intracranially from the facial nerve. Experienta 1985; 41(3):415–417.

31. Moller AR, Jannetta PJ. Hemifacial spasm: results of electrophysiologic recording during microvascular decompression operations. Neurology 1985; 35(7):969–974.

32. Moller AR, Jannetta PJ. Microvascular decompression in hemifacial spasm: intraoperative electrophysiological observations. Neurosurgery 1985; 16(5):612–618.

33. Hopf HC, Lowitzsch K. Hemifacial spasm: location of the lesion by electrophysiological means. Muscle Nerve 1982; 5(9S):S84–S88.

34. Nielsen VK. Electrophysiology of the facial nerve in hemifacial spasm: ectopic/ephaptic excitation. Muscle Nerve 1985; 8(7):545–555.

35. Nielsen VK. Pathophysiology of hemifacial spasm: lateral spread of the supraorbital nerve reflex. Neurology 1984; 34(4):427–431.

36. Nielsen VK. Pathophysiology of hemifacial spasm: ephatic transmission and ectopic excitation. Neurology 1984; 34(4):418–426.

37. Nielsen VK, Jannetta PJ. Pathophysiology of hemifacial spasm: III. Effects of facial nerve decompression. Neurology 1984; 34:891–897.

38. Nielsen VK. Indirect and direct evidence of ephaptic transmission in hemifacial spasm [letter]. Neurology 1986; 36:592.

39. Sanders DB. Ephaptic transmission in hemifacial spasm: a single fiber EMG study. Muscle Nerve 1989; 12:690–694.

40. Esslen E. Der spasmus facialis: eine Parabioseerscheinung. Electrophysiologische Untersuchungen zum Entstehungsmechanismus des Facialisspasmus. Dtsch Z Nervenheilk 1957; 176:149–172.

41. Tankere F, Maisonobe T, Lamas G, Soudant J, Bouche P, Fournier E, Willer JC. Electrophysiological determination of the site involved in generating abnormal muscle responses in hemifacial spasm. Muscle Nerve 1998; 21(8):1013–1018.

42. Loeser JD, Chen J. Hemifacial spasm: treatment by microsurgical facial nerve decompression. Neurosurgery 1983; 13(2):141–146.

43. Esteban A, Molina-Negro P. Primary hemifacial spasm: a neurophysiological study. J Neurol Neurosurg Psychiatry 1986; 49(1):58–63.

44. Roth G, Magistris MR, Pinelli P, Rilliet B. Cryptogenic hemifacial spasm. A neurophysiological study. Electromyogr Clin Neurophysiol 1990; 6:361–370.
45. Eccles JC. The central action of antidromic impulses in motor nerve fibers. Pflugers Arch 1955; 260:385–415.
46. Gasser HS. Recruitement of nerves fibers. Am J Physiol 1938; 121:193–202.
47. Arvanitaki A. Effects evoked in an axon by the activity of a contiguous one. J Neurophysiol 1942; 5:89–108.
48. Nielsen VK, Soso MJ. Amplification of the ephaptic response in hemifacial spasm by collision of impulses [abstr]. Muscle Nerve 1984; 7:S78.
49. Ishikawa M, Ohira T, Namiki J, Kobayashi M, Takase M, Kawase T, Toya S. Electrophysiological investigation of hemifacial spasm after microvascular decompression: F waves of the facial muscles, blink reflexes, and abnormal muscles responses. J Neurosurg 1997; 86:654–661.
50. Ishikawa M, Namiki J, Takase M, Ohira T, Nakamura A, Toya S. Effect of repetitive stimulation on lateral spreads and F waves in hemifacial spasm. J Neurol Sci 1996; 142:99–106.
51. Ishikawa M, Ohira T, Namiki J, Ajimi Y, Takase M, Toya S. Abnormal muscle response (lateral spread) and F wave in patients with hemifacial spasm. J Neurol Sci 1996; 137:109–116.
52. Ishikawa M, Ohira T, Namiki J, Ishihara M, Takase M, Toya S. F-wave in patients with hemifacial spasm: observations during microvascular decompression operations. Neurol Res 1996; 18(1):2–8.
53. Ishikawa M, Ohira T, Namiki J, Gotoh K, Takase M, Toya S. Electrophysiological investigation of hemifacial spasm: F-waves of the facial muscles. Acta Neurochir 1996; 138:24–32.
54. Scolozzi P, Dorfl J, Tribolet N. Microsurgical anatomy of the subtentorial supracerebellar and infracerebellar approach to the trigeminal and facial nerves. J Clin Neurosci 1999; 6:400–407.
55. Wilson CB, Yorke C, Prioleau G. Microsurgical vascular decompression for trigeminal neuralgia and hemifacial spasm. West J Med 1980; 132:481–487.
56. Fairholm D, Wu JM, Liu KN. Hemifacial spasm: results of microvascular relocation. Can J Neurol Sci 1983; 10:187–191.
57. Payner TD, Tew JM Jr. Recurrence of hemifacial spasm after microvascular decompression. Neurosurgery 1996; 38:686–690.
58. Mitsuoka H, Tsunoda A, Okuda O, Sato K, Makita J. Delineation of small nerves and blood vessels with three dimensional fast spin echo MR imaging: comparison of presurgical and surgical findings in patients with hemifacial spasm. Am J Neuroradiol 1998; 19:1823–1829.
59. Martin RG, Grant JL, Peace D, Theiss C, Rhoton AL Jr. Microsurgical relationships of the anterior inferior cerebellar artery and the facial-vestibulocochlear nerve complex. Neurosurgery 1980; 6:483–507.
60. Ouaknine GE. Microsurgical anatomy of the arterial loops in the pontocerebellar angle and the internal acousticus meatus. Samii M, Jannetta PJ, eds. The Cranial Nerves. Berlin: Springer-Verlag, 1981.
61. Sindou M, Fischer C, Derraz S, Keravel Y, Palfi S. Microsurgical vascular decompression in the treatment of hemifacial spasm. A retrospective study of a series of 65 cases and review of the literature. Neurochirurgie 1996; 42:17–28.

62. Kondo A, Ishikawa J, Yamasaki Y, Konishi T. Microvascular decompression of cranial nerves, particularly of the 7th cranial nerve. Neurol Med Chir (Tokyo) 1980; 20:739–751.

63. Piatt JH Jr, Wilkins RH. Treatment of tic douloureux and hemifacial spasm by posterior fossa exploration: therapeutic implications of various neurovascular relationships. Neurosurgery 1984; 14:462–471.

64. Lister JR, Rhoton AL Jr, Matsushima T, Peace DA. Microsurgical anatomy of the posterior inferior cerebellar artery. Neurosurgery 1982; 10:170–199.

65. Tarlov IM. Structure of the nerve root: 1 nature of the junction between the central and peripheral nervous system. Arch Neurol Psychiatry 1937; 37:555–583.

66. Skinner HA. Some histological features of the cranial nerves. Arch Neurol Psychiatry 1931; 25:356–372.

67. Ruby JR, Jannetta PJ. Hemifacial spasm: ultrastructural changes in the facial nerve induced by neurovascular compression. Surg Neurol 1975; 4(4):369–370.

68. Clark GT. The management of oromandibular motor disorders and facial spasms with injections of botulinum toxin. Phys Med Rehabil Clin N Am 2003; 14: 727–748.

69. Boghen DR, Lesser RL. Blepharospasm and hemifacial spasm. Curr Treat Options Neurol 2000; 2:393–400.

70. Defazio G, Abbruzzese G, Girlanda P, Vacca L, Curra A, De Salvia R, Marchese R, Raineri R, Roselli F, Livrea P, Berardelli A. Botulinum toxin A treatment for primary hemifacial spasm: a 10 year multicenter study. Arch Neurol 2002; 59:418–420.

71. Thussu A, Barman CR, Prabhakar S. Botulinum toxin treatment of hemifacial spasm and blepharospasm: objective response evaluation. Neurol India 1999; 47:206–209.

72. Chen RS, Lu CS, Tsai CH. Botulinum toxin A injection in the treatment of hemifacial spasm. Acta Neurol Scand 1996; 94:207–211.

73. Cuevas C, Madrazo I, Magallon E, Zamorano C, Neri G, Reyes E. Botulinum toxin A for the treatment of hemifacial spasm. Arch Med Res 1995; 26:405–408.

74. Ito M, Hasegawa M, Hoshida S, Miwa T, Furukawa M. Successful treatment of hemifacial spasm with selective facial nerve block using doxorubicin (adriamycin) under local anesthesia. Acta Otolaryngol 2004; 124(2):217–220.

75. McLaughlin MR, Jannetta PJ, Clyde BL, Subach BR, Comey CH, Resnick DK. Microvascular decompression of cranial nerves: lessons learned after 4400 operations. J Neurosurg 1999; 90:1–8.

76. Shin JC, Chung UH, Kim YC, Park CI. Prospective study of microvascular decompression in hemifacial spasm. Neurosurgery 1997; 40:730–734.

77. Illingworth RD, Porter DG, Jakubowski J. Hemifacial spasm: a prospective long-term follow up of 83 cases treated by microvascular decompression at two neurosurgical centres in the United Kingdom. J Neurol Neurosurg Psychiatry 1996; 60:72–77.

14

Cerebral Palsy

Jean-Pierre Farmer and Sandeep Mittal

*Division of Pediatric Neurosurgery, McGill University Health Centre,
Montreal, Quebec, Canada*

1. INTRODUCTION

Cerebral palsy comprises a diverse collection of clinical syndromes. These disorders are characterized by abnormalities of posture and movement resulting from an insult to the immature brain. Cerebral palsy remains one of the leading causes of childhood neurological impairment and disability. The characteristic signs are spasticity, movement disorders, muscle weakness, ataxia, and rigidity. Cerebral palsy generally is considered to be a static, nonprogressive encephalopathy, implying that the neurological injury is not an evolving process. However, the clinical expression of cerebral palsy is subject to change as children and their developing nervous system mature. The ability to have extremely immature children survive routinely has in some respect neutralized the benefits of technological advances on reducing the incidence of the disease. Therefore, despite progress in neonatal care, cerebral palsy remains an important clinical problem that has significant effects on function and health-related quality of life of patients and their caregivers. One should also bear in mind that considerable cognitive, psychological, general medical, and social issues are also associated with the disorder. The following chapter aims to outline the epidemiology, pathophysiology, diagnosis, and management of the musculoskeletal manifestations of cerebral palsy.

2. EPIDEMIOLOGY AND DEMOGRAPHICS

Cerebral palsy is a common problem resulting from injury to the developing central nervous system. The motor and postural abnormalities are thought to be associated with prenatal, perinatal, or postnatal events (up to 3 years of life) of varying etiologies that are frequently multifactorial in nature. The overall incidence of cerebral palsy ranges from 1.5 to 3.0 per 1000 live births (1,2). Cerebral palsy inflicts lifelong disabilities on an estimated 500,000 children and adults in the United States (2,3). Worldwide, following an initial modest decline in childhood prevalence, the rate has increased slowly and steadily. This is probably due to not only advances in neonatal care with increased survival of very low birth weight infants but also to improved documentation by national registries among other factors (4). However, causality for the increase in prevalence of cerebral palsy remains to be clearly established. Cerebral palsy cannot be attributed to a single causative factor or event. Rather, multiple etiologic factors are implicated in the development of the disorder that can be classified by both time frame and pathology. Prenatal causes include multiple gestation, chorioamnionitis, maternal infection, antepartum vaginal bleeding, untreated hyperbilirubinemia, and maternal exposure to alcohol. Perinatal factors most commonly identified are fetal anoxia, bradycardia, hemorrhage, and infection. Neonatal causes are prematurity/low-birth weight, germinal matrix hemorrhage, and infection. Early childhood factors include traumatic brain injury, near-drowning, meningitis/encephalitis.

The natural history of cerebral palsy has changed considerably over the last few decades. When appropriate health care is provided, affected children without significant comorbidities may have a near normal life span (5). Ninety-five percent of children with diplegia and 75% of children with quadriplegia survive until the age of 30 years (6). Ninety percent of children with mild mental retardation and 65% of children with severe mental retardation survive until the age of 38 years (6). Overall survival of all children with cerebral palsy until the age of 20 years is 90% (7,8). However, mortality is higher and lifespan shorter in children with quadriparesis, hydrocephalus, lack of basic functional skills, refractory seizures, and profound mental retardation (8,9). Because expected lifespan is longer, particularly in diplegics, a significant emphasis has been placed on quality of life issues in the past 20 years. With a modern multidisciplinary approach, the functional status of children with diplegia and mildly quadriparetic children can tend toward normality. Moreover, severely involved children and their caregivers can still benefit from therapeutic intervention, not only with respect to pain and comfort issues, but also to the use of their upper extremities.

3. PATHOPHYSIOLOGY

Cerebral palsy is defined as a permanent disorder caused by nonprogressive defects or lesions of the immature cerebral motor cortex. A clinical presentation of cerebral palsy may result from an underlying structural abnormality of the brain; early prenatal, perinatal, or postnatal injury due to vascular insufficiency; toxins or infections; or the pathophysiologic risks of prematurity. Evidence suggests that prenatal factors described earlier result in 70–80% of cases of cerebral palsy. In most cases, however, the exact cause is unknown but is most likely multifactorial. The motor skills of children with cerebral palsy improve as they mature, but the rate of improvement is slower compared to unaffected children. The motor impairments are a consequence of various neurological deficits. Central nervous system pathology associated with cerebral palsy includes: cerebral hemorrhage, mechanical spinal cord or brainstem damage, cerebral white matter and cortical hypoxia, and metabolic neuronal cell death from cerebral ischemia (10). A full understanding of the patterns of brain injury seen in children with cerebral palsy mandates a firm grasp of the embryological development of the nervous system. Major events in human brain development and their peak times of occurrence include the following: primary neurulation (week 3–4 of gestation), prosencephalic development (months 2–3 of gestation), neuronal proliferation and migration (months 3–4 of gestation), neuronal circuitry organization (month 5 of gestation to years postnatal), and axonal myelination (birth to years postnatal). It becomes evident that given its complexity and vulnerability, the brain is subject to injury throughout the various stages of growth. Cerebral ischemia prior to the 20th week of gestation may result in a neuronal migration disorder. Periventricular leukomalacia typically occurs following cerebral damage between the 26th and 34th weeks of gestation. Between the 34th and 40th weeks, focal or multifocal cerebral injury is frequently seen. In fact, brain injury seen in premature children consists of multiple lesions including: germinal matrix hemorrhage, intraventricular hemorrhage, posthemorrhagic hydrocephalus, and periventricular leukomalacia (11). Periventricular leukomalacia appears to be the most important determinant of neurologic compromise seen in the very low birth weight infants ($<1500\,g$).

Brain injury due to vascular insufficiency depends on various factors at the time of injury, including vascular distribution to the brain, efficiency and regulation of cerebral blood flow, and biochemical response of brain tissue to decreased oxygenation. The immaturity of the cerebral vasculature likely predisposes the premature infant to a significant risk of developing cerebral palsy. Prior to term, the distribution of fetal circulation to the brain results in the tendency for hypoperfusion to the periventricular white matter. Cerebral hypoperfusion at this point may result in germinal matrix hemorrhages and periventricular leukomalacia, which is classically associated with a spastic diplegic presentation. Often, however, the clinical end result is a combination of these two pathophysiological processes. In contrast, at term, when circulation to the brain closely resembles the mature cerebral vasculature, hypoperfusion mostly targets injury to the watershed areas of

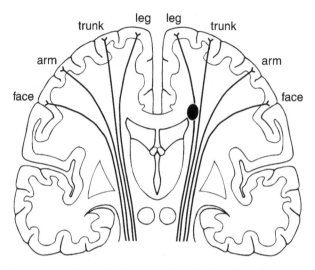

Figure 1 Schematic drawing of projection fibers from the primary motor cortex in relation to the lateral ventricle.

the cortex, resulting in a predominant spastic quadriplegic phenotype. When the basal ganglia are affected, an extrapyramidal presentation with prominent choreoathetoid or dystonic movements is seen. Cerebrovascular injuries at term tend to occur most often in the distribution of the middle cerebral artery, resulting in a spastic hemiplegic phenotype.

Loss of autoregulation of cerebral blood flow in the human newborn occurs with perinatal asphyxia. The extent of injury is thought to be related to regional vascular and metabolic factors and the regional distribution of excitatory synapses. Between weeks 26 and 34 of gestation, the periventricular white matter areas near the lateral ventricles are most susceptible to hypoxic–ischemic injury. Vacuolization and gliosis set in with secondary enlargement of the body of the lateral ventricles. Since these areas carry fibers responsible for the motor control and muscle tone of the legs, a milder injury can result in spastic diplegia (Fig. 1). When larger lesions extend lateral to the area of descending fibers from the motor cortex to involve the centrum semiovale and corona radiata, both the lower and upper extremities may be involved.

3.1. Hypoxic–Ischemic Injury

Periventricular leukomalacia is generally symmetric and thought to be due to ischemic white matter injury in the premature infant. Asymmetric injury to the periventricular white matter can result in one hemibody being more affected than the other. The result mimics a spastic hemiplegia but is best characterized as an asymmetric spastic diplegia and should be distinguished from "double hemiplegia." The germinal matrix capillaries in the periventricular region are particularly vulnerable to hypoxic–ischemic injury due to their location at a vascular border zone between the end zones of the striate and thalamic arteries. In addition, since they are brain capillaries, they have a high requirement for oxidative metabolism. Therefore, another pathophysiological process coexists with ischemic periventricular leukomalacia in these premature children of 24–35 weeks; that is germinal matrix ischemia and intraventricular hemorrhage.

Volpe has classified intraventricular hemorrhage into three grades depending on the extent of ventricular blood (12). Further emphasis is placed on the extent of the intraparenchymal damage seen on cranial ultrasound, which, when present, imparts the greatest prognostic ramifications. In contrast, the extent of intraventricular blood may have more of an incidence on raised intracranial pressure, extension of the germinal matrix damage, and risk of late hydrocephalus. Whether alterations in flow velocity in the anterior cerebral arteries as a result of intracranial hypertension and ventriculomegaly have an effect on the extent of ischemic periventricular leukomalacia is a subject of contention. Clinically, the relative impact of the coexistence of these two pathophysiological processes is that often several months to years later, children exhibit a mixed syndrome. The therapeutic procedures currently available for children have the greatest impact on spasticity and play a limited beneficial role on ataxia (other than if related to hydrocephalus) or dystonia.

Status marmoratus is the neuropathological result of a neonatal hypoxic–ischemic encephalopathy and is thought to affect term infants more than premature infants. This lesion is notable for a marbled appearance due to an abnormal myelin pattern. It involves the basal ganglia and thalamus and results in a dyskinetic phenotype. The underlying brain anomaly in cerebral palsy is thought to be static, whereas the motor impairment and functional consequences evolve with time as the absence of cortical control and the hypotonia yield to an increased influence of the reflex arc via synaptic substitution and dominance of spasticity. By definition, cases due to underlying disorders of a progressive or degenerative nature are excluded when diagnosing cerebral palsy.

4. DIAGNOSIS AND CLINICAL PRESENTATION

Cerebral palsy is a descriptive term, based on clinical observation, rather than a diagnosis informative about etiologic factors, pathology, or prognosis (13). The diagnosis of cerebral palsy is based upon a history of abnormal motor development that is not progressive coupled with a neurological examination (e.g., hypertonicity, increased reflexes, clonus) that localizes the lesion in the brain. In order to establish that a brain abnormality exists in children with cerebral palsy that may, in turn, suggest an etiology and prognosis, neuroimaging is recommended. Magnetic resonance imaging of the head is preferred to computed tomography. Metabolic and genetic studies should be obtained if there are atypical features in the history or on the examination. Detection of a brain malformation in a child with cerebral palsy might also suggest an underlying genetic or metabolic etiology. As cerebral infarction is high in children with hemiplegic cerebral palsy, diagnostic testing for coagulation disorders should be considered. An electroencephalogram is generally not recommended in the initial work-up unless there are features suggestive of epilepsy or a specific epileptic syndrome. Since children with cerebral palsy may have associated cognitive deficits, ophthalmologic and hearing impairments, speech and language disorders, and oral–motor dysfunction, screening for these conditions should be included in the initial assessment (14).

5. CLASSIFICATION

Given the diversity of etiologies of cerebral palsy and the multitude of cerebral territories which can be injured, it follows suit that the ensuing motor syndromes may be highly variable (15). Distinguishing among subtypes of cerebral palsy provides specificity to a broad diagnostic grouping. The topographic distribution of limb involvement and the quality of the movement disorder determine the subtypes.

5.1. Spastic Form

Statistically, $\approx 60\%$ of children will exhibit a predominance of spasticity, either in the form of diplegia or as symmetric or asymmetric quadriparesis. Spasticity is the clinical sign that is most amenable to various medical and surgical therapeutic measures (see the following text). Clinically, these children initially display hypotonia and delayed motor milestones. Gradually, as the spinal reflex arc's influence increases, the predominant picture becomes that of velocity-dependent hypertonia, hyperreflexia, and clonus. On functional examination, these children may have limited sitting ability, poor protective responses, and very little isolation of movements in the lower extremities. These impairments lead to ambulatory difficulties with scissoring gait and equinovarus deformity. Children with the spastic form of cerebral palsy have frequent falls even if global ataxia is not present. This is a reflection of their poor posture and contractures. The motor impairments far exceed the intellectual difficulties.

5.2. Athetoid–Dyskinetic Form

Athetosis and dystonia dominate the clinical picture in 20% of cases. Children then predominantly exhibit slow writhing involuntary movements, which may affect the distal extremities (athetosis) or the proximal limbs and trunk (dystonia). In the pure form, their gait will show both hip and knee hyperextension with an exaggerated step. Children lean backwards and extend the trunk and shoulder girdle as the step is initiated. Involuntary, abrupt jerky movements (chorea) may also occur, particularly with periods of stress and emotions. Rarely, some children may have hemiballistic movements. The motor manifestations exceed the cognitive difficulties in children with the athetoid–dyskinetic form of cerebral palsy.

5.3. Ataxic Form

In ≈10% of children, there is a predominant ataxic form of cerebral palsy. In these patients, extensive cerebellar involvement results in significant gait and balance difficulties, which far exceed the postural problems related to spasticity (see previous text). Even short leg sitting may be arduous because of the imbalance. Weakness, incoordination, intention tremor, wide-based gait, and dysdiadochokinesis dominate the clinical picture. Other than ensuring that accompanying hydrocephalus, when present, is treated, children with the ataxic form of cerebral palsy have limited significant medical or surgical options available to treat their condition. Occupational therapy will provide assistive devices to help these children with their activities of daily living. Physical therapy will help them develop compensatory mechanisms.

5.4. Other Forms

The other subtypes of cerebral palsy account for the remaining 10% of cases. Hemiplegia as a result of an early vascular injury with possible associated migration disorder or as a result of a late middle cerebral artery encephaloclastic event should be distinguished from asymmetric quadraparesis. The former is less amenable to systemic antispasticity therapy than the latter. Most hemiplegics ambulate and adapt well. They are at higher risk of a seizure disorder. Hypotonia, which persists beyond age 3 years, manifests with some spasticity but persistent poor trunk control and an inability for children to carry out graded repetitive motor maneuvers such as squatting. These individuals may use their spasticity positively and need it to support their limited posture. A treatment aiming at eliminating the spasticity in these individuals could be counterproductive.

5.5. Mixed Form

It is clear that the vast majority of children with cerebral palsy present with a mixed clinical picture. The treating team has to determine which of the clinical features predominate in a given individual to be able to tailor therapy.

6. THERAPEUTIC AVENUES

The treatment of cerebral palsy is directed at repair of the injured cerebrum and at the management of the impairments and disabilities resulting from developmental brain injury. At present, there are no clinically meaningful interventions that can successfully repair existing damage to the brain areas that control muscle coordination and movement. However, various interventions are available to diminish the degree of impairment (e.g., muscle spasticity), to increase participation in activities of daily living, and to improve the overall functional performance of these children. Treatment planning requires the determination that excess tone interferes with some aspect of function, comfort, or care, and takes into consideration carefully devised goals that meet the needs of the patient and the caregiver. Management options include physical and occupational therapy, oral medications, chemodenervation with botulinum toxin (Botox®), dorsal rhizotomy, intrathecal baclofen, and orthopedic surgery.

6.1. Physical Therapy

Physical therapy uses several physical and behavioral approaches to diminish disability, improve function, and maintain performance. These approaches are often incorporated within complimentary intervention strategies (see the following text) and aim at lengthening contracted muscles, improving the strength of weakened muscles, increasing the range of motion at restricted joints, improving movement coordination, and developing compensatory strategies to accomplish various gross and fine motor tasks (16). The physiotherapist teaches new skills and, in many cases, helps the children learn to walk, balance, feed, and dress themselves. In other cases, the therapist teaches the child how to use a wheelchair, walker, or other assistive devices. A number of controlled clinical trials have demonstrated that physical therapy can serve both to improve function and to maintain existing function. However, important questions about its use remain: for whom, when, how much, and for how long?

6.2. Speech Therapy

The production of speech, language, and gesture for communication is often affected by cerebral palsy. Communication difficulties associated with cerebral palsy can be multifactorial, arising from motor, intellectual, and/or sensory impairments, and children with this diagnosis can experience mild to severe difficulties in expressing themselves (17). They are often referred to speech and language therapy services to maximize their communication skills and help them to take as independent a role as possible in interaction. Various strategies have been used to treat the communication disorders associated with cerebral palsy. This can include introducing augmentative and alternative communication systems, such as symbol charts or speech synthesizers. This may also include treating children's natural forms of communication. In other cases, teaching alternative ways to communicate, such as sign language or the use of a communication board or other assistive devices, may be of considerable benefit.

6.3. Occupational Therapy

Occupational therapy for cerebral palsy focuses on the development of skills necessary for the performance of activities of daily living (18). Effective use of the upper limb can impact on educational outcomes, participation in activities of daily living, and vocational options for many children with cerebral palsy. Occupational therapy teaches children easier ways to use their arms, hands, and upper bodies more effectively. Therapists concentrate on skills such as feeding, dressing, and hand use. They also teach children how to use assistive technology to make life easier for them. Many tools exist that may enable children with cerebral palsy to obtain significant functional gains.

6.4. Medication Therapy

A variety of oral medications have been used to diminish the sensitivity of local nerves and muscles to control their reactions to environmental stimuli that result in muscle spasticity or involuntary movements (15). The three drugs that are used most often are diazepam, which acts as a general relaxant of the brain and body; baclofen, which blocks signals sent from the spinal cord to contract the muscles; and dantrolene, which interferes with the process of muscle contraction. Given by mouth, these drugs can reduce spasticity for short periods, but their value for long-term control of spasticity has not been clearly demonstrated. They may also trigger significant side effects, such as drowsiness, and their long-term effects on the developing nervous system are largely unknown. Dantrolene sodium (Dantrium) is a muscle relaxant that works by blocking the muscles' ability to contract. Dantrolene exerts its action at the muscular level by inhibiting the release of calcium from sarcoplasmic reticulum and thereby uncoupling excitation and contraction. It can help relieve severe muscle spasms and bring pain relief and increased movement. Baclofen (Lioresol) was introduced in 1967 as an oral medication for the treatment of muscle spasticity. It is a $GABA_B$ agonist that acts at the spinal cord level. Diazepam (Valium) has effects both at the central nervous system and muscle levels. It can be used to help control seizures and to help relieve muscle spasms and spasticity in cerebral palsy sufferers. The benefits of long-term oral medication in children with spasticity are limited either by poor blood–brain barrier penetration (baclofen), by modest long-term benefits (dantrolene), or by numerous side effects (diazepam). In addition, patients with a predominant athetoid form of cerebral palsy may benefit from drugs that help reduce abnormal movements. The most often prescribed drugs belong to a group of anticholinergics including trihexypheni-dyl, benztropine, and procyclidine hydrochloride.

6.5. Botulinum Toxin (Botox®)

Botox is an injectable purified protein derivative that blocks the release of acetylcholine at the neuromuscular junction. It is injected into the muscle belly through surface anatomic localization and spreads by diffusion. This simple, rapid, office-based procedure is generally well tolerated. The first report on the use of therapeutic Botox to treat spasticity in children with cerebral palsy was published in 1993 (19). Recent clinical studies have shown that injecting Botox into the spastic muscles of cerebral palsy sufferers can bring significant relief by causing the muscles to relax. The onset of action related to Botox chemodenervation typically begins within 3–10 days of injection. The duration of effect is usually between 1 and 6 months, with an average of 3 months. Because axonal innervation of the neuromuscular junction is eventually reestablished, multiple injection sessions, usually sepa-rated by at least 12 weeks, are typically needed. Earlier reinjection is discouraged because of the increased risk of developing neutralizing antibo-dies that would render further treatments ineffective (20). The effects of Botox are reversible and there tends to be tachyphylaxis upon repeat injec-tions. Contrary to its use in ophthalmology, the muscles involved in cerebral palsy are bulky and the maximal dose, as determined by the weight of these children, often precludes treating more than one or two muscles such that the effect is incomplete. Casting is required postinjection. Botox injections represent a good adjunct to other treatments when a local residual spasticity problem interferes with progress after the global problem has been dealt with otherwise (see the following text). In addition, it can be used to treat a forearm or hand problem, and to buy time in a youngster (e.g., 2-year-old child) showing tight hip adductors and progressive hip subluxation until more definitive therapy can be provided. It can be used as primary treatment modality if the spasticity problem involves one muscle group (e.g., mild hemiparesis) or as an "outcome predictor" vis-à-vis a given tendon intervention.

6.6. Orthopedic Surgery Interventions

The abnormal muscle tone and imbalances characteristic of spastic cerebral palsy can lead to progressive joint contractures, shortened muscles, and tensional deformities of the hip and foot (21). Soft tissue orthopedic proce-dures should be considered whenever an anatomic structure is at risk as a consequence of the spasticity, with the primary goal of preventing serious bony deformities. Tendon surgery has been a traditional method to treat dis-abling spasticity. It addresses the contractures at the tight joints. Tendon release needs to be done in combination (i.e., triple release) and may need to be repeated as the pathophysiological process in response to the static injury evolves. Casting is required and weakness of the associated muscle is seen following the intervention. Optimal spasticity control needs to be established before and after soft tissue procedures to ensure favorable long-term outcomes. We tend to employ tendon releases more locally after the global spasticity problem is dealt with in severely involved children on a need basis. In addition, children with spastic cerebral palsy may benefit from lengthening procedures of the hip flexors, adductors, hamstrings, and triceps surae. These patients with severe spasticity are usually nonambulators and are at risk of developing scoliosis and hip migration or frank subluxation. These orthopedic problems require careful monitoring and occasional intervention even if antispasticity therapies tend to have a protective effect on the natural history of these conditions.

6.7. Baclofen Pump Implantation and Selective Posterior Rhizotomy

Intrathecal baclofen has been evaluated as a treatment for lower limb muscle spasticity and for general dystonia. Selective posterior rhizotomy has been shown to reduce lower extremity spasticity and thereby improve joint range of motion, gait, and gross motor and functional abilities. These neurosurgical procedures have revolutionized the management of spasticity related to cerebral palsy and are discussed in detail in the ensuing two chapters.

REFERENCES

1. Russman BS, Ashwal S. Evaluation of the child with cerebral palsy. Semin Pediatr Neurol 2004; 11:47–57.
2. Kuban KC, Leviton A. Cerebral palsy. N Engl J Med 1994; 330:188–195.
3. Murphy KP, Molnar GE, Lankasky K. Medical and functional status of adults with cerebral palsy. Dev Med Child Neurol 1995; 37:1075–1084.
4. Rumeau-Rouquette C, Grandjean H, Cans C, du Mazaubrun C, Verrier A. Prevalence and time trends of disabilities in school-age children. Int J Epidemiol 1997; 26:137–145.
5. Strauss DJ, Shavelle RM, Anderson TW. Life expectancy of children with cerebral palsy. Pediatr Neurol 1998; 18:143–149.
6. Crichton JU, Mackinnon M, White CP. The life expectancy of persons with cerebral palsy. Dev Med Child Neurol 1995; 37:567–576.
7. Evans PM, Evans SJ, Alberman E. Cerebral palsy: why we must plan for survival. Arch Dis Child 1990; 65:1329–1333.
8. Hutton JL, Pharoah PO. Effects of cognitive, motor, and sensory disabilities on survival in cerebral palsy. Arch Dis Child 2002; 86:84–89.
9. Strauss DJ, Shavelle RM. Life expectancy of adults with cerebral palsy. Dev Med Child Neurol 1998; 40:369–375.
10. Koman LA, Smith BP, Shilt JS. Cerebral palsy. Lancet 2004; 363:1619–1631.

11. du Plessis AJ, Volpe JJ. Perinatal brain injury in the preterm and term newborn. Curr Opin Neurol 2002; 15:151–157.
12. Blair E, Stanley F. Issues in the classification and epidemiology of cerebral palsy. Ment Retard Dev Disabil Res Rev 1997; 3:184–193.
13. Volpe JJ. Brain injury in the premature infant. Neuropathology, clinical aspects, pathogenesis, and prevention. Clin Perinatol 1997; 24:567–587.
14. Russman BS, Ashwal S. Evaluation of the child with cerebral palsy. Semin Pediatr Neurol 2004; 11:47–57.
15. Murphy N, Such-Neibar T. Cerebral palsy diagnosis and management: the state of the art. Curr Probl Pediatr Adolesc Health Care 2003; 33:146–169.
16. Stiller C, Marcoux BC, Olson RE. The effect of conductive education, intensive therapy, and special education services on motor skills in children with cerebral palsy. Phys Occup Ther Pediatr 2003; 23:31–50.
17. Pennington L, Goldbart J, Marshall J. Interaction training for conversational partners of children with cerebral palsy: a systematic review. Int J Lang Commun Disord 2004; 39:151–170.
18. Steultjens EM, Dekker J, Bouter LM, van de Nes JC, Lambregts BL, van den Ende CH. Occupational therapy for children with cerebral palsy: a systematic review. Clin Rehabil 2004; 18:1–14.
19. Koman LA, Mooney JF, Smith BP, Goodman A, Mulvaney T. Management of spasticity in cerebral palsy with botulinum toxin-A: preliminary investigation. J Pediatr Orthop 1993; 13:489–495.
20. Mahant N, Clouston PD, Lorentz IT. The current use of botulinum toxin. J Clin Neurosci 2000; 7:389–394.
21. Gormley M. Treatment of neuromuscular and musculoskeletal problems in cerebral palsy. Pediatr Rehabil 2001; 4:5–16.

15

Baclofen

Jean-Pierre Farmer and Sandeep Mittal

Division of Pediatric Neurosurgery, McGill University Health Centre, Montreal, Quebec, Canada

1. INTRODUCTION

Spasticity is a motor disorder characterized by a velocity-dependent increase in muscle tone with an exaggerated tendon jerk resulting from hyperexcitability of the stretch reflex (1). Baclofen is a powerful muscle relaxant and antispasmodic agent (2) and has been widely used since the early 1970s to treat spasticity. It was originally synthesized as an antiepileptic medication, but its anticonvulsant activity was found to be negligible. In fact, baclofen has been shown to lower seizure threshold in known epileptic patients. Penn and Kroin first introduced intrathecal baclofen in the treatment of spasticity in 1984 (3). Its first indication was for chronic, medically intractable spasticity of spinal origin (4,5). Indications have since been extended to include: spasticity related to cerebral palsy (6,7), stroke (8,9), generalized dystonia (10,11), traumatic brain injury (12), and chronic pain (13,14). In this chapter, we will review the treatment of spasticity related to cerebral palsy using continuous intrathecal baclofen infusion.

2. BACLOFEN

Baclofen [4-amino-3-(4-chlorophenyl) butanoic acid; Lioresal] is structurally similar to gamma aminobutyric acid (GABA). It binds selectively to pre- and postsynaptic $GABA_B$ receptors to reduce excitatory synaptic transmission.

GABA$_B$ receptors are broadly expressed in the nervous system (brainstem, dorsal horn of the spinal cord, and other central nervous system sites) and have been implicated in a wide variety of neurological and psychiatric disorders (15). The hyperexcitability of the alpha motoneuron and the decrease of presynaptic inhibition of sensory Ia fibers have been well established in the pathophysiologic mechanisms of spasticity (16). The main effect of baclofen is to enhance presynaptic inhibition and thus inhibit monosynaptic and polysynaptic reflexes (17). The precise mechanism of action of this centrally acting skeletal muscle relaxant and antispasmodic agent is not fully understood. Baclofen is capable of inhibiting both monosynaptic and polysynaptic reflexes at the spinal level, possibly by hyperpolarization of afferent terminals, although actions at supraspinal sites may also occur and contribute to its clinical effect. Although baclofen is a synthetic analog of the inhibitory neurotransmitter GABA, there is no conclusive evidence that actions on GABA systems are involved in the production of its clinical effects.

2.1. Oral Baclofen

Baclofen is a white, odorless crystalline powder, which is slightly soluble in water, very slightly soluble in methanol, and insoluble in chloroform. Baclofen tablets are available as 10 and 20 mg tablets for oral administration. Oral baclofen is rapidly and extensively absorbed by more than 80–90% in the stomach and bowel and eliminated primarily by the kidney in unchanged form. Absorption may be dose dependent, being reduced with increasing doses. When given orally, baclofen does not easily penetrate the blood–brain barrier, but is distributed equally to the brain and spinal cord (18). Experimental studies in rats elegantly demonstrated that a significantly restricted distribution of baclofen (less than 1/30 of the blood levels) is found in the brain (19). This poor passage of the drug across the blood–brain barrier better explains the failure of oral medication to produce sufficient relief of spasticity. The problem of insufficient antispastic efficacy (in relation to the incidence of side effects) after systemic delivery may be overcome by direct introduction of the medication in cerebrospinal fluid.

2.2. Intrathecal Baclofen

Injectable baclofen is a sterile, pyrogen-free, isotonic solution free of antioxidants, preservatives, or other potentially neurotoxic additives and is indicated only for intrathecal administration. It is not recommended for intravenous, intramuscular, subcutaneous, or epidural administration. The drug is stable in solution at 37°C and compatible with cerebrospinal fluid. Each milliliter of baclofen injection contains baclofen U.S.P. 500 or 2000 µg. The half-life of intrathecal baclofen is approximately 4 hr (18). Intrathecally administered baclofen acts directly and selectively at the spinal level (20). Following lumbar administration of baclofen, the hydrophilic compound migrates upwards through lumbar subarachnoid space. However, there is considerable reduction of cerebrospinal fluid drug concentration along the spinal canal so that the levels are approximately four times greater in the lumbar cistern than in the cervical subarachnoid space (21). Baclofen injection when introduced directly into the intrathecal space permits effective cerebrospinal fluid concentrations to be achieved with resultant plasma concentrations 100 times less than those occurring with oral administration (22). Since passage across the blood–brain barrier is obviated, intrathecal baclofen can accomplish its unique effects on $GABA_B$ receptors directly in the immediate proximity of the superficial layers of the spinal cord with exponentially lower doses compared to the orally administered drug. Hypersensitivity to oral baclofen is a contraindication for intrathecal baclofen therapy.

3. PUMP TECHNOLOGY

There are currently two programmable pumps available for continuous intrathecal delivery of injectable baclofen. The SynchroMed EL pump (Medtronic Inc., Minneapolis, MN) is available in two reservoir sizes: 10 mL (75 mm diameter; 23 mm thickness) and 18 mL (75 mm diameter; 28 mm thickness). A new model has been introduced, the SynchroMed II, which is also available in two sizes: 20 mL (87.5 mm diameter; 19.5 mm thickness) and 40 mL (87.5 mm diameter; 26.0 mm thickness). The SynchroMed II programmable pump is approved for chronic intrathecal infusion of baclofen for the management of spasticity, for epidural or intrathecal administration of morphine for intractable pain, and for chronic intravascular infusion of floxuridine or methotrexate for the treatment of primary or metastatic cancer. The Medtronic SynchroMed II Programmable Infusion System is comprised of the implantable pump and intrathecal catheters, an external programmer that uses telemetry to regulate the pump, the refill kits, and the catheter access port kit used in diagnostic procedures. The pump precisely delivers a preset prescribed rate of infusion. A Lithion thionyl-chloride battery powers the pumps. The longevity of the pump is based on battery life and device service life, which in turn is a function of the drug infusion rate. The average expected duration of an implantable pump is 7 years. The main disadvantage with the smaller sized pumps is that they have to be refilled twice as often as the larger models. However, the smaller pump may be better suited for children with a small body habitus who have limited soft-tissue mass to cover a subcutaneously implanted pump. Other nonprogrammable implantable delivery systems, such as the Arrow (Arrow International Inc., Minneapolis, MN, U.S.A.), the Isomed (Medtronic Inc., Minneapolis, MN, U.S.A.), the Shiley INFUSAID (Shiley INFUSAID Inc., Boston, MA, U.S.A.), and the Archimedes (Tricumed Medizintechnik GmbH, Kiel, Germany) are available. However, because the manufacturer presets the rate of infusion, these nonprogrammable pumps present a major disadvantage over the programmable delivery systems. With the SynchroMed EL pump, intrathecal baclofen was established to be stable at body temperature for 3 months. Adjustments in drug concentration are made such that the pump is refilled every 3 months. Another advantage of the SynchroMed II pump system is that intrathecal baclofen is confirmed to be stable for a longer period of 6 months. This allows additional flexibility for the patient, family, and treating team.

4. SELECTION OF PATIENTS FOR INTRATHECAL BACLOFEN INFUSION

The overall goal for selected patients is to identify those patients most likely to benefit from treatment while reducing the likelihood of risks, perioperative complications, and long-term side effects. In general, intrathecal baclofen is recommended in patients who have a diagnosis of severe spastic cerebral palsy. Patients chosen to undergo the intrathecal baclofen trial are typically either Group II or III patients (based on NYU Classification; see Chapter 16) with locomotor potential but a contraindication for dorsal rhizotomy (underlying low tone, advanced age, prior spinal fusion, or severe scoliosis) or Groups IV and V. For the more involved children, it is important to screen families for their expectations. Baclofen pumps in these patients can help ease perineal care, sitting posture, reduce body restraints, subluxed hip pain and migration, improve upper extremity dexterity if the patient shows underlying potential preoperatively, as well as bulbar function (dysarthria, swallowing, drooling). Finally, in children with cerebral palsy scheduled for orthopedic spinal fusion, prior baclofen pump implantation can increase fusion efficacy by reducing trunk spasticity and lead to better overall comfort. Baclofen at low doses has little action against dystonia or athetosis but can reduce tardive dyskinesia. Baclofen at high doses (1000–2000 µg/day) has a beneficial effect on dystonia, but pump refills are frequent, at least prior to the availability of the second generation SynchroMed II pumps. If family expectations are realistic, an intrathecal baclofen screening trial may be in order.

5. PREOPERATIVE EVALUATION

The systematic approach to patient selection would then lead the treating team rule out any contraindications for intrathecal baclofen pump implantation. A history of oral baclofen intolerance and poorly controlled seizure disorder represent absolute and relative contraindications for intrathecal baclofen, respectively. The presence of prior lumbosacral spinal fusion could preclude the trial. However, if the indications are fairly clear, one could proceed directly to surgery via laminectomy at a level above the fusion to access the spinal canal given the high rate of positive screening tests (see following text). Prior to screening for a response to intrathecal baclofen, an attempt should be made to slowly titrate or discontinue concomitant oral antispasmodic drugs. This is done to avoid the risk of overdose or adverse drug interactions with intrathecal baclofen. Rapid or abrupt tapering of oral baclofen may result in seizures or hallucinations.

6. SCREENING TEST

All children are admitted for 3–4 days prior to pump implantation to be screened for responsiveness to, and safety of, intrathecal baclofen administration. The screening test must be conducted in a fully monitored environment (to include an apnea monitor and pulse oximetry). In children with disabling spasticity, the baclofen boluses can be administered by repeated lumbar punctures or through repeated injections into a lumbar subarachnoid catheter. We prefer to insert a lumbar catheter in the operating room under sedation with either midazolam or triple sedation (meperidine, hydroxyzine, and droperidol). Most children can be managed with a laryngeal mask and do not require endotracheal intubation. In cases of severe scoliosis, intraoperative fluoroscopy is used for catheter insertion. The following day, an initial bolus of 25 µg of baclofen (diluted to a final concentration of 50 µg/ mL) is delivered intrathecally. The onset of action of intrathecal baclofen in patients with cerebral spasticity is seen within 30–60 minutes after delivery of the bolus. The greatest effect of baclofen on spasticity occurs between 2 and 8.5 hours, with a maximal effect at 4 hours after intrathecal baclofen injection (23). We use a validated measure, the modified Ashworth Scale, to assess spasticity and to quantify the effect of the intrathecal test dose. A pediatric physiotherapist carries out the formal evaluation of spasticity and spasms at 2-hourly intervals after baclofen injection. A positive response consists of a significant decrease in muscle tone, frequency, and/or severity of spasms. Commonly, the clinical response is suboptimal and a second bolus injection of 50 µg (1 mL of the 50 µg/mL solution) is given 24 hours after the first. Again, the formal evaluation is completed by the physical therapist. If the clinical response is again less than desired, a third bolus injection of 75 µg in a volume of 1.5 mL is administered in the thecal space. The patient is observed for an interval of 4–8 hours. If the response remains inadequate, a final bolus screening dose of 100 µg in 2 mL may be administered 24 hours later. Adverse effects related to the screening test doses were reported to be less than 5% in one series (17). In our experience, the vast majority of patients will demonstrate a significant positive response to an intrathecal injection of 50 µg. Once the patient is judged to benefit from intrathecal baclofen infusion, the next step is pump implantation at a future date. We value the baclofen screening test, even if our successful response rate approaches 100%, because it helps us predict the starting basal rate at time of implantation. It also helps families see the potential benefits of intrathecal baclofen prior to committing them to the frequent hospital visits mandated by the treatment modality. In exceptional cases, we will implant a pump without the screening test if the patient has a history of extensive spinal fusion rendering the test technically difficult, as long as the indications and expectations are appropriate.

7. PUMP IMPLANTATION

Patients who successfully completed the initial screening test for intrathecal baclofen proceed to undergo implantation of a programmable pump, usually after a minimum 2-week delay to allow the puncture site of the screening test to heal. Following general anesthesia, the patient is placed in lateral decubitus position. The lumbosacral, flank, and anterior abdominal wall are sterilized using a chlorhexidine and 70% alcohol solution. A single prophylactic dose of gentamycin (20 mg/kg) and cefazolin (50 mg/kg) is given intravenously prior to skin incision. A 1.5–2 cm midline incision is centered over the L3–L4 interspace. The incision is undermined to the level of the lumbodorsal fascia. In small children, we perform a keyhole laminect-omy to have a dural opening tailored to the size of the catheter in order to avoid cerebrospinal fluid leakage. In addition, if a cervicothoracic approach is chosen because of prior spinal fusion, then the procedure is completed in two steps. The infusion catheter is first inserted in prone position; the patient is then turned in lateral decubitus position for the pump implantation and catheter connection. A 14-guage Tuohy needle is inserted into the lumbar subarachnoid space at the L3–L4 until there is good cerebrospinal fluid flow. With the needle still in position, the infusion catheter is threaded into the subarachnoid space and guided cephalad. Catheter tip location at the mid-thoracic region is confirmed by intraoperative fluoroscopy. The guide wire is removed and the infusion catheter is secured to the dorsal fascia using the V-wing anchor supplied in the kit. Once cerebrospinal fluid drains from the distal end of the tubing, we proceed with creating a subcutaneous pocket to house the pump. A 7 cm transverse abdominal incision is made just lateral to the umbilicus. Care is taken to ensure that the pocket is well below the last rib and above the iliac crest and is large enough to accommodate the pump with minimal tension on the suture line. Complete hemostasis also helps to reduce the risk of postoperative seroma formation. The catheter is then pulled through a subcutaneous tunnel into the anterior abdominal wall. This catheter is then trimmed with care taken to measure the length of the excess tubing. The pump is then introduced into the subcutaneous pocket, ensuring the proper orientation of the reservoir fill port. We prefer to use the polyeth-ylene terephthalate mesh pouch supplied by the manufacturer as it helps to stabilize the pump in the subcutaneous pocket. The distal end of the catheter is then secured onto the catheter port of the pump and the catheter strain-relief sleeve is properly anchored. Excess catheter tubing is coiled behind the pump, which is then secured within the pocket using either the mesh or, on alternate models, the suture loops. Once all connections are secured, we ensure meticulous hemostasis and proceed with wound closure.

7.1. Subfascial Implantation of Pump

Some authors favor a subfascial implantation of intrathecal baclofen pumps to reduce the potential for skin breakdown and to improve the cosmetic appearance of the implantation site (24). We prefer the subcutaneous implantation method for three main reasons. First, since gastroesophageal reflux is a common problem in this patient population, we are concerned about further restricting the intraabdominal volume using a subfascial implantation. Second, access to the reservoir fill port is usually more difficult with a subfascial pump insertion. Finally, at the time of refill, needle introduction through the fascia is quite painful, whereas in a subcutaneous implantation, it is generally well tolerated using topical anesthetics alone.

7.2. Preparation of Pump

Prior to implantation, careful preparation of the pump is mandatory. This is accomplished in three steps. First, it is necessary for the pump to be tested in vitro, under sterile conditions. This is accomplished by purging the 0.36 mL of sterile water already contained within the reservoir at the time of purchase. The pump test purge occurs over approximately 15 min and it is important to respect the entire time needed by the pump to accomplish this in order to avoid overdosage (25). The next step consists of exchanging the sterile water for the baclofen solution. The baclofen concentration used depends on the child's response to the screening dose of baclofen, and hence the projected infusion rate. The final step is dead-space purging. At the end of surgery, the implanted pump is purged over 40 min to prime the combined dead-space of both the pump and the implanted catheter. The pump has a dead-space of 0.23 or 0.26 mL depending on the model, as specified by the manufacturer, between the reservoir and pump outlet. The implanted catheter dead-space is calculated from its length as follows: volume = length of catheter inserted (in cm) $\times$ 2.22 μL/cm. This means that following the 40 min dead-space purge, once the intrathecal continuous infusion is started, the patient will actually be receiving intrathecal baclofen in the recovery room when emerging from anesthesia in pain and exhibiting exacerbation of the spasticity. The treating physician can then titrate the rate of infusion prior to discharge from hospital.

8. INTRATHECAL BACLOFEN THERAPY

Patients must be monitored closely in a fully equipped and staffed environment during the dose-titration period immediately following implant. Resuscitative equipment should be readily available for use in case of life-threatening or intolerable adverse effects, particularly in the 4–6 hours following the intraoperative bolus.

8.1. Postimplantation Dose Titration Period

We use the dose of baclofen that gave a positive effect during the screening test to help us determine the initial total daily dose of baclofen injection following implantation. We commonly use two times the screening dose and administer it over a 24-hours period. Generally, no dose increases are given in the first 24 hours until a steady state is achieved. After the first 24 hours, the daily dose is slowly increased by 5–15% only once every 24 hours, until the desired clinical effect is achieved. If there is a lack of an important clinical response to increases in the daily dose, pump malfunction or catheter-related problems must be ruled out. Plain radiographs assessing catheter position and pump connection site are obtained during hospitalization. Patients are typically discharged from the hospital on the third or fourth postoperative day once they achieve significant reduction in spasticity following incremental dosing during the titration period. The families subsequently return for postoperative wound check and maintenance dose adjustments.

8.2. Maintenance Therapy

The maintenance dose very often needs to be adjusted during the first few months of therapy while patients and their families adjust to dramatic changes resulting from elimination of spasticity. Our goal is to maintain muscle tone as close to normal as possible. We also aim to minimize the frequency and severity of spasms while avoiding intolerable side effects. During periodic refills of the pump, the daily dose may be increased 10–40%, but no more than 40%, to maintain adequate symptom control. Likewise, the daily dose may be reduced by 10–20% if patients experience adverse effects. Most patients require gradual increases in dose over time to maintain optimal response during chronic therapy. A sudden large dose escalation characteristically suggests a catheter-related pump malfunction. Maintenance dosage for long-term continuous infusion of baclofen injection has a wide range (from 12 to 1500 μg/day). However, most patients obtain substantial benefits on 300–800 μg/day. Determination of the optimal baclofen infusion rate obviously requires individual titration. The lowest dose with an optimal response should be used. For those patients implanted with programmable pumps who have achieved relatively satisfactory control on continuous infusion, further benefit may be attained using more complex schedules of baclofen injection delivery. For example, patients who have increased spasms at night may require a 20% increase in their hourly infusion rate. Changes in flow rate should be programmed to start 2 hours before the time of the desired clinical effect.

8.3. Baclofen Tolerance

Although intrathecal baclofen is safe and effective in the majority of patients, tolerance has been reported in approximately 10% of patients during long-term treatment (26–28). Tolerance is defined as the condition requiring gradual dose increases of a substance to obtain the same therapeutic effect. This physiological tolerance usually occurs in the first months of intrathecal baclofen delivery and normally stabilizes within the first year after pump implantation. However, in some cases of long-term baclofen infusion, a decreasing effect is seen, which persists even with progressive dose increases (29). After ruling out mechanical problems in the system, arachnoiditis, or an impaired cerebrospinal fluid circulation, this phenomenon suggests the presence of tolerance to baclofen. It has been shown that continuous, persistent binding of $GABA_B$ receptors by baclofen results in a decreased response to the medication (30). The mechanisms by which tolerance develops have not been fully elucidated. It appears that refractoriness to the escalating doses of intrathecal baclofen could be due to downregulation of the $GABA_B$ receptors or intracellular changes (31). The number of receptors decreases after repeated drug infusion, causing the loss of efficacy of baclofen (30,32). Other authors report an interaction between $GABA_B$ receptor and opioid receptor systems within the spinal cord (33). There is insufficient experience to establish clear guidelines for the management of baclofen tolerance. However, "a drug holiday" consisting of the gradual reduction of baclofen injection over a 2-week period and switching to alternative methods of spasticity management should be considered. After a few weeks, sensitivity to baclofen may return, and baclofen injection may be restarted at the initial continuous infusion dose. Two groups (34,35) successfully employed a therapy based on "baclofen holiday" for 15 days in conjunction with a bridge infusion of intrathecal morphine to treat baclofen tolerance.

9. COMPLICATIONS

Continuous intrathecal baclofen infusion is associated with a significant number of potential complications in all patient groups (Table 1). Complication rates following this procedure have been reported to be relatively low. Common adverse effects may be related to the drug itself, due to local problems with the surgical procedure or mechanical problems concerning the pump or catheter (36). The main risks of intrathecal baclofen infusion are symptoms related to overdose or withdrawal; the latter is more important because of the associated severe effects on clinical status and the possibility of death, but it is responsive to rapid intervention.

Table 1 Complications of Intrathecal Baclofen Pump

Baclofen withdrawal
  Nausea
  Headache
  Weakness
  Light-headedness
  Fever
  Pruritus
  Hypotension
  Paresthesias
  Altered mental status
  Rebound spasticity
  Seizures
  Rhabdomyolysis
  Multiorgan system failure
  Death
Baclofen toxicity
  Dizziness
  Somnolence
  Respiratory depression
  Seizures
  Altered mental status
  Coma
Hardware failure
  Catheter kinking
  Catheter breakage/puncture
  Catheter disconnection
  Catheter migration
  Mechanical failure of pump
Infection
  Hardware infection
  Wound infection

9.1. Baclofen Withdrawal

Delivery of an incorrect dose of baclofen can lead to serious sequelae including drowsiness, nausea, headache, muscle weakness, light-headedness, and return of pretreatment spasticity. Intrathecal baclofen withdrawal syndrome is a very rare, potentially life-threatening complication caused by an unexpected cessation of intrathecal baclofen. Baclofen withdrawal most commonly occurs as a result of a problem with the delivery system. Abrupt discontinuation of intrathecal baclofen, regardless of the cause, results in a clinical spectrum that includes high fever, pruritus, hypotension, paresthesias, altered mental status (dysphoria, visual, auditory and tactile hallucinations, paranoia), exaggerated rebound spasticity, seizures, and muscle rigidity that in rare cases may advance to rhabdomyolysis, multiple organ-system failure and death (37–39). Prevention of abrupt discontinuation of intrathecal baclofen requires meticulous attention to programming and monitoring of the infusion system, refill scheduling and procedures, and pump alarms. Patient and family education remains critical in preventing serious consequences of baclofen withdrawal resulting from catheter-related complications. Caregivers should be advised of the importance of keeping scheduled refill visits and should be educated on the early symptoms of baclofen withdrawal. In order to avoid the development of withdrawal, adequate doses of GABA agonist agents should be administered immediately prior to, and following, baclofen pump removal (40). However, oral baclofen replacement may not be an effective method to treat or prevent intrathecal baclofen withdrawal syndrome. Our management algorithm includes an early recognition of syndrome, proper intensive care management, high-dose benzodiazepines, and prompt analysis of intrathecal pump with reinstitution of intrathecal baclofen.

9.2. Baclofen Toxicity

Baclofen overdose may occur during the screening test, postimplant dose titration, and whenever intrathecal baclofen infusion has been interrupted or reintroduced. Signs and symptoms of baclofen toxicity include: drowsiness, light-headedness, dizziness, somnolence, respiratory depression, seizures, and altered level of consciousness progressing to coma (38). Baclofen antagonists are not available, but physostigmine may improve the lethargy and cardiorespiratory depression associated with mild overdoses (41). Overdose primarily arises from drug test doses or human error during refill and programming of the pump. Overdose from pump malfunction has not been reported. We described our experience with postoperative reversible coma occurring in five children related to inadvertent intrathecal baclofen bolus due to improper pump preparation technique as outlined earlier (25). Typical management strategies for systemic baclofen overdose are directed toward stopping further drug administration, reducing drug load, and continued supportive care. Appropriate care of these patients requires awareness of the clinical patterns of toxicity and mechanics of the pump delivery system. However, in emergency situations, when a programmer is unavailable, emptying the reservoir can stop the pump because an empty reservoir leads to automatic stalling of the pump's motor (42). In cases of massive intrathecal overdose of baclofen, removal of 30–50 mL of cerebrospinal fluid by lumbar puncture has shown beneficial effects in reducing central nervous system baclofen load (43). When available, the catheter access side port on the pump may be used to gain direct access to cerebrospinal fluid. Admission to an intensive care facility has been recommended for patients demonstrating clinical signs of toxicity. Clinicians must remain aware of potential acute withdrawal symptoms once baclofen is successfully removed and titrate judiciously.

9.3. Hardware Failure

Catheter complications, including kinking, breaking, puncturing, occluding (partially or completely), disconnecting, dislodging, and migrating were previously very common, occurring in up to 50% of cases (26). Current generation silastic catheters are larger, stronger, and thick-walled, and have translated into fewer catheter-related problems (44). As mentioned earlier, with recurrence of spasticity, one needs to determine whether tolerance to baclofen has occurred or whether there is failure of the drug delivery system. Therefore, mechanical failure of the pump and other components of the system must be excluded. Plain radiographs of the infusion system are obtained in anteroposterior and lateral views and compared with those obtained immediately after implantation. These usually easily demonstrate any obvious breaks or disconnections (Fig. 1). Catheter migration out of the intrathecal space is also easily seen on plain x-rays. An unusual case of subdural catheter migration was recently documented by obtaining a computed tomography (CT) scan following injection of a water-soluble radioopaque solution by the side port of the pump (45). Alternatively, radionuclide flow studies could also be used to assess catheter patency, pump function, and evaluate for leaks adjacent to the pump reservoir (46).

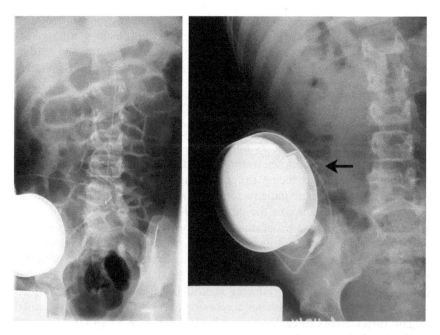

Figure 1 Anteroposterior plain radiographs obtained immediately after baclofen pump implantation (*left*) and 3 months postoperatively (*right*). The catheter has migrated out of the spinal canal and has looped around the pump (*arrow*).

9.4. Infection

Postoperative infection is a major concern for any neurosurgical intervention, but is especially cumbersome in the context of an implanted device. A rare but potentially fatal complication is infection of the pump or the catheter that connects it to the subarachnoid space. This may occur from direct microbial inoculation at time of surgery, back wound contamination in the early postoperative period, or contamination at the time of refilling of the pump. Rarely, it is caused by hematogenous contamination of the device. One of the main causes leading to pump infection in spasticity patients is skin breakdown over the bulky device. Infections of central nervous system delivering pumps are dominated by organisms of low virulence. The microorganisms most frequently implicated in baclofen pump infections are the coagulase-negative *Staphylococcus epidermidis*, *Staphylococcus aureus*, gram-negative enteric bacteria, and anaerobic diphtheroids (47). Some of these organisms demonstrate unique features that appear to facilitate the colonization and subsequent infection of a pump (48). Local infection of the wound or subcutaneous pump pocket has been reported in up to 20% of cases. According to clinical experience, a Staphylococcal infection of an implanted device mandates removal of the foreign material and appropriate systemic antimicrobial therapy. Boviatsis and colleagues described their experience in treating three patients with documented baclofen pump infection with intrapocket administration of antibiotics (47). Using this conservative approach, they achieved high drug levels within the subcutaneous pocket and were able to eradicate the deep-seated infection while maintaining the integrity of the pump. Another group reported successful intrareservoir gentamycin injection for treating pump infection with Pseudomonas aeruginosa without the need for pump extraction (49). Rarely, pathogens may infect the cerebrospinal fluid. Because success rates with intravenously administered antibiotic drugs for the treatment of meningitis have been low, intrathecal administration of antibiotic agents is often advocated to eradicate the pathogen. A few patients were successfully treated by providing uninterrupted intrathecal coadministration of the baclofen and antimicrobial agent given either through the reservoir or the side port (49–52). Finally, determining the concentration of baclofen in the cerebrospinal fluid via lumbar puncture may also provide additional information. We have had a single wound infection in a patient whose urine was colonized with *Pseudomonas aeruginosa* and who had urinary incontinence. The mechanism of pump infection was direct wound contamination via the diaper. This initiall required excision of the catheter and later on the pump. For that reason, our protocol now includes preoperative urine culture and gentamycin treatment or prophylaxis prior to implantation, depending on the results of the culture. This is in addition to the cephazolin prophylaxis.

9.5. Procedure-Related Adverse Effects

A further consideration is that various side effects can be related to the technical complications. Occasionally, cerebrospinal fluid leakage may occur, resulting in a subcutaneous collection. This can be managed conservatively if it is not associated with clinical symptoms of spinal headache, pain, or inhibiting proper wound healing. With severe or symptomatic leakage, it may be necessary to reintroduce the infusion catheter at a higher spinal level. Occasionally, a pocket seroma or hematoma may develop in the postoperative period. The subcutaneous collection usually disappears with repeated aspiration and applying a pressure dressing over the pump using an elastic bandage. Pump inversion has been documented as a cause of inability to cannulate the refill port of the pump. This typically occurs in larger patients or if the pump is not tightly anchored to the fascia. We have seen one case of caudal migration of the pump to the groin leading to femoral vein compression in the sitting restrained position, which required repositioning of the pump.

10. OUTCOME

Intrathecally delivered baclofen via programmable pumps has been used as a treatment for severe spasticity resistant to oral medications since 1984 (3). Several studies have since demonstrated the effectiveness for spasticity associated with spinal spasticity and multiple sclerosis (5,53–55). Intrathecally administered baclofen is effective in reducing the positive manifestations of spasticity including tone, spasms, and reflex activity. Significant reductions in spasm-related pain can also be achieved. The overall reduction in spasticity leads to improvement in ability to transfer and ease of nursing care in the majority of patients. Significant improvements are also noted in terms of mobility. Benefits are most notable in bedridden patients who are able to sit comfortably in a wheelchair following pump implantation. The decrease in spasticity in these patients also leads to improved skin care, hygiene, reduction of pain, and improved patient transfers. Therefore, despite the high incidence of complications, patient satisfaction remains elevated in the majority of cases as a result of improved function and quality of life (36,56).

Intrathecal baclofen appears most beneficial in severe spastic tetraparetics or tetraplegics. Ambulatory patients can also benefit from an improved gait but are less often treated because they usually rely upon their spasticity for support during ambulation. In addition, children with secondary dystonia can be treated with intrathecal baclofen (11). However, continuous baclofen administration does not have any positive impact in children with athetosis or ataxia. In addition to improvements in locomotion, continuous intrathecal baclofen infusion positively affects the progression of hip subluxation in children with cerebral palsy. A recent study noted no deterioration or improvement of hip migration 1 year after intrathecal baclofen therapy in over 90% of cases (57).

Impaired oral motor function and speech, associated with inadequate feeding, nutrition, growth, and communication, are prevalent in children with spasticity (58). Some aspects of speech and communication seem to show improvement following intrathecal baclofen administration (58,59). There are also considerable improvements in saliva control, appetite, and self-feeding. In some children receiving intrathecal baclofen, bowel movement frequency also decreases significantly. Several studies have indicated that intrathecal baclofen provides relief of central pain in patients with spasticity (60). Patients with persistent neuropathic pain of peripheral origin and with unsatisfactory pain relief with spinal cord stimulation may also benefit from intrathecal baclofen infusion (61).

10.1. Our Experience

Between November 1999 and June 2004, we implanted baclofen pumps in 38 children (29 boys, 9 girls). Spasticity was related to cerebral palsy in 33 children and to other underlying neurological disorders in the remaining five children. These included one child each with a Dandy–Walker malformation, holoprosencephaly, spina bifida, postmeningitic hydrocephalus, and metabolic encephalopathy. Patients were categorized according to age-related severity of functional locomotive impairment using a grading scale based on the NYU classification system (see Chapter 16 on selective posterior rhizotomy). None of the patients was classified in Group I (independent ambulators). Five children who required assistive mobility devices were in Group II and three patients were in Group III. Five nonambulatory patients were classified in Group IV and 25 children (65.8%) had severely limited mobility despite use of assistive devices (Group V). All patients had a positive intrathecal baclofen screening test by day 4. The mean age at surgery was 10.3 years (range, 3.9–19.7 years). Patients were followed for an average of 2.1 years (range, 3 months to 6.4 years). The mean dosage of intrathecal baclofen was 284 µg/day (range, 75–2000 µg/day). When subgrouping the children into those that had predominant spasticity ($N = 33$) and those with predominant dystonia ($N = 5$), we saw a significant difference in the daily requirements of intrathecal baclofen. Whereas children with predominant spasticity required an average of 162 µg/day of intrathecal baclofen (range, 75–300 µg/day), patients with predominant dystonia required a maintenance infusion of 992 µg/day on average (range, 320–2000 µg/day). Similar to other series, our main complications were hardware-related and included catheter migration in two children, erosion of anchoring device in one, cerebrospinal fluid leakage due to splicing of the silastic catheter in one, caudal migration of the pump in one, and shortened pump life in two. Other side effects included truncal hypotonia in two patients, seroma formation in six, and reversible coma in the recovery room in four. Only one patient had an infection of the infusion system, which required removal of the baclofen pump. He was colonizing *Pseudomonas aeroginosa* in his urine and contaminated his lower lumbar wound from leakage around his diaper. Since then, we have implemented a protocol with urine culture 72 hr prior to pump implantation. If the preoperative urine culture is positive, a full course of intravenous gentamycin is administered in addition to the preoperative cefazolin prophylaxis. If the culture is negative, then gentamycin and cefazolin prophylaxis is given at induction only. It is too early to comment on the benefits of this modification recommended by our institutional infectious diseases service.

Postoperative assessments showed no change in the functional grading. We are currently studying the beneficial effects on upper extremity function and activities of daily living with our occupational therapy colleagues and should be in a position to report on this matter in the near future.

11. CONCLUSIONS

In our spasticity program, dorsal rhizotomies were available as a treatment modality 8 years prior to baclofen pumps. Approximately one third of patients evaluated at our multidisciplinary clinic exhibited interfering spasticity but were not felt to meet rhizotomy eligibility criteria either because of underlying low tone in higher functioning patients or because of scoliosis and limited expected gains in the face of major surgery in more involved children. The availability of the intrathecal baclofen pump system allows us to offer a modulable treatment of spasticity for this population using a treatment, which is less invasive than selective posterior rhizotomy. The attendant complications of infusion pumps and the cost to the family and society in general make us insist on the development of strict selection criteria. A child who fulfills the selection criteria for dorsal rhizotomy should be offered a "one time only" relief of his or her spasticity with selective posterior rhizotomy first.

REFERENCES

1. Lance JW. Symposium synopsis. Feldman RG, Young RR, Koella WP, eds. Spasticity: Disordered Motor Control. Chicago, IL: Year Book Medical Publications, 1980:485–500.
2. Krach LE. Pharmacotherapy of spasticity: oral medications and intrathecal baclofen. J Child Neurol 2001; 16:31–36.
3. Penn RD, Kroin JS. Intrathecal baclofen alleviates spinal cord spasticity. Lancet 1984; 1:1078.
4. Ochs G, Naumann C, Dimitreejevic M, Sindou M. Intrathecal baclofen therapy for spinal origin spasticity: spinal cord injury, spinal cord disease, and multiple sclerosis. Neuromodulation 1999; 2:108–119.

5. Plassat R, Perrouin Verbe B, Menei P, Menegalli D, Mathe JF, Richard I. Treatment of spasticity with intrathecal Baclofen administration: long-term follow-up, review of 40 patients. Spinal Cord 2004; 42:686–693.
6. Tilton AH. Management of spasticity in children with cerebral palsy. Semin Pediatr Neurol 2004; 11:58–65.
7. Hodgkinson I, Sindou M. Traitement neurochirurgical de la spasticité: indications chez l'enfant. Neurochirurgie 2003; 49:408–412.
8. Francisco GE. Intrathecal baclofen therapy for stroke-related spasticity. Top Stroke Rehabil 2001; 8:36–46.
9. Meythaler JM, Guin-Renfroe S, Brunner RC, Hadley MN. Intrathecal baclofen for spastic hypertonia from stroke. Stroke 2001; 32:2099–2109.
10. Dachy B, Dan B. Electrophysiological assessment of the effect of intrathecal baclofen in dystonic children. Clin Neurophysiol 2004; 115:774–778.
11. Albright AL, Barry MJ, Shafton DH, Ferson SS. Intrathecal baclofen for generalized dystonia. Dev Med Child Neurol 2001; 43:652–657.
12. Turner MS. Early use of intrathecal baclofen in brain injury in pediatric patients. Acta Neurochir Suppl 2003; 87:81–83.
13. Slonimski M, Abram SE, Zuniga RE. Intrathecal baclofen in pain management. Reg Anesth Pain Med 2004; 29:269–276.
14. Taira T, Hori T. Clinical application of drug pump for spasticity, pain, and restorative neurosurgery: other clinical applications of intrathecal baclofen. Acta Neurochir Suppl 2003; 87:37–38.
15. Simeone TA, Donevan SD, Rho JM. Molecular biology and ontogeny of gamma-aminobutyric acid (GABA) receptors in the mammalian central nervous system. J Child Neurol 2003; 18:39–48.
16. Katz RT. Réévaluation des mécanismes physiopathologiques qui génèrent le réflexe d'étirement: de nouvelles hypothèses sur la physiopathologie de la spasticité. Ann Readapt Med Phys 2001; 44:268–272.
17. Albright AL. Baclofen in the treatment of cerebral palsy. J Child Neurol 1996; 11:77–83.
18. Sallerin B, Lazorthes Y. Baclofène intrathécal. Études expérimentales et pharmacokinétiques. Neurochirurgie 2003; 49:271–275.
19. Deguchi Y, Inabe K, Tomiyasu K, Nozawa K, Yamada S, Kimura R. Study on brain interstitial fluid distribution and blood–brain barrier transport of baclofen in rats by microdialysis. Pharm Res 1995; 12:1838–1844.
20. Gracies JM, Nance P, Elovic E, McGuire J, Simpson DM. Traditional pharmacological treatments for spasticity. Part II: General and regional treatments. Muscle Nerve 1997; 6(suppl):S92–S120.
21. Kroin JS, Ali A, York M, Penn RD. The distribution of medication along the spinal canal after chronic intrathecal administration. Neurosurgery 1993; 33:226–230.
22. Albright AL, Shultz BL. Plasma baclofen levels in children receiving continuous intrathecal baclofen infusion. J Child Neurol 1999; 14:408–409.
23. Pohl M, Rockstroh G, Ruckriem S, Mehrholz J, Pause M, Koch R, Strik H. Time course of the effect of a bolus dose of intrathecal baclofen on severe cerebral spasticity. J Neurol 2003; 250:1195–1200.

24. Kopell BH, Sala D, Doyle WK, Feldman DS, Wisoff JH, Weiner HL. Subfascial implantation of intrathecal baclofen pumps in children: technical note. Neurosurgery 2001; 49:753–756.

25. Anderson KJ, Farmer JP, Brown K. Reversible coma in children after improper baclofen pump insertion. Paediatr Anaesth 2002; 12:454–460.

26. Penn RD, Kroin JS. Long-term intrathecal baclofen infusion for treatment of spasticity. J Neurosurg 1987; 66:181–185.

27. Coffey JR, Cahill D, Steers W, Park TS, Ordia J, Meythaler J, Herman R, Shetter AG, Levy R, Gill B. Intrathecal baclofen for intractable spasticity of spinal origin: results of a long-term multicenter study. J Neurosurg 1993; 78: 226–232.

28. Meythaler JM, Steers WD, Tuel SM, Cross LL, Haworth CS. Continuous intrathecal baclofen in spinal cord spasticity. A prospective study. Am J Phys Med Rehabil 1992; 71:321–327.

29. Nielsen JF, Hansen HJ, Sunde N, Christensen JJ. Evidence of tolerance to baclofen in treatment of severe spasticity with intrathecal baclofen. Clin Neurol Neurosurg 2002; 104:142–145.

30. Wallace M, Yaksh TL. Long-term spinal analgesic delivery: a review of the preclinical and clinical literature. Reg Anesth Pain Med 2000; 25:117–157.

31. Abel NA, Smith RA. Intrathecal baclofen for treatment of intractable spinal spasticity. Arch Phys Med Rehabil 1994; 75:54–58.

32. Akman MN, Loubser PG, Donovan WH, O'Neill ME, Rossi CD. Intrathecal baclofen: does tolerance occur?. Paraplegia 1993; 31:516–520.

33. Hara K, Saito Y, Kirihara Y, Yamada Y, Sakura S, Kosaka Y. The interaction of antinociceptive effects of morphine and GABA receptor agonists within the rat spinal cord. Anesth Analg 1999; 89:422–427.

34. Vidal J, Gregori P, Guevara D, Portell E, Valles M. Efficacy of intrathecal morphine in the treatment of baclofen tolerance in a patient on intrathecal baclofen therapy (ITB). Spinal Cord 2004; 42:50–51.

35. Soni BM, Mani RM, Oo T, Vaidyanathan S. Treatment of spasticity in a spinal cord-injured patient with intrathecal morphine due to intrathecal baclofen tolerance—a case report and review of literature. Spinal Cord 2003; 41:586–589.

36. Gooch JL, Oberg WA, Grams B, Ward LA, Walker ML. Complications of intrathecal baclofen pumps in children. Pediatr Neurosurg 2003; 39:1–6.

37. Mohammed I, Hussain A. Intrathecal baclofen withdrawal syndrome—a life-threatening complication of baclofen pump: a case report. BMC Clin Pharmacol 2004; 4:6.

38. Dario A, Tomei G. A benefit-risk assessment of baclofen in severe spinal spasticity. Drug Saf 2004; 27:799–818.

39. Coffey RJ, Edgar TS, Francisco GE, Graziani V, Meythaler JM, Ridgely PM, Sadiq SA, Turner MS. Abrupt withdrawal from intrathecal baclofen: recognition and management of a potentially life-threatening syndrome. Arch Phys Med Rehabil 2002; 83:735–741.

40. Greenberg MI, Hendrickson RG. Baclofen withdrawal following removal of an intrathecal baclofen pump despite oral baclofen replacement. J Toxicol Clin Toxicol 2003; 41:83–85.

41. Muller-Schwefe G, Penn RD. Physostigmine in the treatment of intrathecal baclofen overdose. Report of three cases. J Neurosurg 1989; 71:273–275.

42. Yeh RN, Nypaver MM, Deegan TJ, Ayyangar R. Baclofen toxicity in an 8-year-old with an intrathecal baclofen pump. J Emerg Med 2004; 26:163–167.

43. Delhaas EM, Brouwers JR. Intrathecal baclofen overdose: report of 7 events in 5 patients and review of the literature. Int J Clin Pharmacol Ther Toxicol 1991; 29:274–280.

44. Penn RD, York MM, Paice JA. Catheter systems for intrathecal drug delivery. J Neurosurg 1995; 83:215–217.

45. Pasquier Y, Cahana A, Schnider A. Subdural catheter migration may lead to baclofen pump dysfunction. Spinal Cord 2003; 41:700–702.

46. O'Connell M, Wong TZ, Forkheim KE, Jain M, Shipes SW, Fuchs HE. Comparison of Tc99m-DTPA and Indium-111 DTPA studies of baclofen pump function. Clin Nucl Med 2004; 9:578–580.

47. Boviatsis EJ, Kouyialis AT, Boutsikakis I, Korfias S, Sakas DE. Infected CNS infusion pumps. Is there a chance for treatment without removal? Acta Neurochir 2004; 146:463–467.

48. von Eiff C, Peters G, Heilmann C. Pathogenesis of infections due to coagulase-negative staphylococci. Lancet Infect Dis 2002; 2:677–685.

49. Galloway A, Falope FZ. Pseudomonas aeruginosa infection in an intrathecal baclofen pump: successful treatment with adjunct intra-reservoir gentamicin. Spinal Cord 2000; 38:126–128.

50. Bennett MI, Tai YM, Symonds JM. Staphylococcal meningitis following Synchromed intrathecal pump implant: a case report. Pain 1994; 56:243–244.

51. Samuel M, Finnerty GT, Rudge P. Intrathecal baclofen pump infection treated by adjunct intrareservoir antibiotic instillation. J Neurol Neurosurg Psychiatry 1994; 57:1146–1147.

52. Zed PJ, Stiver HG, Devonshire V, Jewesson PJ, Marra F. Continuous intrathecal pump infusion of baclofen with antibiotic drugs for treatment of pump-associated meningitis. Case report. J Neurosurg 2000; 92:347–349.

53. Albright AL, Gilmartin R, Swift D, Krach LE, Ivanhoe CB, McLaughlin JF. Long-term intrathecal baclofen therapy for severe spasticity of cerebral origin. J Neurosurg 2003; 98:291–295.

54. Campbell WM, Ferrel A, McLaughlin JF, Grant GA, Loeser JD, Graubert C, Bjornson K. Long-term safety and efficacy of continuous intrathecal baclofen. Dev Med Child Neurol 2002; 44:660–665.

55. Fitzgerald JJ, Tsegaye M, Vloeberghs MH. Treatment of childhood spasticity of cerebral origin with intrathecal baclofen: a series of 52 cases. Br J Neurosurg 2004; 18:240–245.

56. Albright AL. Neurosurgical treatment of spasticity and other pediatric movement disorders. J Child Neurol 2003; 18(suppl 1):S67–S78.

57. Krach LE, Kriel RL, Gilmartin RC, Swift DM, Storrs BB, Abbott R, Ward JD, Bloom KK, Brooks WH, Madsen JR, McLaughlin JF, Nadell JM. Hip status in cerebral palsy after one year of continuous intrathecal baclofen infusion. Pediatr Neurol 2004; 30:163–168.

58. Bjornson KF, McLaughlin JF, Loeser JD, Nowak-Cooperman KM, Russel M, Bader KA, Desmond SA. Oral motor, communication, and nutritional status of

children during intrathecal baclofen therapy: a descriptive pilot study. Arch Phys Med Rehabil 2003; 84:500–506.

59. Mason C, Gilpin P, McGowan S, Rossiter D. The effect of intrathecal baclofen on functional intelligibility of speech. Int J Lang Commun Disord 1998; 33(suppl):24–25.

60. Slonimski M, Abram SE, Zuniga RE. Intrathecal baclofen in pain management. Reg Anesth Pain Med 2004; 29:269–276.

61. Lind G, Meyerson BA, Winter J, Linderoth B. Intrathecal baclofen as adjuvant therapy to enhance the effect of spinal cord stimulation in neuropathic pain: a pilot study. Eur J Pain 2004; 8:377–383.

16

Rhizotomy

Jean-Pierre Farmer and Sandeep Mittal

Division of Pediatric Neurosurgery, McGill University Health Centre, Montreal, Quebec, Canada

1. INTRODUCTION

Cerebral palsy is the term chosen to describe a heterogeneous group of non-progressive syndromes of posture and motor impairment that result from perinatal insults to the developing central nervous system (1). Cerebral palsy is an important neurological disorder and represents the most common cause of severe physical disability in childhood (2). The predominant types of cerebral palsy are classified as spastic, athetoid-dyskinetic, ataxic, hypotonic, or mixed. In recent years there have been a number of advances in the understanding of predisposing and protective factors in the development of cerebral palsy in infants (3). Opportunities for prevention of cerebral palsy may develop from an improved understanding of etiologic factors and their mechanisms of operation. Similar progress has been made in the evaluation of treatments for cerebral palsy and the effects of these treatments on the individual's impairment, function, and disability. Selective posterior rhizotomy has become a widely used neurosurgical technique for the treatment of lower extremity spasticity in children with cerebral palsy. The procedure aims to relieve the velocity-dependent hypertonicity, predominantly seen in the lower limbs, and to improve motor function in ambulatory children or younger children with emerging locomotor function.

2. HISTORICAL BACKGROUND

In 1889, two surgeons, Abbe and Bennett, independently described sensory nerve root section for the treatment of chronic pain in a limb (4,5). Foerster was the first to systematically examine sensory rhizotomies as a treatment for the relief of debilitating spasticity. In 1913, he published a report on a series of 159 patients who obtained relief from spasticity following dorsal rhizotomy; 88 of these individuals had congenital spasticity (6). Foerster also first proposed intraoperative electrical stimulation to identify the segmental level and distinguish between ventral and dorsal roots during the lesioning process. Despite these impressive results, dorsal rhizotomies did not gain wide acceptance because of the severe morbidity associated with this "radical" technique. In the mid-1960s, Gros et al. developed the concept of partial section of each sensory root in an attempt to limit the sensorimotor complications (7). He showed that significant benefits result from partial rhizotomies. Unsatisfied with their ability to control which muscles responded favorably to surgery, Gros and colleagues subsequently incorporated electromyography (EMG) to the procedure to permit identification of rootlets innervating more dysfunctional muscle groups. Sindou then proposed a surgical technique that transected the sensory fibers of nerve roots at the level of the posterior radiculomedullary junction whose myotome contained spastic muscles (DREZotomy) (8). In 1976, Fasano et al. made the observation that a one-for-one compound motor action potential was seen in response to sensory root stimulation with 30–50 Hz trains (9). He developed a series of criteria based on the "abnormality" of evoked motor responses to electrical stimulation. Fasano and colleagues believed that these abnormal response patterns identified rootlets that were abnormal and should be sectioned. In the 1980s, Peacock and Arens moved the operative site to the lumbosacral canal, allowing a more secure identification of the segmental level (10). Thus the midsacral roots could be confidently identified and preserved during the lesioning, lowering the risk of urologic complications. Most centers in North America continue to employ variations of the techniques originally described by Fasano and Peacock.

3. RATIONALE UNDERLYING SELECTIVITY OF POSTERIOR RHIZOTOMY

Since Sherrington's landmark experimental studies (11), the understanding of the mechanisms of spasticity has evolved considerably. In 1967, DeCandia and coworkers studied spinal reflexes in cats in which they showed that they could abolish reflexive motor responses when they stimulated sensory nerves (12). Fasano and colleagues made the observation that motor responses were in fact not eliminated by sensory root stimulation in the context of loss of upper motor neurons (9). Previously, the work of Sindou elegantly documented the location in humans of the 1A sensory fibers of nerve roots as they entered the dorsal horn of the spinal cord (8). The afferent 1A action potentials are the presumptive mediators of the hyperactive reflex arcs responsible for spasticity. The interneuronal pool within the spinal cord functions to modulate the pattern of alpha motoneuron activation in response to afferent stimuli (13,14). In the normal spinal cord, the 1A afferents and other joint, muscle, and cutaneous receptor afferents normally exert inhibitory tone on the interneurons, which exert an inhibitory influence on the alpha motoneurons, making them less susceptible to activation by afferent action potentials. Innervation to the spinal cord interneuronal pool is supplied by descending fiber tracts, from the cerebrum and various segmental spinal afferents (15). These modulatory influences are severely disrupted following injury to the descending upper motor neuron tracts as seen with brain or spinal cord injury. As a result, an imbalance occurs whereby sensory 1A fibers exert a much greater effect on the interneuronal pool. This dysregulated state results in an overall decrease in alpha motoneuron inhibition. It is thought that the interneuronal pool becomes maximally reactive to stimulatory afferent action potentials such as delivered by the 1A fibers coming from the muscle spindles (16). The premise of current deafferentation techniques is that they "reset" the influences exerted on the interneuronal pool back in to balance by decreasing the amount of afferent input.

It is postulated that lumbosacral dorsal rootlets that evoke "abnormal" reflex activity in lower extremity muscles upon direct, repetitive, high-frequency stimulation are involved in a dysfunctional spinal reflex. Abnormalities in these reflex circuits are believed to produce spasticity, which in turn impairs ambulation. These "abnormal" rootlets should therefore be selected for sectioning. Similarly, dorsal rootlets with "normal" reflex responses must be spared since they presumably do not participate in the abnormal circuitry. Targeting which 1A afferents should be cut requires identification of those fibers that synapse at alpha motor neuron fields that have lost the descending regulatory control. This forms the theoretical basis for selective posterior rhizotomy. However, there is continuing disagreement regarding the criteria and methodology for selection of the rootlets to be lesioned. The ability of EMG-guided dorsal rhizotomy to reliably outline populations of spinal rootlets that are maximally involved in a dysfunctional circuitry and maintenance of spasticity has become a matter of controversy. The debate regarding the utility of electrophysiological recording has centered around the lack of technical standardization (17,18), the variability of motor responses in response to repetitive nerve root stimulation (19,20), the effect of anesthetics on spinal reflexes (21,22), the variability of segmental innervation of lower extremity muscles (23), and the observation of sustained contractions following stimulation in patients without spasticity (24–26). Moreover, the validity of any of the criteria of "abnormality' used has been challenged (27,28). The skepticism has been further heightened by anecdotal reports of favorable results obtained with random partial rhizotomy (29). Those who doubt the reliability have questioned the overall impact of intraoperative stimulation on the success of the operation. In our opinion, spread of muscle response to the contralateral limb and/or upper extremity remains a valid criterion to define a posterior nerve rootlet that feeds into a disinhibited spinal circuit involved in uncontrolled spasticity. Although sustained contractions following 50 Hz stimulation have been observed in a few nonspastic patients (24,25), none of these children demonstrated contralateral or suprasegmental propagation. We, like others (30), believe that concerns about the value of intraoperative monitoring have resulted in part from inconsistent intraoperative conditions, from misinterpretation of the electrophysiological information, and from the paucity of well-defined functional outcome measures. Using the criteria of contralateral and suprasegmental spread as the primary lesioning parameter, we clearly demonstrated that motor responses obtained by repetitive orthodromic stimulation of posterior roots are consistent and easily reproducible by EMG (31). We showed that the absolute grade variation in response of 0 or 1 occurred in 93% of roots stimulated and, further, a correlation of greater than 90% occurred in pattern of spread of stimulation between physiotherapy and EMG at our center. Our results reinforced the concept that contralateral and upper extremity spread is a valuable approach to delineate sensory rootlets involved in aberrant modulation of spinal cord reflexes. We therefore advocate the routine use of intraoperative electrophysiological monitoring during selective posterior rhizotomy. By "selectively" lesioning the posterior rootlets involved most in the spastic process, a significant reduction of spasticity coupled with preservation of sensation, voluntary muscle control, and bladder function can be achieved.

4. PREOPERATIVE EVALUATION

Every child considered for neurosurgical treatment of spasticity should be evaluated using a multidisciplinary approach. Our childhood spasticity team consists of the following medical professionals: a neurosurgeon, a neurologist, an orthopedic surgeon, a physiotherapist, an occupational therapist, and a nurse clinician. The preoperative assessment begins with a thorough review of the patient's prenatal, perinatal, and postnatal history. In particular, evidence of hypoxic/ischemic events, gestational age, birth weight, multiple gestation, intraventricular hemorrhage, maternal/fetal infection, and seizure are elucidated. A complete developmental profile should be obtained including the patient's fine motor and locomotor impairments, language skills, and assistance required for performing activities of daily living. Prior treatments for spasticity and orthopedic surgeries should also be reviewed in detail. A careful neurological examination is clearly essential for proper determination of signs of spasticity, including increased muscle tone, hyperactive deep tendon reflexes, and ankle clonus. The child's ability to walk, stand, crawl, and sit should be assessed. Videotaping is helpful not only for initial evaluation using validated measurement tools but also to document changes in the patient's condition over time. Abnormal posturing, such as equinus deformity of the ankles, tiptoe walking, and scissoring of the lower extremities, will help determine whether spasticity plays a significant role on the patient's motor performance. The absence of movement disorders such as athetosis and dystonia must be ascertained. Radiologic studies include magnetic resonance imaging of the head and spine and plain radiographs of the lumbosacral spine and hip. Magnetic resonance imaging of the head and spine is useful to rule out progressive cerebral or spinal pathologies. Lumbosacral spine x-rays will demonstrate the presence of lumbar hyperlordosis, scoliosis, spondylolysis, spondylolisthesis, and congenital anomalies. Radiographs of the hip will reveal the degree of subluxation and dislocation and may affect the timing of neurosurgical intervention.

4.1. Functional Outcome Measurements

At our center, all patients receive a comprehensive standardized assessment protocol preoperatively, at 6 and 12 months postoperatively, and at yearly intervals thereafter. Functional outcome measures consist of quantitative determinations of lower extremity spasticity, passive range of motion, developmental motor skills, gross motor function, fine motor skills, and evaluation of activities of daily living. A pediatric physiotherapist, who is previously trained in the use of the standardized evaluation tools, takes measurements using a consistent technique. The children are examined without braces, orthoses, or walking aids. All developmental motor skill assessments are videotaped for analysis of the performance and scoring.

4.2. Evaluation of Spasticity and Range of Motion

The spasticity of the hip adductors, hamstrings, and ankle plantar flexors is assessed by a modification of the Ashworth scale using a 5-point grading system based on the NYU Tone Scale (32). A muscle that offers normal resistance to passive limb movement is assigned grade 0. Grade 1 is given if the limb is floppy with less than normal tone. Grades 1, 2, and 3 are designated as mildly, moderately, and severely increased tone, respectively corresponding to the severity of resistance to passive movement and impairment of function. Passive range of motion is measured for hip abduction from midline with the hip and knee extended (normal, 45°). Knee extension is measured in supine position (normal, 0°), and ankle dorsiflexion is assessed with the knee in extension and the subtalar joint of the foot in neutral position (normal, 20°). The joint angle is measured at maximal range of movement with the use of a protractor goniometer.

4.3. Evaluation of Developmental Motor Skills

The method we use to assess developmental positions and transitional movements is taken in part from the functional assessment section of the Rusk Institute of Rehabilitation/NYU Rhizotomy Evaluation Form (33). The specific developmental positions and transitional movements analyzed were previously identified as functional skills that young ambulatory children with spastic cerebral palsy have difficulty executing. In addition, analysis of the quality of alignment in each static developmental position is added to the assessment to quantify qualitative changes in posture after selective posterior rhizotomy.

Five developmental positions are used to determine the effect of selective dorsal rhizotomy on the child's stability and the quality of alignment in the static positions. These include long sitting, bench sitting, side sitting (right and left), half kneeling (right and left), and standing. During the assessment, each position is first demonstrated for the child by a clinician. The patient is then asked to assume the position and verbal cues are given to elicit the best performance. The ability to maintain the position independently is graded on a scale of 1–5. Grade 1 is given if the child cannot be maintained in position; grade 2 is assigned when the child requires full external support from the therapist to maintain the position. Grades 3 and 4 are given if the patient requires bilateral or unilateral upper extremity support to maintain position, respectively. Finally, children that can maintain the position independently are assigned grade 5. To quantify changes in the quality of alignment, the position of relevant body segments (head, trunk, elbows, hips, knees, ankle, and feet) is assessed in each developmental position. An extensive grading system is used to measure quality of alignment at each of the body segments, as appropriate, in the five developmental positions. The segmental scores for each static position are summed for a total alignment score. A mean score is used for the developmental positions in which both the right and left sides were assessed.

Five developmentally-based transitional movements are evaluated to assess the gains in the level of performance following selective posterior rhizotomy. These include transition from supine to long sitting, supine to side sitting, floor to bench sitting, floor to standing, and tall kneeling to half kneeling. During the assessment, each movement is first demonstrated for the child by a clinician. The patient is then asked to perform the movement and verbal cues are given to elicit the best performance. All transitional movements are graded on a 5-point scale. Grade 1 is assigned to a child who cannot be placed in position, and grade 2 to a child who cannot observably participate in transition but in whom the therapist can complete the entire movement. Grade 3 is given to a patient who requires assistance to complete the limb movement and uses furniture to assist into position; and grade 4 is given when the child completes the movement but requires assistance from the therapist or furniture. Finally, grade 5 is assigned if the patient is able to complete the transition movement independently.

4.4. Evaluation of Motor Function

The Gross Motor Function Measure (GMFM) is a criterion-referenced observational measure that was developed and validated to assess children with cerebral palsy (34). The 88 items of the GMFM are measured by observation of the child and scored on a 4-point ordinal scale. The items are weighted equally and grouped into five dimensions: A = lying and rolling (17 items); B = sitting (20 items); C = crawling and kneeling (14 items); D = standing (13 items); and E = walking, running, and jumping (24 items). Scores for each dimension are expressed as a percentage of the maximum score for that dimension. The total score is obtained by averaging the percentage scores across the five dimensions. As indicated by Russell and colleagues (34), a change of 6% in the total score or within a dimension of the GMFM is considered to be clinically important in children with cerebral palsy having undergone a surgical intervention.

4.5. Measurement of Fine Motor Skills and Patterns

Functional outcome measures of fine motor skills consist of administration of the Peabody Developmental Motor Scales (PDMS) test by pediatric occupational therapists, who are experienced in the use of this standardized evaluation tool.

The 1983 version of the PDMS is a criterion and norm-referenced scale (35). Normative data were established with 617 typically developing children aged 0–83 months. The PDMS was developed to establish the developmental skill level of a child, to identify skills that are not developed or are emerging, and then to provide suggestions for program planning. It is a standardized instrument with established reliability and validity (36–38) and consists of gross motor and fine motor scales, which can be administered and scored separately. The gross motor scale contains 170 items divided into 17 age levels, with 10 items at each level. It consists of tasks that require precise movement of the large muscles of the body. The items are classified into five skill categories: A = reflexes, B = balance, C = nonlocomotor, D = locomotor, and E = receipt and propulsion of objects. The fine motor scale consists of 112 items divided into 16 age levels, with six or eight items at each level. It evaluates tasks that require precise movement of the small muscles of the body. The items of the fine motor scale are classified into four skill categories: A = grasping, B = hand use, C = eye–hand coordination, and D = manual dexterity. Norms are provided for each skill category at each age level as well as for total scores.

The fine motor scale of the PDMS is an independent scale that measures upper extremity skills in more common daily fine motor tasks. This scale identifies children whose fine motor skills are delayed or aberrant relevant to a normative group. The fine motor scale of the PDMS also enables the examiner to measure performance across time or before and after intervention. It provides a system that enables the examiner to measure changes that are quite small and thus not likely to be detected using traditional measures (35).

The PDMS employs a 3-point scoring system that enables identification of emerging skills and measurement of progress in children who are slow in acquiring new skills. A score of 0 is assigned if the child cannot or will not attempt the item, or the attempt does not show that the skill is emerging. A score of 1 is given if the child's performance shows a clear resemblance to the item criterion but does not fully meet the criterion. Finally, a score of 2 is given if the child performs the item according to the specified item criterion. The scores are summed for a cumulative raw score for each of the four fine motor skills. The addition of individual skill scores provides the total raw score. Using the PDMS conversion tables, raw scores can be converted into age-equivalent scores, percentile ranks, and four normalized standard scores (z-scores, T-scores, developmental motor quotients, and scaled scores). For the present study, raw data were transformed into age-equivalent, percentile, and z-scores.

Normative scores indicate the child's age-related fine motor skills. Comparison of the child's total fine-motor standard scores with those of the norming population enables the examiner to determine whether the child's motor performance is like that of his or her chronological age peers. Age-equivalents are scores that indicate the age group in which an obtained score is average independent of the child's actual age. They provide a useful index for measuring the year-to-year improvement in performance. Percentile ranks are scores that specify the percentage of the norming sample that scored below a given raw score. They provide a clear measure of how a child's performance compares with the performance of other children in the norming sample. Percentile ranks can also be used to describe relative improvement in performance. If the child is improving at the same rate as the rest of the age group, his or her percentile rank will remain the same. If performance has not improved or has decreased, the child's percentile rank will go down from one age to the next. Finally, z-scores are standardized scores that result from transforming sets of raw scores into distributions with a mean of 0 and a standard deviation of 1. If the child's z-score is $+1.0$ or greater, or -1.0 or less, this suggests that the performance is different from the mean of the norming population. If the z-score is $+1.5$ or greater, or -1.5 or less, the difference is considered to be significant.

4.6. Evaluation of Activities of Daily Living

Functional performance outcome measures consist of administration of the Pediatric Evaluation of Disability Inventory (PEDI) questionnaire. Pediatric occupational therapists that are highly experienced in managing children with cerebral palsy and experienced in the use of the standardized evaluation tools take measurements using a consistent technique. The PEDI is a parental report questionnaire used for chronically ill and disabled children aged 0.5–7.5 years (39). The reliability and validity of the PEDI have been well demonstrated (39–41). It is now recognized as a standardized instrument for evaluating functional performance. In children with cerebral palsy, its sensitivity to change in motor function following selective dorsal rhizotomy has also been studied (42–44).

The PEDI, a judgment-based tool, is administered in the form of a structured interview with the child's parents in conjunction with clinical observation by the therapist. All patients are pretested, parents are interviewed, and therapists complete a questionnaire. The PEDI measures both capability and performance of functional activities in daily life situations in three domains (39). The functional performance capacity (197 discrete items) explores the patient's ability to perform various tasks. The caregiver assistance domain (20 complex functional activities) describes the amount of assistance a child requires to complete a skill. The environmental modifications domain (20 complex functional activities) details the adaptive equipment a child needs to perform a given task. Each domain is further divided into categories of mobility, self-care, and social skills. Individual items of the questionnaire measure distinct aspects of self-care, bowel and bladder control, mobility and transfers, and communication and social function. The self-care (81 items) and mobility (66 items) dimensions of the functional skills and caregiver assistance domains of the PEDI are parameters that measure function in more concrete daily activity tasks.

Two different scoring systems are used in the PEDI. For the functional skills domain, a score of 0 is assigned if the child is unable, or limited in capability, to perform the 132 discrete items of functional skills. Conversely, a score of 1 is given if the child is capable of performing the functional task, or if the item had been previously mastered and that functional skills had progressed beyond this level. For the caregiver assistance domain, a 6-point ordinal scale is used to grade the 20 complex functional activities: $0 =$ complete dependence (total assistance); $1 =$ maximal assistance; $2 =$ moderate assistance; $3 =$ minimal assistance; $4 =$ with supervision, prompting, or monitoring; and $5 =$ complete independence. The scores for each PEDI domain are summed for a total raw score for each of the two dimensions (self-care and mobility) in both the functional skills and caregiver assistance domains. Using the PEDI conversion tables (39), raw scores for individual items and content areas are transformed into normative and scaled scores.

Normative scores indicate the child's age-related functional skills and caregiver assistance levels, based on a mean of 50 and a standard deviation of 10. Scores outside the 10–90 range are recorded as <10 or >90. Also, as the normative or standard scores show how close the child is to the normal population of the same age, they are not available for patients 7.5 years or older. Scaled scores indicate the child's individual performance and increasing levels of function along a 0–1 continuum of task difficulty.

4.7. Patient Subgrouping

All patients are categorized preoperatively according to age-related severity of functional locomotive impairment using a grading scale based on the NYU classification system as outlined in Table 1 (32). Children in Group I (independent ambulators) are thought to have the best chance of improving appearance and efficiency of walking. Patients requiring assistive mobility devices (Group II) are anticipated to improve quality of locomotion and decrease level of assistance required for ambulation. Children classified in Group III (reciprocal and nonreciprocal quadruped crawlers) are expected to improve their functional ability with the ultimate goal of ambulating with braces or assistive devices. Generally, nonambulatory patients in Group IV and V (severely limited mobility despite use of assistive devices) do not obtain functional motor gains despite elimination of spasticity with SPR. Consequently, these severely disabled children are offered alternative therapies, such as intrathecal baclofen pump implantation or tendon lengthenings, in order to improve ease of care taking and facilitate positioning.

Table 1 Preoperative Locomotive Abilities[a] and Expected Outcomes Following SPR

	Preoperative function	Postoperative goals
Group I	Walks without assistive devices	Improve appearance and efficiency of walking
Group II	Walks with assistive mobility devices (canes, crutches, walkers, etc.)	Improve quality of walking and decrease amount of assistance required for ambulation
Group III	Quadruped crawlers; reciprocal or nonreciprocal (i.e., bunny hoppers)	Improve ability to move through development sequence; walk with assistive devices
Group IV	Commando or belly crawlers; wheelchair bound	Improve ease of care taking; facilitate function in sitting position
Group V	No locomotive abilities; fully dependent	Improve ease of care taking; facilitate positioning in adaptive equipment

[a]Based on the NYU Classification System.
Source: From Ref. 32.

5. SURGICAL TREATMENT

The surgical procedure for selective posterior rhizotomy is straightforward if completed in an ordered stepwise fashion. Since 1992, we have performed selective posterior rhizotomies on 175 patients through a narrow L1–S2 laminotomy with no significant postoperative complications.

5.1. Anesthetic Conditions and Preparation

All patients are anesthetized with a mixed technique of sufentanyl (0.2–0.5 µg/kg/hr) and propofol (1–10 mg/kg/hr) infusions along with nitrous oxide (70%). A short-acting nondepolarizing neuromuscular blocker, rocuronium, is used only at induction. Its effects are dissipated at the onset of stimulation. Care is taken that all infusions achieve a steady state that is maintained throughout the stimulation protocol. Secondary tachycardia and hypertension is managed by delaying the stimulation sequence for 5 min. Postoperative analgesia is delivered by morphine infusion (4 µg/kg/hr) containing 0.125% bupivacaine for 72 hours through an epidural catheter placed under direct vision at the time of surgery. A bladder catheter is placed and removed only 24 hours after the epidural catheter is removed. Recording electrodes are placed and verified for conductance. Adhesive skin electrodes are placed bilaterally (see following text).

5.2. Laminotomy and Identification of Dorsal Roots

Patient position is very important. Surgery is performed with patients in prone position with the hips and shoulders slightly elevated on bolsters. The patient's back is kept in neutral position, the feet are supported by pillows, and the arms are placed upwards. Care is taken to ensure freedom of the abdominal wall between widely spaced bolsters to reduce epidural venous engorgement. Skin preparation is done with chlorhexidine and 70% alcohol solution. The spinous processes and laminae of L1 through S2 are exposed through a midline lumbosacral skin incision. Beginning at the caudal margin of the last lamina, the interlaminar ligament is separated from the inferior border of the lamina, and the epidural space is entered using a small periosteal elevator or curette. Using a craniotome, the small footplate is inserted under the lamina into the spinal canal midway between the base of the spinous process and the articular surface of the joint and advanced through the laminar levels in one step. The same procedure is repeated on the opposite side. In this manner, a multilevel, narrow laminotomy (1.5 cm) may be performed safely. The laminar plate is gently retracted from the underlying epidural fat. Bleeding from the cut edges of the bone is controlled with bone wax. The high speed drill is used to make laminar and spinous process holes for subsequent reattachment, and the laminar flap is hinged at T12–L1, wrapped in bacitracin-soaked gauze. The epidural fat is swept laterally with narrow Gelfoam strips (Pharmacia & Upjohn Co., Kalamazoo, MI) and the dura is opened in the midline. Multiple traction sutures tied to the muscular layer help to fully expose the cauda equina in its entirety. The spinal level of individual roots is determined by counting from the lowest root in the cul-de-sac using bony landmarks, foraminae, size variations of the roots, and by stimulating the motor roots of S2 and S1 orthodromically. At the level of the neural foramina, the motor root lies anterior and cephalad in the foramen. The motor and sensory roots should separate easily by placing a microdissector in the cleft and allowing gravity to move the motor root ventrally away from the sensory root retained by the dissector (Fig. 1). Electrical stimulation of posterior roots is performed to determine a "threshold" for a motor response. Once the electrophysiological monitoring protocol, as described in the following text, is completed, the roots are divided into rootlets. Based on their evoked stimulation responses, the rootlets are sectioned using the criteria defined below. At the end of the procedure, the subarachnoid space is irrigated to remove any blood. The dura is closed in a water-tight manner and the laminotomy flap is reattached to the surrounding laminae and suspended using a 3-point fixation at each level. Beside the two laminar sutures, a figure-of-eight suture is passed through a spinous process hole and incorporated in the reflected periosteum to allow the latter to overlay the fracture lines and facilitate osteogenesis. An epidural catheter is placed for postoperative analgesia.

5.3. Electrophysiological Monitoring

In all cases, a neurophysiologist, a neurophysiology technician, and a physical therapist are present in the operating room during stimulation. Electrical stimulation of roots and rootlets is done using two insulated unipolar electrodes (Aesculap Inc., Bethlehem, PA, U.S.). The cathode is placed proximally along the course of the dorsal root, and the anode is placed 1 cm distally for orthodromic stimulation (Fig. 1). Stimulation of the dorsal roots is obtained by elevating them from the cerebrospinal fluid pool starting on the right side from S2 to L2. The initial round of stimulations determines the "threshold" for motor response using a 1 msec duration stimulus. The stimulus strength is adjusted to give a maximal dorsal root potential, but care is taken to keep the stimulus intensity low enough to prevent current spread to adjacent roots. The highest "threshold" stimulus intensity for all sensory roots is used as a basis for the intensity of the tetanic stimulus. The entire dorsal root is then restimulated at two-to-four times the highest "threshold" intensity with a 1 sec 50 Hz stimulus train (Trial 1). The current intensity usually varies from 6 to 12 mA (median, 8 mA). The posterior root is then separated into three to seven rootlets. The threshold run as well as tetanus stimulation is carried out in the same dorsal root sequence—from S2 to L2 starting on the right.

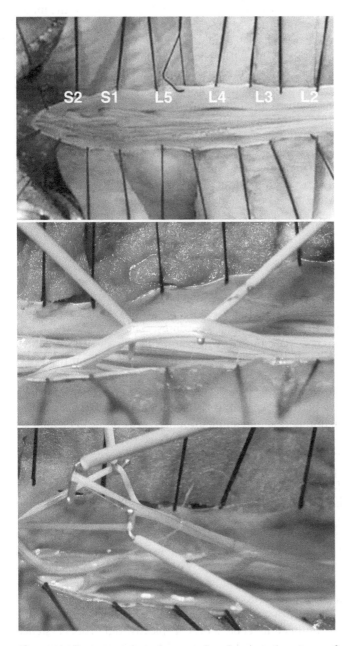

Figure 1 Intraoperative photographs showing the steps of selective posterior rhizotomy: exposure and identification of the L2–S2 dorsal spinal roots (*upper*), separation of the dorsal roots from the ventral roots (*middle*), and division of the spinal root into rootlet fascicles and intraoperative electromyographic testing (*lower*).

Both the neurophysiologist and the physical therapist assess the motor responses to electrical stimulation of dorsal roots and rootlets. Recording of the compound muscle action potential (CMAP) is done using a multi-channel electromyograph (Viking II, Nicolet Biomedical Inc., Madison, WI, U.S.) with silver chloride surface electrodes placed on the quadriceps, hamstrings, and gastrocnemius muscle groups bilaterally and monitored over a 2 second time frame. Upper extremity motor responses are recorded either from the deltoid or biceps muscle. Thus, up to eight muscle groups are monitored simultaneously (Fig. 2). Clinical pattern of muscle response is observed and palpated by the physiotherapist with particular attention placed on contractions in muscle groups other than those monitored by the neurophysiologist (e.g., hip adductors, toe flexors). Rootlets are sectioned based on extent of "abnormality" of their clinical and EMG motor responses to electrical stimulation.

5.4. Lesioning Criteria

The response to tetanic stimulation is used to determine which rootlet to cut. The decision to transect or preserve individual rootlets is made on the basis of three pieces of information. The first is the electrophysiological response monitored through the eight-channel recordings. The second criterion is the behavioral response (i.e., muscle contraction in the legs) documented by the physiotherapist. Behavioral responses are used to confirm the EMG response pattern, to define contractions in unmonitored muscle groups, and to assist with trouble shooting if no electrical response is observed (e.g., rootlet in refractory period). As well, if the physiotherapist signals rigidity, we delay further manipulation and stimulation by 5–10 minute. The final set of criteria includes: (i) the root level being stimulated (less aggressive lesioning at L4 and S2); (ii) the number of rootlets severed at previous levels; (iii) the strength and quality of evoked responses; and (iv) the congruence of the intraoperative information with the clinical status of the patient (i.e., low tone, massive scissoring, degree of hip subluxation). The motor response of each root and rootlet is recorded and assigned a grade of 0, 1+, 2+, 3+, or 4+, as described by Phillips and Park (45), and also employed by other authors (19,20). This scale grades the response with regards to its level of segmental and contralateral spread and whether it is "abnormally" sustained. We use a slightly modified grading scheme such that grade 0 represents an unsustained response (normal response) and grade 4+ is assigned to a sustained response with contralateral spread, as well as spread to the upper extremities as outlined in Table 2 (45). Typically, only roots assigned a grade 4+ response are divided into rootlets. The intensity and pattern of clinical and EMG motor responses to every stimulation (of roots and rootlets) contribute to the decision regarding sectioning or preservation of individual rootlets. In addition, some restrictions in the lesioning pattern

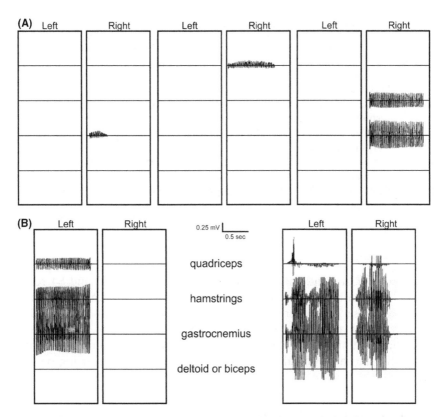

Figure 2 Intraoperative EMG recordings following stimulation of individual dorsal roots with a 1-second 50-Hz constant current at the threshold level of 8.0 mA in a 5-year-old diplegic child. CMAP were recorded from surface electrodes placed on various muscle groups of the lower and upper extremity bilaterally. (**A**) *Left:* Unsustained CMAP following stimulation of the right S2 dorsal root. This "normal" response was assigned a grade 0 (see Table 1 for grading scheme). *Center*: Sustained CMAP in the target segmental level following stimulation of the right L3 dorsal root. The grade of 1+ was assigned to this response. *Right*: Sustained electrophysiological response in adjacent segmental level after right S2 nerve root stimulation (Grade 2+). (**B**) *Left*: Following stimulation of the left L5 dorsal root, sustained activity spreading to multiple myotomes of the ipsilateral limb was recorded (Grade 3+). (*Right*) Diffusion of the response to the contralateral lower extremity following stimulation train of the left S1 dorsal root. The maximally "abnormal" grade 4+ was assigned to this EMG response pattern.

are carefully observed. In all patients, no more than two-thirds of dorsal S2 rootlets are cut on one side and no more than 50% of both S2 sensory roots combined are cut (to minimize risk of bladder dysfunction) (46), less than half of the sensory L4 root are severed [to preserve knee stability as

Table 2 Grading Scale of Motor Response[a]

Grade	Motor response following 1-second 50-Hz stimulus train to dorsal root or rootlet
0	Unsustained CMAP in any muscle ("normal" response)
1+	Sustained CMAP from muscles innervated by the segmental level of the stimulated dorsal rootlet
2+	Same as grade 1+ with CMAP in muscles innervated by an adjacent segmental level
3+	Same as grade 2+ with CMAP in muscles innervated by multiple multiple ipsilateral levels
4+	Same as grade 3+ with motor response in the contralateral leg or upper extremity

[a]Modified from Ref. 23.

suggested by Gros and colleagues (7)], and sectioning of S3 and S4 roots is avoided. Contrary to other authors (26,47,48), the pattern of sustained motor response (e.g., incremental, multiphasic, or clonic) and H-reflex recovery curves are not used as criteria for rootlet lesioning. An identical procedure of stimulation followed by lesioning is performed on all sensory rootlets in the same dorsal root sequence, from S2 to L2 starting on the right.

5.5. Postoperative Care and Follow-Up

Following dorsal rhizotomy, patients are allowed to sit in a chair on the fourth postoperative day. Children receive intensified inpatient rehabilitation devoted to muscle reeducation and strengthening for 6 weeks. Thereafter, they continue with standard physiotherapy involving stretching and strengthening exercises for lower extremities at their local center 3 hours per week. One hour of occupational therapy per week is also recommended for the first year. Postoperative stability and control of lower limbs is further enhanced by judicious use of orthotics. All patients undergo detailed assessments pre-operatively and at 6 and 12 months postoperatively, with yearly evaluations thereafter.

6. OUTCOME

Reduction of spasticity has predictable benefits, but does not automatically lead to functional improvements. Since the fundamental aim of spasticity-relieving surgical techniques is to improve function, proper assessment of treatment effect must include functional outcome measurements.

6.1. Spasticity

Decreased spasticity has been demonstrated qualitatively up to 12 years after selective posterior rhizotomy (24,49–53). Quantitative assessments of spasticity, using myometry, dynamometry, or the Ashworth scale or some variation of this scale, have been reported in 16 studies to date (32,54–68). This includes three randomized controlled trials which showed significant reduction of spasticity after selective dorsal rhizotomy and physiotherapy compared with a control group of patients having physiotherapy alone (59–61). Only two studies performed quantitative assessments at 5 years after rhizotomy (29,54). In agreement with these earlier studies, our results demonstrate that lower limb spasticity is significantly reduced at 1 year postrhizotomy (Fig. 3). This beneficial effect is maintained at 3 and 5 years following surgery.

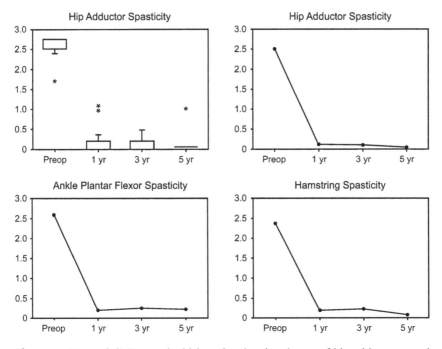

Figure 3 (*Upper left*) Box and whisker plot showing degree of hip adductor muscle spasticity, the primary outcome measure for spasticity. Each box defines the interquartile range, the line in each box represents the median, and the vertical bars represent the 5th and 95th percentile values. The decrease in adductor spasticity from before rhizotomy to 1, 3, and 5 years after rhizotomy was found to be statistically significant (Friedman test, $p < 0.001$). *Represent outliers above the 95th percentile or below the 5th percentile values. Line plots showing the degree of muscle spasticity in the hip adductors (*upper right*), ankle plantar flexors (*lower left*), and hamstrings (*lower right*). Assessments of muscle spasticity were made using the 5-point NYU Tone Scale prior to rhizotomy, and at 1, 3, and 5 years following rhizotomy.

6.2. Strength

Quantitative examination of lower limb strength has been reported in only six studies (29,54,58,61,67,69). Two long-term studies showed a tendency for further strengthening between 1 and 5 years after selective posterior rhizotomy (29,54). We have used five static developmental positions and five transitional movements taken from the Rusk Institute of Rehabilitation/ NYU Rhizotomy Evaluation Form (32) to measure the postural stability, transition, and quality of alignment. This is a nonvalidated tool for assessing motor function. As noted in Figure 4, significant improvement in the total alignment score, a primary outcome measure, is seen up to 5 years

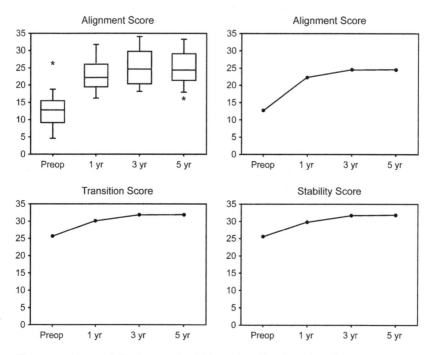

Figure 4 (*Upper left*) Box and whisker plot showing the alignment score, the primary outcome measure of motor function. Each box defines the interquartile range, the line in each box represents the median, and the vertical bars represent the 5th and 95th percentile values. Alignment score from before rhizotomy to 1, 3, and 5 years after rhizotomy was found to be statistically significant (Friedman test, $p < 0.001$). *Represent outliers above the 95th percentile or below the 5th percentile values. Line plots showing the alignment (*upper right*), transition (*lower left*), and assistance (*lower right*) scores. Functional assessments of the five developmental positions and five transitional movements were done using the Rusk/NYU motor function evaluation scale prior to rhizotomy, and at 1, 3, and 5 years following rhizotomy.

postsurgery. Since a large proportion of children in this study were able to maintain the sitting positions and perform the transition movements independently prior to rhizotomy, the transition and stability scores, although improved postsurgery, do not increase as much as the alignment score. Given the above results, it is believed that the children were able to effectively utilize the decrease in spasticity following selective dorsal rhizotomy in order to improve their performance of developmental motor skills.

6.3. Range of Motion

Range of movement in the lower limbs has been previously examined quantitatively, using goniometry, in 10 prospective case series (29,32,54, 55,64,65,67,70–72) and two randomized controlled studies (60,61). All studies have indicated greater range of motion in the lower extremity joints tested from 9 months to 2 years after selective posterior rhizotomy. Only two studies demonstrated an increase in range at 1 year postsurgery, which was maintained up to 5 years following rhizotomy (29,54). In addition to improved range of movement, several authors have also shown increased stride length and velocity using instrumented gait analysis in ambulatory patients (26,56,60,72–79). Among these studies, only two had follow-up longer than 2 years (54,74). In our group of patients, we found that passive range of motion is significantly improved up to 5 years following rhizotomy (Fig. 5).

6.4. Gross Motor Function

Several investigators have reported beneficial effects of selective posterior rhizotomy on quantitative parameters assessing functional limitations involving sitting ability (80–82), ambulation (57,59,61,62,65,67,70,83), and motor function (29,49,82,84). However, almost all these studies used nonvalidated outcome assessment measures. The validated tool most widely used to assess motor function has been the GMFM score, which measures independent functional skills. It is also an indirect reflection of the ability of spasticity to interfere with normal motor activity (34). Six studies, including two randomized controlled trials, have reported statistically significant increases in GMFM scores following rhizotomy (54,56,60–62,66). Only one of these studies had follow-up data beyond 2 years (54). Figure 6 demonstrates that a statistically and clinically significant improvement in motor function occurred in all dimensions of the GMFM at 1, 3, and 5 years postsurgery. In our patients, this was especially evident in the two dimensions involving lower limb function (Fig. 7).

A milder preoperative disability predicts better outcome. As noted earlier, all patients were classified into one of five groups according to their preoperative locomotive abilities. Children with mild to moderate degree of ambulatory dysfunction (Groups I, II, and III) represented 94.4%

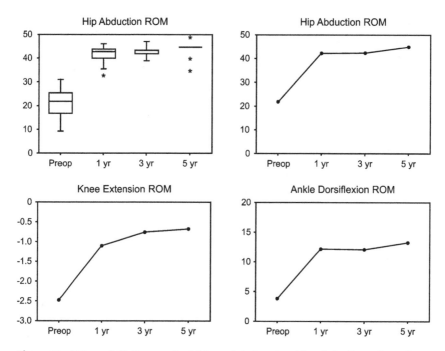

Figure 5 (*Upper left*) Box and whisker plot showing hip abduction, the primary outcome measure for range of motion. Each box defines the interquartile range, the line in each box represents the median, and the vertical bars represent the 5th and 95th percentile values. Hip abduction range of movement from before rhizotomy to 1, 3, and 5 years after rhizotomy was found to be statistically significant (Friedman test, $p < 0.001$). *Represent outliers above the 95th percentile or below the 5th percentile values. Line plots showing the extent of joint range of motion upon hip abduction (*upper right*), knee extension (*lower left*), and ankle dorsiflexion (*lower right*). Assessments of joint range of motion were measured using a goniometer prior to rhizotomy, and at 1, 3, and 5 years following rhizotomy.

(67 of 71) of the study population (54). More detailed analysis of these three subgroups revealed that patients with milder motor deficits (Groups I and II, independent and dependent ambulators) were more likely to improve ambulatory function at 3 and 5 years following surgery than those who were unable to walk (Group III, 4-point crawlers) (Fig. 7). Therefore, children who exhibit a better baseline ambulatory function may potentially benefit the most from selective posterior rhizotomy. On the other hand, severely disabled, nonambulatory patients (Groups IV and V) are unlikely to have any worthwhile improvement in motor function despite adequate elimination of lower extremity spasticity. This is in agreement with Russell and coworkers (34) who determined that, when controlled for age, the amount of change in GMFM scores is dependent on the severity of the child's cerebral palsy.

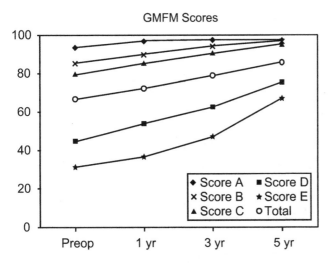

Figure 6 Line plots showing the level of motor function. Assessments of motor function were done using the GMFM scores prior to rhizotomy, and at 1, 3, and 5 years following rhizotomy. Dimensions A, B, and C predominantly examine upper extremity function, whereas dimensions D and E of the GMFM principally reflect lower extremity motor function.

Paradoxically, children with better ambulatory function (Group I) are often not referred for an evaluation (or deferred referral) because of the misconception that their potential for significant gains is low. Indeed, in our own group of patients, the total GMFM baseline score for independent ambulators was 84.3%. However, we noted a mean change in dimensions D and E from patients in Group I of 13.0% and 25.8%, respectively, at the 5 years follow-up compared to preoperative values (Fig. 7). Furthermore, we have found that the greatest degree of family satisfaction with respect to outcome is seen in the independent ambulating patient subgroup (unpublished data) because the family feels that the child is no longer stigmatized as "being different" when introduced in a cohort of children of the same age.

6.5. Fine Motor Skills and Patterns

Whereas primary gains should be expected in lower extremity function following dorsal rhizotomy, improvements in upper extremity function have been noted by many authors anecdotally. Suprasegmental effects of selective dorsal rhizotomy have been studied in both orthopedic and functional fields. In several reports, comments have been made about improvements in upper extremity function after selective posterior rhizotomy. Quantitative assessments have been done infrequently, using multiple different assessment measures, and with variable results. As the optimal goal of spasticity-relieving

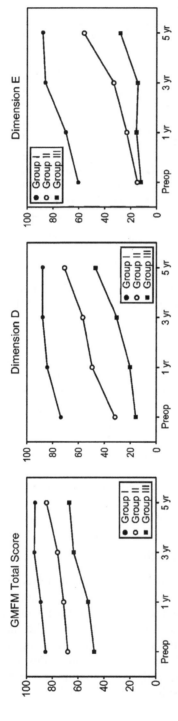

Figure 7 Line plots comparing total GMFM scores (*left*), dimension D (*center*), and dimension E (*right*) between the study patients according to the preoperative level of functioning. Patients were subdivided into five groups according to their preoperative locomotive abilities. Dimensions D and E primarily relate to lower extremity motor function and are the primary outcome measures of the GMFM.

surgical methods is primarily to improve function, assessment of treatment effect must include functional outcome measurements. A number of different tools have been used to examine the effects of SPR on upper extremity function. Folio and Fewell (35) constructed the PDMS to accomplish several purposes, including: (a) identification of children with delayed motor development; (b) identification of a child's unique strengths and needs; (c) assessment of motor development over time in response to intervention; and (d) identification of motor objectives and intervention strategies. The PDMS was therefore designed for use as both a discriminative and an evaluative measure. This developmental, sequential test provides a comprehensive assessment of a child's gross and fine motor patterns and skills in relation to adaptive capacities. The items tested require the child to use his or her motor capacity to adapt to specific situations. The large number of items provides a greater opportunity for the child to demonstrate abilities and for the examiner to program effectively (35). In this manner, the child's strengths and weaknesses can be analyzed thoroughly and accurately.

Previous studies have reported a decrease in upper extremity spasticity following selective posterior rhizotomy (24,66,68,85). However, reduction of upper limb spasticity, while having predictable benefits, does not automatically translate into improved fine motor function. Several investigators have reported beneficial effects of selective dorsal rhizotomy on qualitative parameters assessing functional limitations involving upper limb range of motion (24,86) and grasp strength (64). Fifteen different prospective case series have reported suprasegmental effects of selective rhizotomy. In seven studies, the suprasegmental benefits were described qualitatively, the most common being improvement in the upper limbs (24,49,50,53,65,67,86). Quantitative assessments using nonvalidated tools have been reported in six studies (64,87–91). These prospective studies have shown improved block stacking, with variable effects on upper limb tone and manipulation patterns. Two recent studies, using a validated, quantitative tool to measure upper limb function, reported beneficial effects on upper extremity skills following SPR (87,92). Finally, improved cognitive function was noted in one prospective study using the validated Woodcock–Johnson Psychoeducational battery (93). However, only of these quantitative studies had follow-up data beyond 1 year after dorsal rhizotomy (87).

As noted by Buckon and colleagues (64), children with cerebral palsy frequently have unstable force generation and inefficient sensory feedback during upper limb manipulation. This impairs their ability to develop the learned motor programs necessary to execute smooth, precise hand movements. We therefore focused on fine motor coordination and analyzed upper extremity skills from a developmental and functional perspective in this study. Standardized, validated, objective tests of fine motor skills and patterns were used to determine if selective posterior rhizotomy results in functional upper extremity use. We clearly demonstrated that the PDMS

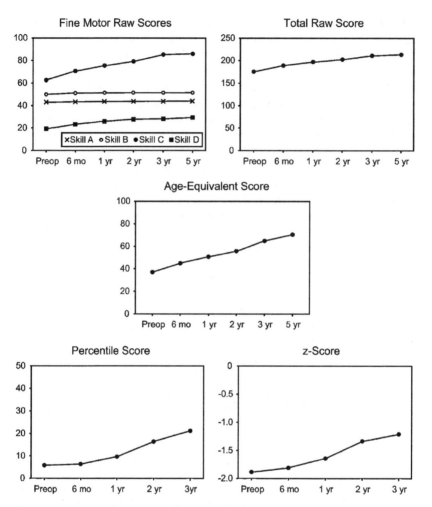

Figure 8 Line plots showing the raw scores for each of the four categories (*upper left*), the total raw score (*upper right*), the age-equivalence (*center*), the percentile rank (*lower left*), and the *z*-scores (*lower right*) of the fine motor skills section of the PDMS scores. Quantitative evaluations of upper extremity performance were made using a comprehensive standardized assessment of the PDMS measured prior to rhizotomy, at 6 and 12 months postoperatively, and at yearly intervals thereafter. The fine motor scale evaluates tasks that require precise movement of the small muscles of the body and is classified into four skill categories: skill A evaluates grasping, skill B measures hand use, skill C evaluates eye-hand coordination, and skill D quantifies manual dexterity. The addition of the four individual skill scores provides the total raw score. Using the PDMS conversion tables, raw scores were converted into age-equivalent scores. As normative scores show how close the child is to the normal population of the same age, they were not available for patients 7 years or older at follow-up. Since none of the children was under 7 years at the 5-year assessment, the percentile rank and *z*-scores were available up to the 3-year follow-up.

is capable of identifying longitudinal changes (up to 5 years postrhizotomy) in fine motor function in children with spastic cerebral palsy (Fig. 8). This is in contrast to lower extremity gains, which reach significance at the 1 year follow-up and are maintained subsequently but without any further significant improvements after 1 year following dorsal rhizotomy. Furthermore, eye–hand coordination and manual dexterity, where the clinically relevant improvements occur, are skills that have a major impact on the quality of life of affected children. Selective posterior rhizotomy allows them to reach low-normal level of function, which even the higher functioning group of children with spastic cerebral palsy does not reach preoperatively.

In our recent study (87), children with mild to moderate degree of ambulatory dysfunction (Groups I, II, and III) represented 97.8% of the study population (44 of 45 patients). More detailed analysis of these three subgroups revealed that children with milder motor deficits (Group I and II, independent and dependent ambulators) were more likely to improve fine motor skills at 3 and 5 years following surgery than those who were unable to walk preoperatively (Group III, 4-point crawlers) (Fig. 9). Therefore, children who have some baseline ambulatory function may potentially benefit the most from selective posterior rhizotomy. On the other hand, severely disabled, nonambulatory patients (Groups IV and V) are unlikely to have any worthwhile improvement in functional performance (both upper and lower extremities) despite adequate elimination of spasticity. In addition, these severely affected children often have poor motor power globally. Therefore, we are in full agreement with von Koch et al. (94), who state that the upper extremity spasticity and blunted fine motor skills seen in quadriplegic children may be addressed more readily with intrathecal baclofen by placement of the catheter higher in the spinal cord. However, our study clearly shows that for higher functioning children, excellent results in upper extremity fine motor control can be achieved with selective dorsal rhizotomy, which remains the therapeutic gold standard for children who meet preoperative criteria. A comparative study between selective posterior rhizotomy and intrathecal baclofen looking specifically at upper extremity gains would be interesting, although perhaps very difficult to organize given the growing body of literature demonstrating that the two operations are better suited for distinct subgroups of children with spastic cerebral palsy (94). Our results explicitly indicate that one should not favor baclofen pump implantation over SPR because of a theoretical misconception that dorsal rhizotomy only addresses lower extremity impairments.

6.6. Activities of Daily Living

Once reduction of spasticity, improved joint range of motion, and increased motor strength are optimized through selective posterior rhizotomy, the therapists can focus on daily activities (such as oral-facial hygiene, groom-

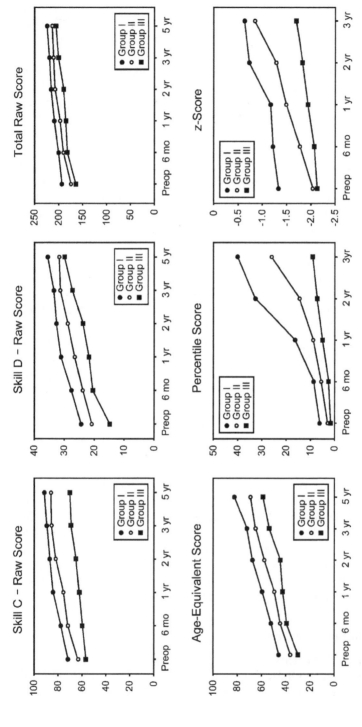

Figure 9 Line plots comparing raw scores of skill C (*upper left*) and skill D (*upper center*), total raw scores (upper right), age-equivalence (*lower left*), percentile ranks (*lower center*), and z-scores (*lower right*) of the PDMS between the study patients according to preoperative level of functioning. Patients were subdivided into five groups according to their preoperative locomotive abilities. As normative scores show how close the child is to the normal population of the same age, they were not available for patients 7 years or older at follow-up. Since none of the children were under 7 years at the 5-year assessment, the percentile rank and z-scores were available up to the 3-year follow-up.

ing, and feeding) with particular emphasis on upper and lower extremity dressing and toileting. Mobility issues are further addressed, such as independent sitting and moving in bed; transfer onto a chair, toilet, bathtub, or car; and indoor and outdoor walking skills. These functional skills, which serve as the foundation to all activities of daily living, ultimately translate into a reduction in caregiver demands for patients with cerebral palsy and thus improve patient independence.

The PEDI was used as an interview tool to elicit parental assessments of what the child actually does achieve on average. Administration of the PEDI in this way has been suggested to be more effective than professional assessments based on the PEDI because, owing to its administration in the clinical environment, the therapist is unable to observe the child's performance of certain functional skills at home (41). However, comparisons of scoring by parents and that of therapists have shown them to manifest a high level of agreement (39,41).

Several investigators have reported beneficial effects of selective posterior rhizotomy on quantitative parameters assessing functional limitations involving sitting ability (80–82), ambulation (57,59,61,62,65,67,70,83), and motor function (29,49,82,84). However, almost all the studies used nonvalidated outcome assessment tools. The WeeFIM has been used in two prospective studies, which showed significant improvements in activities of daily living after selective posterior rhizotomy (70,92). The quantitative, validated tool most widely used to assess activities of daily living in children is the PEDI. Four prospective case series have used the PEDI and reported statistically significant improvements in the self-care and mobility domains following dorsal rhizotomy (42,44,88,95). However, only one of these studies had follow-up data beyond 2 years after selective rhizotomy (44). Our results show that important gains in functional performance are seen as early as 6 months after dorsal rhizotomy (Figs. 10 and 11). Furthermore, these clinically significant benefits continue to occur up to 5 years following rhizotomy (Figs. 10 and 11).

Children with mild to moderate degree of ambulatory dysfunction (Groups I, II, and III) represented 97.6% (40 of 41) of the study population (44). More detailed analysis of these three subgroups revealed that patients with milder motor deficits (Groups I and II, independent and dependent ambulators) were more likely to improve functional performance at 3 and 5 years following surgery than those who were unable to walk preoperatively (Group III, 4-point crawlers) (Fig. 12). Therefore, children that have some baseline ambulatory function may potentially benefit the most from selective dorsal rhizotomy. On the other hand, severely disabled, nonambulatory patients (Groups IV and V) are likely to have more modest improvements in activities of daily living despite adequate elimination of lower extremity spasticity. Dorsal rhizotomy in these functional groups is associated with more complications. The modest gains are likely to be equally achievable in

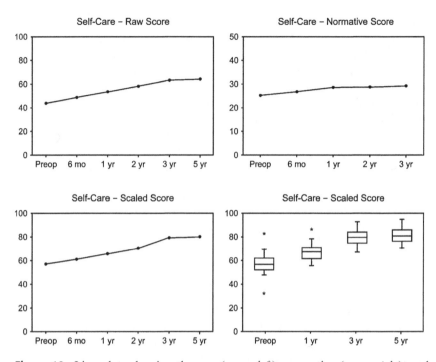

Figure 10 Line plots showing the raw (*upper left*), normative (*upper right*), and scaled (*lower left*) scores of the self-care dimension of the functional skills domain of the PEDI. Quantitative evaluations of self-care skills were made using a comprehensive standardized assessment of the PEDI measured prior to rhizotomy, at 6 and 12 months postoperatively, and at yearly intervals thereafter. As the normative scores show how close the child is to the normal population of the same age, they were not available for patients 7.5 years or older at follow-up. Since none of the children were under 7.5 years at the 5-year assessment, normative scores (*upper right*) were available up to the 3-year follow-up. Box and whisker plot (*lower right*) showing the scaled scores of the self-care dimension of the functional skills domain of the PEDI. Each box defines the interquartile range, the line in each box represents the median, and the vertical bars represent the 5th and 95th percentile values. The increase in self-care skill from before rhizotomy to 1, 3, and 5 years after rhizotomy was found to be statistically significant (Friedman test, $p < 0.001$). *Represent outliers above the 95th percentile or below the 5th percentile values.

these more involved children with a less invasive and reversible treatment—intrathecal baclofen pump implantation (see chap. 15).

6.7. Hip Deformity

We (unpublished data), and others (96,97), have noted stabilization of progressive hip deformity following selective posterior rhizotomy provided

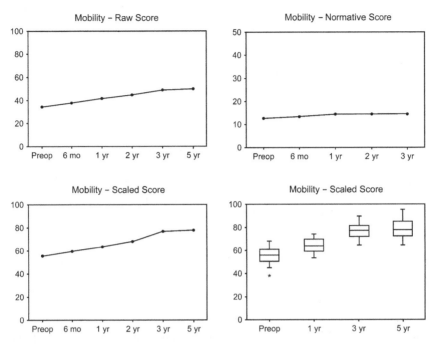

Figure 11 Line plots showing the raw (*upper left*), normative (*upper right*), and scaled (*lower left*) scores of the mobility dimension of the functional skills domain of the PEDI. Box and whisker plot (*lower right*) showing the scaled scores of the mobility dimension of the functional skills domain of the PEDI. The increase in functional mobility from before rhizotomy to 1, 3, and 5 years after rhizotomy was found to be statistically significant (Friedman test, $p < 0.001$).

that the prerhizotomy Reimer index does not exceed 50%. Therefore, if the child meets all other criteria and the index is less than 50%, dorsal rhizotomy is recommended. If all criteria are met but the subluxation is greater than 50%, orthopedic hip surgery should precede rhizotomy by 6–12 months.

6.8. Bladder Function

In an attempt to preserve sphincter control, several groups have tried to better identify pudendal afferents (46,98–102). In our experience, in addition to identifying pathologic reflex circuits for interruption, EMG-guided rhizotomy also enables accurate identification of sacral nerve roots involved in bowel and bladder control. It remains critical to limit lesioning of dorsal S2 rootlets and avoid sectioning S3 and S4 roots in selective posterior rhizotomy. Using these lesioning criteria, all children who were toilet trained prior to dorsal rhizotomy remained so after surgery. Those who were not became toilet trained postoperatively. Finally, detailed urodynamic studies done

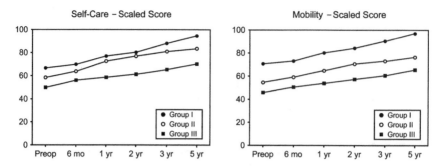

Figure 12 Line plots comparing scaled scores of self-care (*left*) and mobility (*right*) domains between the study patients according to preoperative level of functioning. Patients were subdivided into five groups according to their preoperative locomotive abilities. Scaled scores of the self-care and mobility dimensions of the PEDI primarily relate to functional performance and are the primary outcome measures of the PEDI.

pre- and postoperatively on our patients showed that a large number of patients have markedly elevated bladder pressures preoperatively and low bladder capacities and poor compliance as would be expected of a spastic bladder. The bladder pressures were in the range that would cause upper urinary tract and renal diseases in the long run. Following surgery, bladder pressure and capacity, as well as compliance, tend towards minimally acceptable values for age (46).

6.9. Adjunctive Orthopedic Procedures

The management of spasticity in cerebral palsy is complex and best handled by a multidisciplinary team. Neurosurgical and orthopedic treatment options for spastic cerebral palsy are diverse and are complementary rather than mutually exclusive. Analysis of outcome measures does not suggest that adjuvant orthopedic procedures during the follow-up period have a significant impact on spasticity, range of motion, or motor function. Indeed, statistically and clinically significant durable gains in all functional measures occurred at the 1-year assessment, prior to any orthopedic intervention (54). Also, in our patients, one could argue that the significant ongoing improvements seen in dimensions D and E of the GMFM at 3 and 5 years postrhizotomy (Fig. 6) could be partly influenced by orthopedic interventions. However, we note that only 6 of 71 patients (8.5%) underwent an orthopedic procedure before the 3-year assessment, and that only 9 (12.7%) children needed lower extremity botulinum toxin injections prior to the 3-year assessment. Even when these patients are excluded from analysis of dimensions D and E, a significant gain remains at the 3 and 5 years follow-up compared to baseline and 1-year values (54). In fact, the mean change in dimension D is

24.5% at 3-year and 31.3% at 5-year assessment compared to preoperative scores. For dimension E of the GMFM, the mean increase is 21.4% and 33.9% at 3 and 5 years follow-up, respectively. Whereas there is no doubt that orthopedic interventions can procure further gains to the children, they will usually have reached their goals and made their significant gains prior to the introduction of these adjuvant modalities in the armamentarium.

7. COMPLICATIONS

The long-term safety and efficacy of selective posterior rhizotomy has been rigorously studied. However, as with any major surgical intervention, potential side effects and complications can result following dorsal rhizotomy. These can occur in the intraoperative, early postoperative, and late postoperative periods (Table 3).

7.1. Intraoperative Complications

A potential hazard during selective dorsal rhizotomy is aspiration pneumonia. Children with advanced cerebral palsy are especially at higher risk of aspiration pneumonia because of their increased tendency to have gastroesophageal reflux. Euler and colleagues (103) reported that 18 of 19 children with a history of gastroesophageal reflux had episodes of aspiration pneumonia. Abbott (104) reported a 12% (5 of 60 patients) incidence of aspiration pneumonia intraoperatively, with three children requiring postoperative mechanical ventilation. Patients undergoing selective posterior rhizotomy are also at risk of developing respiratory complications. A child born prematurely or with a history of bronchopulmonary dysplasia has a fivefold increased risk of reactive airway disease compared to the general pediatric population (105). A threefold increased risk is seen with a child with a history meconium aspiration (106). Also, since neuromuscular block-

Table 3 Complications of Selective Posterior Rhizotomy

Intraoperative period	Early postoperative period	Late postoperative period
Hypotonia	Aspiration pneumonia	Kyphosis/scoliosis
Bronchospasm	Sensory loss	Lumbar hyperlordosis
	Dysesthesia	Spondylosis
	Neurogenic bladder	Spondylolisthesis
	Ileus	Lumbar spinal stenosis
	Urinary tract infection	Muscle contracture
	CSF leakage	Hip dislocation
	Wound infection	Persisting neurogenic bladder
	Subdural hematoma	
	Headache	

ing agents cannot be used during nerve root stimulation to allow for adequate electrophysiological monitoring of the "abnormal" circuits, this aggravates any inherent tendency toward bronchospasm. Abbott (104) reported that 13 of 60 patients (22%) had experienced bronchospasm during surgery, with five cases requiring aborting the surgery. Other groups have reported a lower incidence of pulmonary complications (107,108). Protective measures such as perioperative administration of bronchodilators and H_2 blockers have been suggested by some to reduce the risk of aspiration pneumonia and bronchospasm. We have not encountered any problems with pulmonary complications, possibly because of our selection bias towards higher-functioning children where lung disease is less prevalent. Additionally, the use of propofol in our protocol has allowed us to eliminate the need for bronchodilators which we were using routinely on early cases.

7.2. Early Postoperative Complications

Reduction of spasticity is apparent immediately following selective dorsal rhizotomy. Patients often complain of "weakness" in the immediate post-operative period. This is related to the unmasking of underlying hypotonia previously hidden by superimposed global spasticity. Postoperative weakness was reported by Peter and Arens (109) in 26 of 110 children who underwent dorsal rhizotomy. A transient functional decline due to weakness following surgery was experienced in 2 of 25 patients reported by Peacock and Staudt (77). Significant lower extremity weakness must be excluded prior to considering for selective dorsal rhizotomy. The postoperative hypotonia seen in most patients remains transient and underscores the necessity of intensified inpatient rehabilitation devoted to muscle re-education and strengthening following dorsal rhizotomy.

Potential postoperative sensory abnormalities include sensory loss, dysesthesia, and, rarely, hyperesthesia. Most large series report persistent sensory loss in 4–10% of children after dorsal rhizotomy (108–110). The sensory deficits typically resolve or improve significantly in the majority of cases. They tended to be more frequent in the late 1980s and early 1990s, when the lesioning rate was reported in certain cases to be around 70–80% of rootlets and frequently where two adjacent dorsal roots could be sectioned completely if the responses were abnormal. Most centers currently lesion at 40–60% (44% in our group). Furthermore, we have taken the habit of always preserving at least the most normal one or two rootlets at each level (31). Using this approach, sensory changes are limited to restless leg syndrome for the first 3 weeks at the end of a hard day of physiotherapy in approximately 30% of patients. This responds well to a small diazepam dose at bedtime and never exceeds 3 weeks following surgery. No patients have chronic sensory changes or dysesthesias. Older children who are collaborative will do very well with proprioceptive testing postoperatively.

An increased incidence of bladder dysfunction is seen in children with cerebral palsy (111,112). We noted that 23 of 35 patients who underwent preoperative urodynamic testing showed abnormal bladder capacity, pressure-specific volumes, and full resting pressure (46). This patient population is at high risk for postrhizotomy neurogenic bladder and therefore, formal urodynamic testing should be performed in all children who have a history of urologic dysfunction (enuresis, stress incontinence, or dribbling). We reported three cases of urinary retention (4.3%) requiring intermittent catheterization for up to 14 days following selective posterior rhizotomy (54). This avoidable complication occurred early in the series and has since been avoided by cutting no more than two-thirds of dorsal S2 rootlets (and 50% combined S2) and by leaving the indwelling urinary catheter an additional 24 hours after discontinuation of epidural morphine. Abbott and coworkers developed a technique for identifying and preserving the afferent sacral roots containing cutaneous branches of the pudendal nerve, thereby decreasing the risk of postoperative micturition and perhaps potential sexual dysfunction (98).

Other early postoperative complications reported in children after selective dorsal rhiztomy include cerebrospinal fluid leakage, meningitis, wound infection, ileus, emesis, constipation, subdural hematomas, and headache (24,104,108).

7.3. Late Postoperative Complications

Spinal deformities such as spondylosis, spondylolisthesis, lumbar spinal stenosis, and lumbar hyperlordosis have been reported in children who undergo spinal surgery including dorsal rhizotomy. The incidence of spinal abnormalities following a multilevel lumbosacral laminectomy has been determined by Peter and colleagues (113). They found that 19 of 99 patients developed isthmic spondylolysis or grade I spondylolisthesis following five-level lumbosacral laminectomies for selective posterior rhizotomy. Six of the 19 children with grade I spondylolisthesis remained asymptomatic without evidence of further slipping on follow-up examination. The majority of these patients was ambulatory and active and the authors postulated that the laminectomy, associated lordosis, and increased mobility after rhizotomy contributed to the postoperative deformity of the spine. Lumbar spinal stenosis was reported by Gooch and Walker (114) in two patients who underwent dorsal rhizotomy for spastic diplegia 4 years after L1–S2 laminectomy and 2 years after L2–S2 laminotomy, respectively. Both patients required decompression to relieve their symptoms. Severe lumbar lordosis was seen in two nonambulatory children with spastic quadriplegia with significant trunk weakness following dorsal rhizotomy (115). An analysis of scoliosis rates in the first 100 of our patients suggests that the rate is low (6%) and that the degree of scoliosis is very mild and not requiring

bracing in this group of ambulatory children. We are in the process of looking at the rate of hyperlordosis with lateral films of the spine. Only one
patient needed decompressive laminectomy for spinal stenosis 12 years following dorsal rhizotomy. She was noted to have a congenitally narrow canal
at the time of the rhizotomy procedure 12 years earlier. A limited two-level
laminectomy using ultrasonographic localization of the conus medullaris as
described by Park and colleagues (116) is postulated to reduce the long-term
risk of spinal abnormalities. The rate of complications and of spinal deformity complications is so low with a narrow laminoplasty that we have been
hesitant to convert to a 1–2 level technique described by Park and colleagues
(116). We are not certain if the potential gains of a smaller exposure might
be offset by the inability to stimulate all rootlets prior to deciding which
ones will be lesioned (which is not possible with the conus operation given
the limited space). We strongly believe in the benefits of intraoperative
stimulation in our decision making and prefer to decide for a given root
when all rootlets have been stimulated and patterns of spread analyzed.
Our other concern with the operation at the conus is the need for a wider
exposure and a laminectomy at that level, which is the junction of the rigid
thoracic and mobile lumbar segments. Long-term orthopedic consequences,
if any, need to be analyzed in a controlled fashion to clarify this important
subject.

Tendon releases, transfers, and lengthenings may be required for some
patients with progressive joint immobility due to fixed contractures, despite
the elimination of spasticity following dorsal rhizotomy. Abbott et al. (32)
reported that 8 of 250 children required tendon lengthenings after selective
dorsal rhizotomy. Carroll and colleagues published a 65% incidence of
orthopedic procedures in 112 patients who underwent selective dorsal rhizotomy. Finally, progressive hip migration requiring derotation osteotomies was described in seven children 1 year after rhizotomy (118). Heim
and coworkers used the Reimers migration percentage as a quantitative
measure of hip stability in 45 children before and after selective dorsal rhizotomy (97). They found that 80% (72 of 90 hips) remained unchanged, 9%
improved, and 11% worsened radiographically. Four patients required unilateral derotational femoral osteotomies for persistent or worsening hip subluxation. We have found, comparing 88 hips preoperatively and at 1 year
postsurgery, that the Reimer index is stable in 75%, improved in 20%, and
worse in 5% (unpublished data). Those who worsened had an index exceed-
ing 50% and would now be offered "prophylactic" hip surgery prior to dorsal
rhizotomy if they met the eligibility criteria.

8. CONCLUSIONS

Lumbosacral selective posterior rhizotomy has become a standard neurosurgical procedure for the management of carefully selected children with

the spastic form of cerebral palsy. The intent of surgery is to permanently eliminate lower limb spasticity while improving muscle strength and range of motion. Children with spastic diplegia also show significant functional gains in ambulation, gross and fine motor skills, and in performing activities of daily living as measured by validated tools. Selected children may also show stabilization of progressive hip subluxation and augmentation of bladder capacity. Finally, suprasegmental benefits have also been reported, including improved upper limb coordination and function, positive changes in oral-motor skills, and enhancement of visual attention, cognitive function, and language skills. In an effort to optimize the balance between elimination of spasticity and preservation of strength, most centers employ intraoperative electrophysiological monitoring to reliably outline populations of spinal rootlets that are maximally involved in a dysfunctional circuitry and maintenance of velocity-dependent hypertonicity. The procedure, based upon, or modified from, the original techniques described by Fasano and Peacock, consists of selectively cutting dorsal rootlets from L2 to S2, thereby eliminating the aberrant myotatic reflex impulse. The challenge remains to objectively determine how these promising interventions can alter long-term function and quality of life outcomes in children with spastic cerebral palsy. We believe that rigorous analysis of standardized quantitative functional outcome measurements, especially those looking at enhancement of function rather than suppression of spasticity is critical for defining the most relevant benefits of the EMG-guided procedure.

REFERENCES

1. Bax MCO. Terminology and classification of cerebral palsy. Dev Med Child Neurol 1964; 6:295–296.
2. Kuban KC, Leviton A. Cerebral palsy. N Engl J Med 1994; 330:188–195.
3. Peterson MC, Palmer FB. Advances in prevention and treatment of cerebral palsy. MRDD Res Rev 2000; 7:30–37.
4. Abbe R. A contribution to surgery of the spine. Med Rec NY 1889; 35: 149–152.
5. Bennett WH. A case in which acute spasmodic pain in the left lower extremity was completely relieved by subsural division of the posterior rootlets of certain spinal nerves. Med Chir Trans 1889; 72:329–348.
6. Foerster O. On the indications and results of the excision of posterior spinal nerve roots in men. Surg Gynecol Obstet 1913; 16:463–474.
7. Gros C, Ouknine G, Vlahovitch B, Frerebeau P. La radicotomie sélective postérieure dans le traitement neurochirurgical de l'hypertonie pyramidale. Neurochirurgie 1967; 13:505–518.
8. Sindou M. Étude de la jonction radicolu-médullaire postérieure. La radicellotomie postérieure sélective dans la chirurgie de la douleur. Doctoral dissertation, Lyon, 1972.

9. Fasano VA, Barolat-Romana G, Ivaldi A, Sguazzi A. La radicotomie postér-
    ieure fonctionnelle dans le traitement de la spasticité cérébrale. Neurochirurgie
    1976; 22:23–34.
10. Peacock WJ, Arens LJ. Selective posterior rhizotomy for the relief of spasticity
    in cerebral palsy. S Afr Med J 1982; 62:119–124.
11. Sherrington CS. Decerebrate rigidity and reflex coordination of movements.
    J Physiol 1898; 22:319–337.
12. DeCandia M, Provini L, Taborikova H. Mechanisms of the reflex discharge
    depression in the spinal motoneurone during repetitive orthodromic stimula-
    tion. Brain Res 1967; 4:284–291.
13. Lundberg A. Convergence of excitatory and inhibitory action on interneur-
    ones in the spinal cord. UCLA Forum Med Sci 1969; 11:231–265.
14. Yanagisawa N, Tanaka R, Ito Z. Reciprocal Ia inhibition in spastic hemiple-
    gia of man. Brain 1976; 99:555–574.
15. Gilbert M, Stelzner DJ. The development of descending and dorsal root con-
    nections in the lumbosacral spinal cord of the postnatal rat. J Comp Neurol
    1979; 184:821–838.
16. Katz RT. Réévaluation des mécanismes physiopathologiques qui génèrent le
    réflexe d'étirement: de nouvelles hypothèses sur la physiopathologie de la spas-
    ticité. Ann Readapt Med Phys 2001; 44:268–272.
17. Logigian EL, Shefner JM, Goumnerova L, Scott RM, Soriano SG, Madsen J.
    The critical importance of stimulus intensity in intraoperative monitoring for
    partial dorsal rhizotomy. Muscle Nerve 1996; 19:415–422.
18. Steinbok P, Kestle JR. Variation between centers in electrophysiologic techni-
    ques used in lumbosacral selective dorsal rhizotomy for spastic cerebral palsy.
    Pediatr Neurosurg 1996; 25:233–239.
19. Warf BC, Nelson KR. The electromyographic responses to dorsal rootlet sti-
    mulation during partial dorsal rhizotomy are inconsistent. Pediatr Neurosurg
    1996; 25:13–19.
20. Weiss IP, Schiff SJ. Reflex variability in selective dorsal rhizotomy. J Neuro-
    surg 1993; 79:346–353.
21. Chabal C, Jacobson L, Little J. Effects of intrathecal fentanyl and lidocaine on
    somato-sensory evoked potentials, the H reflex, and clinical responses. Anesth
    Analg 1988; 67:509–513.
22. Grossi P, Arner S. Effect of epidural morphine on the Hoffman-reflex in man.
    Acta Anesthesiol Scand 1984; 28:152–154.
23. Phillips LH, Park TS. Electrophysiologic mapping of the segmental anatomy
    of the muscles of the lower extremity. Muscle Nerve 1991; 14:1213–1218.
24. Cohen AR, Webster HC. How selective is selective posterior rhizotomy? Surg
    Neurol 1991; 35:267–272.
25. Steinbok P, Langill L, Cochrane DD, Keyes R. Observations on electrical
    stimulation of lumbosacral nerve roots in children with and without lower
    limb spasticity. Childs Nerv Syst 1992; 8:376–382.
26. Storrs BB, Nishida T. Use of the 'H' reflex recovery curve in selective posterior
    rhizotomy. Pediatr Neurosci 1988; 74:178–184.

27. Hays RM, McLaughlin JF, Bjornson KF, Stephens K, Roberts TS, Price R. Electrophysiological monitoring during selective dorsal rhizotomy, and spasticity and GMFM performance. Dev Med Child Neurol 1998; 40:233–238.

28. Landau WM, Hunt CC. Dorsal rhizotomy, a treatment of unproven efficacy. J Child Neurol 1990; 5:174–178.

29. Gul SM, Steinbok P, McLeod K. Long-term outcome after selective posterior rhizotomy in children with spastic cerebral palsy. Pediatr Neurosurg 1999; 31:84–95.

30. Peacock WJ, Nuwer MR, Staudt LA. Dorsal rhizotomy: to monitor or not to monitor. J Neurosurg 1994; 80:769–771.

31. Mittal S, Farmer JP, Poulin C, Silver K. Reliability of intraoperative electrophysiological monitoring in selective posterior rhizotomy. J Neurosurg 2001; 95:67–75.

32. Abbott R, Johann-Murphy M, Shiminski-Maher T, Quartermain D, Forem SL, Gold JT, Epstein FJ. Selective dorsal rhizotomy: outcome and complications in treating spastic cerebral palsy. Neurosurgery 1993; 33:851–857.

33. Johann-Murphy M, Bier TC, Shakin R, et al. NYU rhizotomy evaluation form: reliability study. Pediatr Phys Ther 1993; 5:69–74.

34. Russell DJ, Rosenbaum PL, Cadman DT, Gowland C, Hardy S, Jarvis S. The Gross Motor Function Measure: a means to evaluate the effects of physical therapy. Dev Med Child Neurol 1989; 31:341–352.

35. Folio MR, Fewell RR. Peabody Developmental Motor Scales and Activity Cards. Austin, TX: PRO-ED, 1983.

36. Stokes NA, Deitz JL, Crowe TK. The Peabody Developmental Fine Motor Scale: an interrater reliability study. Am J Occup Ther 1990; 44:334–340.

37. Palisano RJ, Kolobe TH, Haley SM, Lowes LP, Jones SL. Validity of the Peabody Developmental Gross Motor Scale as an evaluative measure of infants receiving physical therapy. Phys Ther 1995; 75:939–951.

38. Schmidt LS, Westcott SL, Crowe TK. Interrater reliability of the gross motor scale of the Peabody Developmental Motor Scales with 4- and 5-year-old children. Pediatr Phys Ther 1993; 5:169–175.

39. Haley SM, Coster J, Faas RM. A content validity study of the Pediatric Evaluation of Disability Inventory. Pediatr Phys Ther 1991; 3:177–184.

40. Feldman AB, Haley SM, Coryell J. Concurrent and construct validity of the Pediatric Evaluation of Disability Inventory. Phys Ther 1990; 70:602–610.

41. Nichols DS, Case-Smith J. Reliability and validity of the Pediatric Evaluation of Disability Inventory. Pediatr Phys Ther 1996; 8:15–24.

42. Bloom KK, Nazar GB. Functional assessment following selective posterior rhizotomy in spastic cerebral palsy. Childs Nerv Syst 1994; 10:84–86.

43. Dudgeon BJ, Libby AK, McLaughlin JF, Hays RM, Bjornson KF, Roberts TS. Prospective measurement of functional changes after selective dorsal rhizotomy. Arch Phys Med Rehabil 1994; 75:46–53.

44. Mittal S, Farmer JP, Al-Atassi B, Montpetit K, Gervais N, Poulin C, Benaroch TE, Cantin MA. Functional performance following selective posterior rhizotomy: long-term results determined using a validated evaluative measure. J Neurosurg 2002; 97:510–518.

45. Phillips LH, Park TS. Electrophysiologic studies of selective posterior rhizotomy patients. Park TS, Phillips LH, Peacock WJ, eds. Neurosurgery: State of the Art Reviews: Management of Spasticity in Cerebral Palsy and Spinal Cord Injury. Philadelphia, PA: Hanley & Belfus, 1989:459–469.

46. Houle AM, Vernet O, Jednak R, Pippi Salle JL, Farmer JP. Bladder function before and after selective dorsal rhizotomy in children with cerebral palsy. J Urol 1998; 160:1088–1091.

47. Peacock WJ, Staudt LA. Spasticity in cerebral palsy and the selective posterior rhizotomy procedure. J Child Neurol 1990; 5:179–185.

48. Vaughan CL, Berman B, Peacock WJ. Cerebral palsy and rhizotomy. A 3-year follow-up evaluation with gait analysis. J Neurosurg 1991; 74:178–184.

49. Arens LJ, Peacock WJ, Peter J. Selective posterior rhizotomy: a long-term follow-up study. Childs Nerv Syst 1989; 5:148–152.

50. Fasano VA, Broggi G, Zeme S. Intraoperative electrical stimulation for functional posterior rhizotomy. Scand J Rehabil Med Suppl 1988; 17:149–154.

51. Fraioli B, Zamponi C, Baldassarre L, et al. Selective posterior rootlet section in the treatment of spastic disorders of infantile cerebral palsy: immediate and late results. Acta Neurochir Suppl 1984; 33:539–541.

52. Peter JC, Arens LJ. Selective posterior lumbosacral rhizotomy in teenagers and young adults with spastic cerebral palsy. Br J Neurosurg 1994; 8:135–139.

53. Schijman E, Erro MG, Meana NV. Selective posterior rhizotomy: experience of 30 cases. Childs Nerv Syst 1993; 9:474–477.

54. Mittal S, Farmer JP, Al-Atassi B, Gibis J, Kennedy E, Galli C, Courchesnes G, Poulin C, Cantin MA, Benaroch TE. Long-term functional outcome after selective posterior rhizotomy. J Neurosurg 2002; 97:315–325.

55. Fukuhara T, Najm IM, Levin KH, Luciano MG, Brant MSCL. Nerve rootlet to be sectioned for spasticity resolution in selective dorsal rhizotomy. Surg Neurol 2000; 54:126–133.

56. Sacco DJ, Tylkowski CM, Warf BC. Nonselective partial dorsal rhizotomy: a clinical experience with 1-year follow-up. Pediatr Neurosurg 2000; 32:114–118.

57. Lazareff JA, Garcia-Mendez MA, De Rosa R, Olmstead C. Limited (L4-S1, L5-S1) selective dorsal rhizotomy for reducing spasticity in cerebral palsy. Acta Neurochir 1999; 141:743–751.

58. Engsberg JR, Olree KS, Ross SA, Park TS. Spasticity and strength changes as a function of selective dorsal rhizotomy. J Neurosurg 1998; 88:1020–1026.

59. McLaughlin JF, Bjornson KF, Astley SJ, Graubert C, Hays RM, Roberts TS, Price R, Temkin N. Selective dorsal rhizotomy: efficacy and safety in an investigator-masked randomized clinical trial. Dev Med Child Neurol 1998; 40:220–232.

60. Wright FV, Sheil EM, Drake JM, Wedge JH, Naumann S. Evaluation of selective dorsal rhizotomy for the reduction of spasticity in cerebral palsy: a randomized controlled trial. Dev Med Child Neurol 1998; 40:239–247.

61. Steinbok P, Reiner AM, Beauchamp R, Armstrong RW, Cochrane DD, Kestle J. A randomized clinical trial to compare selective posterior rhizotomy plus physiotherapy with physiotherapy alone in children with spastic diplegic cerebral palsy. Dev Med Child Neurol 1997; 39:178–184.

62. Hodgkinson I, Berard C, Jindrich ML, Sindou M, Mertens P, Berard J. Selective dorsal rhizotomy in children with cerebral palsy. Results in 18 cases at one year postoperatively. Stereotact Funct Neurosurg 1997; 69:259–267.

63. Steinbok P, Kestle JR. Variation between centers in electrophysiologic techniques used in lumbosacral selective dorsal rhizotomy for spastic cerebral palsy. Pediatr Neurosurg 1996; 25:233–239.

64. Buckon CE, Sienko Thomas S, Aiona MD, Piatt JH. Assessment of upperextremity function in children with spastic diplegia before and after selective dorsal rhizotomy. Dev Med Child Neurol 1996; 38:967–975.

65. Steinbok P, Gustavsson B, Kestle JR, Reiner A, Cochrane DD. Relationship of intraoperative electrophysiological criteria to outcome after selective functional posterior rhizotomy. J Neurosurg 1995; 83:18–26.

66. McLaughlin JF, Bjornson KF, Astley SJ, Hays RM, Hoffinger SA, Armantrout EA, Roberts TS. The role of selective dorsal rhizotomy in cerebral palsy: critical evaluation of a prospective clinical series. Dev Med Child Neurol 1994; 36:755–769.

67. Steinbok P, Reiner A, Beauchamp RD, Cochrane DD, Keyes R. Selective functional posterior rhizotomy for treatment of spastic cerebral palsy in children. Review of 50 consecutive cases. Pediatr Neurosurg 1992; 18:34–42.

68. Lazareff JA, Mata-Acosta AM, Garcia-Mendez MA. Limited selective posterior rhizotomy for the treatment of spasticity secondary to infantile cerebral palsy: a preliminary report. Neurosurgery 1990; 27:535–538.

69. Engsberg JR, Ross SA, Park TS. Changes in ankle spasticity and strength following selective dorsal rhizotomy and physical therapy for spastic cerebral palsy. J Neurosurg 1999; 91:727–732.

70. Nishida T, Thatcher SW, Marty GR. Selective posterior rhizotomy for children with cerebral palsy: a 7-year experience. Childs Nerv Syst 1995; 11: 374–380.

71. Staudt LA, Nuwer MR, Peacock WJ. Intraoperative monitoring during selective posterior rhizotomy: technique and patient outcome. Electroencephalogr Clin Neurophysiol 1995; 97:296–309.

72. Boscarino LF, Ounpuu S, Davis RB, Gage JR, DeLuca PA. Effects of selective dorsal rhizotomy on gait in children with cerebral palsy. J Pediatr Orthop 1993; 13:174–179.

73. Wong AM, Chen CL, Hong WH. Motor control assessment for rhizotomy in cerebral palsy. Am J Phys Med Rehabil 2000; 79:441–450.

74. Subramanian N, Vaughan CL, Peter JC, Arens LJ. Gait before and 10 years after rhizotomy in children with cerebral palsy spasticity. J Neurosurg 1998; 88:1014–1026.

75. Thomas SS, Aiona MD, Pierce R, Piatt JH. Gait changes in children with spastic diplegia after selective dorsal rhizotomy. J Pediatr Orthop 1996; 16:747–752.

76. Adams J, Cahan LD, Perry J, Beeler LM. Foot contact pattern following selective dorsal rhizotomy. Pediatr Neurosurg 1995; 23:76–81.

77. Peacock WJ, Staudt LA. Functional outcomes following selective posterior rhizotomy in children with cerebral palsy. J Neurosurg 1991; 74:380–385.

78. Cahan LD, Adams JM, Perry J, Beeler LM. Instrumented gait analysis after selective dorsal rhizotomy. Dev Med Child Neurol 1990; 32:1037–1043.

79. Vaughan CL, Berman B, Staudt LA, Peacock WJ. Gait analysis of cerebral palsy children before and after rhizotomy. Pediatr Neurosci 1988; 14: 297–300.

80. Yang TF, Chan RC, Wong TT, Bair WN, Kao CC, Chuang TY, Hsu TC. Quantitative measurement of improvement in sitting balance in children with spastic cerebral palsy after selective posterior rhizotomy. Am J Phys Med Rehabil 1996; 75:348–352.

81. Beck AJ, Gaskill SJ, Marlin AE. Improvement in upper extremity function and trunk control after selective posterior rhizotomy. Am J Occup Ther 1993; 47:704–707.

82. Berman B, Vaughan CL, Peacock WJ. The effect of rhizotomy on movement in patients with cerebral palsy. Am J Occup Ther 1990; 44:511–516.

83. Marty GR, Dias LS, Gaebler-Spira D. Selective posterior rhizotomy and soft-tissue procedures for the treatment of cerebral diplegia. J Bone Joint Surg Am 1995; 77:713–718.

84. Montgomery PC. A clinical report of long term outcomes following selective posterior rhizotomy: implications for selection, follow-up, and research. Phys Occup Ther Pediatr 1992; 12:69–87.

85. Peacock WJ, Arens LJ, Berman B. Cerebral palsy spasticity. Selective posterior rhizotomy. Pediatr Neurosci 1987; 13:61–66.

86. Albright AL, Barry MJ, Fasick MP, Janosky J. Effects of continuous intrathecal baclofen infusion and selective posterior rhizotomy on upper extremity spasticity. Pediatr Neurosurg 1995; 23:82–85.

87. Mittal S, Farmer JP, Al-Atassi B, Montpetit K, Gervais N, Poulin C, Cantin MA, Benaroch TE. Impact of selective posterior rhizotomy on fine motor skills. Long-term results using a validated evaluative measure. Pediatr Neurosurg 2002; 36:133–141.

88. Dudgeon BJ, Libby AK, McLaughlin JF, Hays RM, Bjornson KF, Roberts TS. Prospective measurement of functional changes after selective dorsal rhizotomy. Arch Phys Med Rehabil 1994; 75:46–53.

89. Beck AJ, Gaskill SJ, Marlin AE. Improvement in upper extremity function and trunk control after selective posterior rhizotomy. Am J Occup Ther 1993; 47:704–707.

90. Lewin JE, Mix CM, Gaebler-Spira D. Self-help and upper extremity changes in 36 children with cerebral palsy subsequent to selective posterior rhizotomy and intensive occupational and physical therapy. Phys Occup Ther Pediatr 1993; 13:25–42.

91. Kinghorn J. Upper extremity functional changes following selective posterior rhizotomy in children with cerebral palsy. Am J Occup Ther 1992; 46:502–507.

92. Loewen P, Steinbok P, Holsti L, MacKay M. Upper extremity performance and self-care skill changes in children with spastic cerebral palsy following selective posterior rhizotomy. Pediatr Neurosurg 1998; 29:191–198.

93. Craft S, Park TS, White DA, Schatz J, Noetzel M, Arnold S. Changes in cognitive performance in children with spastic diplegic cerebral palsy following selective dorsal rhizotomy. Pediatr Neurosurg 1995; 23:68–74.

94. von Koch CS, Park TS, Steinbok P, Smyth M, Peacock WJ. Selective posterior rhizotomy and intrathecal baclofen for the treatment of spasticity. Pediatr Neurosurg 2001; 35:57–65.

95. Nordmark E, Jarnlo GB, Hagglund G. Comparison of the Gross Motor Function Measure and Paediatric Evaluation of Disability Inventory in assessing motor function in children undergoing selective dorsal rhizotomy. Dev Med Child Neurol 2000; 42:245–252.

96. Heim RC, Park TS, Vogler GP, Kaufman BA, Noetzel MJ, Ortman MR. Changes in hip migration after selective dorsal rhizotomy for spastic quadriplegia in cerebral palsy. J Neurosurg 1995; 82:567–571.

97. Park TS, Vogler GP, Phillips LH, Kaufman BA, Ortman MR, McClure SM, Gaffney PE. Effects of selective dorsal rhizotomy for spastic diplegia on hip migration in cerebral palsy. Pediatr Neurosurg 1994; 20:43–49.

98. Deletis V, Vodusek DB, Abbott R, Epstein FJ, Turndorf H. Intraoperative monitoring of the dorsal sacral roots: minimizing the risk of iatrogenic micturition disorders. Neurosurgery 1992; 30:72–75.

99. Huang JC, Deletis V, Vodusek DB, Abbott R. Preservation of pudendal afferents in sacral rhizotomies. Neurosurgery 1997; 41:411–415.

100. Lang FF, Deletis V, Cohen HW, Velasquez L, Abbott R. Inclusion of the S2 dorsal rootlets in functional posterior rhizotomy for spasticity in children with cerebral palsy. Neurosurgery 1994; 34:847–853.

101. Smyth MD, Peacock WJ. The surgical treatment of spasticity. Muscle Nerve 2000; 23:153–163.

102. Sweetser PM, Badell A, Schneider S, Badlani GH. Effects of sacral dorsal rhizotomy on bladder function in patients with spastic cerebral palsy. Neurourol Urodyn 1995; 14:57–64.

103. Euler AR, Byrne WJ, Ament ME, Fonkalsrud EW, Strobel CT, Siegel SC, Katz RM, Rachelefsky GS. Recurrent pulmonary disease in children: a complication of gastroesophageal reflux. Pediatrics 1979; 63:47–51.

104. Abbott R. Complications with selective posterior rhizotomy. Pediatr Neurosurg 1992; 18:43–47.

105. Bader D, Ramos AD, Lew CD, Platzker AC, Stabile MW, Keens TG. Childhood sequelae of infant lung disease: exercise and pulmonary function abnormalities after bronchopulmonary dysplasia. J Pediatr 1987; 110:693–699.

106. Swaminathan S, Quinn J, Stabile MW, Bader D, Platzker AC, Keens TG. Long-term pulmonary sequelae of meconium aspiration syndrome. J Pediatr 1989; 114:356–361.

107. Van de Wiele BM, Staudt LA, Rubinstien EH, Nuwer M, Peacock WJ. Perioperative complications in children undergoing selective posterior rhizotomy: a review of 105 cases. Paediatr Anaesth 1996; 6:479–486.

108. Steinbok P, Schrag C. Complications after selective posterior rhizotomy for spasticity in children with cerebral palsy. Pediatr Neurosurg 1998; 28:300–313.

109. Peter JC, Arens LJ. Selective posterior lumbosacral rhizotomy for the management of cerebral palsy spasticity. A 10-year experience. S Afr Med J 1993; 83:745–747.

110. Fasano VA, Broggi G, Zeme S, Lo Russo G, Sguazzi A. Long-term results of posterior functional rhizotomy. Acta Neurochir Suppl 1980; 30:435–439.

111. Reid CJ, Borzyskowski M. Lower urinary tract dysfunction in cerebral palsy. Arch Dis Child 1993; 68:739–742.
112. McNeal DM, Hawtrey CE, Wolraich ML, Mapel JR. Symptomatic neurogenic bladder in a cerebral-palsied population. Dev Med Child Neurol 1983; 25:612–616.
113. Peter JC, Hoffman EB, Arens LJ. Spondylolysis and spondylolisthesis after five-level lumbosacral laminectomy for selective posterior rhizotomy in cerebral palsy. Childs Nerv Syst 1993; 9:285–287.
114. Gooch JL, Walker ML. Spinal stenosis after total lumbar laminectomy for selective dorsal rhizotomy. Pediatr Neurosurg 1996; 25:28–30.
115. Crawford K, Karol LA, Herring JA. Severe lumbar lordosis after dorsal rhizotomy. J Pediatr Orthop 1996; 16:336–339.
116. Park TS, Gaffney PE, Kaufman BA, Molleston MC. Selective lumbosacral dorsal rhizotomy immediately caudal to the conus medullaris for cerebral palsy spasticity. Neurosurgery 1993; 33:929–933.
117. Carroll KL, Moore KR, Stevens PM. Orthopedic procedures after rhizotomy. J Pediatr Orthop 1998; 18:69–74.
118. Greene WB, Dietz FR, Goldberg MJ, Gross RH, Miller F, Sussman MD. Rapid progression of hip subluxation in cerebral palsy after selective posterior rhizotomy. J Pediatr Orthop 1991; 11:494–497.

Index

T - #0170 - 101024 - C0 - 229/152/19 [21] - CB - 9780824729509 - Gloss Lamination